Hot Health Care Careers:

30 Occupations With Fast Growth and Many New Job Openings

College & Career Press
Chicago, Illinois

1/18

Editorial Staff

Andrew Morkes, Publisher/Editorial Director
Amy McKenna, Additional Editorial Assistance
Salvatore Concialdi, Cover Design

Cover photos courtesy of Adobe Stock. Photos.com, Thinkstock

Library of Congress Cataloging-in-Publication Data
Names: Morkes, Andrew, author. | McKenna, Amy, 1969- author.
Title: Hot health care careers : 30 occupations with fast growth and many
    new job openings/ by Andrew Morkes and Amy McKenna.
Description: 2nd edition. | Chicago, Illinois : College & Career Press,
    [2017] | Revision of: Hot health care careers. c2007. | Includes
    bibliographical references and index.
Identifiers: LCCN 2016058541 | ISBN 9780974525181 (alk. paper)
Subjects: LCSH: Medical personnel--Vocational guidance.
Classification: LCC R690 .H68 2017 | DDC 610.69--dc23 LC record available at
    https://lccn.loc.gov/2016058541

Published and distributed by
College & Career Press, LLC
PO Box 300484
Chicago, IL 60630
amorkes@chicagopa.com
www.cccpnewsletters.com

Printed in the United States of America

17-02

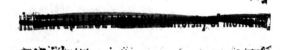

TABLE OF CONTENTS

Also Available From College & Career Press:

They Teach That in College!?: A Resource Guide to More Than 100 Interesting College Majors, 3rd Edition (ISBN-13: 978-0-9829210-8-1), $14.99

Provides information about interesting and cutting-edge college majors (including Alternative Fuels, Commercial Space Operations, Computational Finance, Film Scoring, Human-Centered Design and Engineering, Mechatronics Systems Engineering, and Social Media) unknown to many counselors, educators, and parents. Features profiles of more than 100 college majors, course listings, potential employers, contact information for colleges and universities that offer these programs, and interviews with more than 70 educators. Majors and programs available at the associate, baccalaureate, and graduate levels at more than 500 colleges and universities throughout the United States and Canada are covered. Voted one of the "Best 11 Books of the Year" by *Voice of Youth Advocates*.

CAM Report newsletter (ISSN: 0745-4341; published 20 times annually)

A career resource newsletter for guidance and education professionals and the students they serve. Features articles about emerging and fast-growing careers; tips on writing resumes and acing interviews; advice on landing a job and internships; and much more.

Subscription Rates: 1 year/$75 (20 issues); 2 years/$140 (40 issues); 3 years/$210 (60 issues)

College Spotlight newsletter (ISSN 1525-4313, published six times during the school year)

A college resource newsletter geared toward guidance and education professionals and the students they serve. Provides advice on selecting, applying to, evaluating, and entering college, as well as information on non-college alternatives for today's high school graduates.

Subscription Rates: 1 year/$29.99 (9 issues); 2 years/$54.99 (18 issues); 3 years/$69.99 (27 issues)

Nontraditional Careers for Women and Men: More Than 30 Great Jobs for Women and Men With Apprenticeships Through PhDs (ISBN-13: 978-0-9745251-9-8), $14.99

Features 22 nontraditional careers for women in the book, including Aircraft Pilots, Architects, Automotive Service Mechanics, Carpenters, Chief Executives, Chiropractors, Civil Engineers, Construction Inspectors, Construction Managers, Cost Estimators, Electrical and Electronics Engineers, Electricians, Engineering Technicians, Firefighters, Industrial Engineers, Police Officers, and Software Engineers. This book also features 9 fast-growing careers in which fewer than 20 percent of males are employed, such as Dental Hygienists, Elementary and Middle School Teachers, Health Information Management Specialists, Occupational Therapists, Paralegals, Registered Nurses, and Special Education Teachers. Features nearly 35 interviews. *Booklist* says that *Nontraditional Careers for Women and Men* is "recommended for public libraries and college/university career centers."

Hot Jobs: More Than 25 Careers With the Highest Pay, Fastest Growth, and Most New Job Openings (ISBN-13: 978-0-9745251-6-7), $14.99

Features more than 25 hot careers, including Civil Engineers, Computer Support Specialists, Computer Systems Analysts, Construction Managers, Market Research Analysts, Medical Scientists, Personal Financial Advisors, Pharmacists, Physical Therapists, Registered Nurses, and Software Engineers. Provides nearly 40 interviews with professionals and educators, photographs, and useful sidebars. *Midwest Book Review* says that *Hot Jobs* is "a fine pick for anyone with an eye out for their career."

Visit www.collegeandcareerpress.com to read introductions, tables of contents, and sample chapters or copies (newsletters) for these and other publications.

Check out The Morkes Report career and college blog at www.ccpnewsletters.com/college-and-career-planning

FOREWORD

By Benjamin D. Anderson, M.B.A., Chief Executive Officer, Kearny County Hospital, and named to *Becker's Hospital Review*'s "25 Healthcare Leaders Under 40" list in 2015

To those considering their next career steps: consider my story and the lessons learned...

I was born in northern California and raised by a single mother amidst intense poverty. At our most vulnerable point, we received medication and food from a ministry focused on the care of homeless people, an experience I will never forget.

These formative experiences played a major role in my decision to find ways to improve the lives of underserved, distressed people. As a college student, I developed a mentoring program benefiting the lowest-performing students at an inner-city middle school. As a graduate student, I founded an organization that assisted at-risk high school students with enrollment in colleges across the United States. After graduate school, I recruited physicians to remote areas in rural Northern California, Oregon, and Alaska. Ultimately, I chose health care administration as a career because it is mission-driven and tied to the community. I believe the community is where change takes place. I want to be in the community visibly working to improve the delivery of health care to all people, with special attention to those who are most vulnerable.

During my time as a medical staffing consultant, I attended a health conference in Bend, Oregon. While there, I invited several rural hospital CEOs to have dinner with me. I was interested in learning about their career paths and what influenced their decision to choose health care administration as a vocation. As I listened to them, I was both impressed and intrigued by the complexity of their work. It seemed to me, especially in underserved areas, that the health of a society was closely tied to the condition of its local hospital. Consequently, I learned that hospital CEOs were positioned to leverage their resources and influence to positively impact their communities, way outside the walls of their health care facilities. At 28 years old, and with the urging of my new dinner friends, I set a clear goal to spend the remainder of my career in health care administration.

Having never worked in a hospital, I knew I was a nontraditional candidate who faced a steep learning curve. If this career would be a reality for me, I would need to be mentored by experienced rural hospital CEOs. So for 90 days, I committed my early morning hours (before work) to "cold-calling" the CEOs of high-performing hospitals in specific geographic locations and asking them for advice. With each call, I briefly stated my name, background, and professional goal, asking for their insights as to how to accomplish it. I was not looking for instant gratification or a "free ride." I genuinely desired their wisdom. To my surprise, they expressed interest in coaching me. I later learned that they rarely received such interest from people my age. Apparently, "Millennials" were not known among some circles in preceding generations for their willingness to work hard or seek counsel from older, more experienced professionals. Within several months of beginning this approach, I interviewed for and accepted my first hospital CEO position. I was 29 years old.

I quickly learned that I was entering the industry during a time of historic and rapid change. National health care costs were rising at such a rapid rate that they were enveloping resources that were needed for other social services. And yet, the increased expenses were not commensurate with better health outcomes, while a growing gap of working Americans could no longer afford care at all. Put simply, we could not afford the broken system being funded.

The response to this complicated dilemma is a multifaceted challenge the Institute for Healthcare Improvement calls "The Triple Aim"—simultaneously improving the health of the population, enhancing the experience and outcomes of the patient, and reducing per capita cost of care for the benefit of communities. This is both challenging and gratifying because I have an opportunity to think innovatively and lead others toward a purpose of serving humanity.

Our industry is full of health care administrators who are filling the roles of plant managers. They are focused on finding ways for hospitals to be sustainable in a system where we are incentivized to give more care instead of more effective care. In the future, the most impactful health care leaders will not only be well educated; they will be radically innovative with insatiable social consciences. They will be community developers who are disguised in health care uniforms. They will be compassionate and humble, but unafraid to work hard in pursuit of social justice. They will assertively leverage their education and influence to advocate for marginalized people who are suffering and unable to speak for themselves.

Health care in the twenty-first century is not for the weak or the faint of heart. But those mission-focused people who are seeking a vocation with true purpose will find themselves challenged in exhilarating ways. In the midst of your efforts, you will experience long-lasting encouragement and joy. As a health care leader, my every workday is full of opportunities to help people help other people, to leverage resources to meet the needs of humanity. If you feel you are called to such a life, I invite you to spend a day with us at Kearny County Hospital in Lakin, Kansas.●

INTRODUCTION

Health care jobs are a popular career option for students who enjoy helping others and learning about the latest cutting-edge technology and diagnostic and treatment methods. The health care industry consistently enjoys strong employment growth, and here are several reasons why this field is an excellent career option.

✔ The U.S. Department of Labor (USDL) predicts that employment in the health care and social assistance industry will grow by 19 percent from 2014 to 2024—more than triple the average employment growth for all industries.

✔ No other industry will add more jobs than the health care field from 2014-24. In fact, the USDL predicts that the growing elderly population and technological breakthroughs will help generate more than 3.6 million new jobs between 2014 and 2024.

✔ Seven of the top 20 careers that will add the most new positions through 2024 are in the health care industry.

✔ 19 of the top 25 fastest-growing careers through 2024 are health care-related.

✔ Unlike jobs in many other fields, most health care careers are difficult to offshore to other countries because they require "face time" with patients.

So, the prognosis for health care careers is excellent, and you should consider becoming a health care professional. To help you in your career exploration, the editors of *Hot Health Care Careers* have identified 30 careers that will grow most quickly and add the most new jobs during the next decade. These careers offer exciting opportunities for people with a variety of skill sets and educational backgrounds—from a high school diploma and on-the-job training, to a bachelor's or master's degree, to a medical degree, dental degree, or doctorate. The following paragraphs provide more information on the sections in each career article and other features in the book.

The **Fast Facts** sidebar appears at the beginning of each article. It provides a summary of recommended high school classes and personal skills; the minimum educational requirements to enter the field; the typical salary range; employment outlook; and acronyms and identification numbers for the following government classification indexes: the Occupational Information Network (O*NET)-Standard Occupational Classification System (SOC) index and the National Occupational Classification (NOC) Index. The O*NET-SOC index has been created by the U.S. government; the NOC index is Canada's career classification system. Readers can use the identification numbers listed in this section to obtain further information about a career. Digital editions of the O*NET-SOC (https://www.onetonline.org) and NOC (http://noc.esdc.gc.ca/English/home.aspx) are available online.

6 Great Reasons to Pursue a Career in the Health Care Industry

1. The growing elderly population will continue to create employment opportunities for decades. In fact, about 87 million Americans—or 25 percent—will be age 65 and older by 2050, according to the Organization for Economic Cooperation and Development. This adds up to many opportunities for health care workers, since the elderly often need more medical assistance than those in younger demographic groups.

2. Advances in technology—including the government-mandated digitization of health records, the use of computers and data analytics software in medical research (bioinformatics), and new medical equipment and apps—will create demand for a variety of health care workers.

3. Most health care careers cannot be outsourced to foreign countries because they require "face time" with patients.

4. Health care positions are broadly distributed throughout the United States, and sometimes are the only viable jobs in economically depressed areas.

5. The industry offers excellent opportunities for women; other industries that are male-dominated, such as construction, have suffered employment declines or slower growth than the health care field.

6. The industry offers a wide variety of career options for those with educational backgrounds ranging from a high school diploma to a medical degree. If you get bored or "burned-out" with one career, you can always pursue additional education to become qualified for a new position.

The **Overview** section provides a capsule summary of work duties, educational requirements, the number of people employed in the field, and employment outlook.

The Job provides a detailed overview of primary and secondary job duties and typical work settings.

The **Requirements** section features four subsections: **High School** (which lists recommended high school classes), **Postsecondary Training** (which lists required post-high school training requirements to prepare for the field), **Certification and Licensing** (which details voluntary certification and mandatory licensing requirements, when applicable), and **Other Requirements** (which lists key personal and professional skills for success in the field).

Exploring provides suggestions to young people about how they can explore the field while in school. Examples include books and magazines, websites, information interviews, membership in clubs and other organizations, hands-on activities, competitions, and summer and after-school programs.

The Elephant in the Room: the Affordable Care Act

The Patient Protection and Affordable Care Act—which is often referred to as "Obamacare" or the "Affordable Care Act" (ACA)—was passed in 2010. The Act provided coverage to 15 to 20 million previously uninsured Americans. Approximately 48.6 million people—or 15.7 percent of the U.S. population—were uninsured before the ACA was passed, according to the U.S. Census Bureau. A 2015 study by the Centers for Disease Control found that the uninsured rate had fallen to 9.2 percent under the ACA, the lowest uninsured rate in 50 years. In addition to increasing the number of people who had health care, the Act also created many new opportunities for nurses, physicians, health care managers, and allied health professionals.

Yet, despite these successes, rising insurance premiums and poorly performing exchanges in some states, among other issues, prompted some to question the effectiveness of the ACA. As we publish this book, the Trump Administration has announced plans to revise or repeal/replace the Act, which has created a significant degree of uncertainty about coverage and what features will be included in the revised or new health care legislation.

One thing is certain: demand will continue to be strong for health care professionals. It's hard to imagine (but possible) that insurance coverage would be eliminated for the 15 to 20 million Americans covered under the ACA, but Congress is currently developing alternative plans. Whether the revised ACA or new plan is better than the current ACA will only be known with time. Regardless of what happens with the ACA, the U.S. population continues to grow and medical advances allow more people to be treated for what were once life-threatening conditions. These developments will fuel demand for health care professionals.

Employers lists the number of people employed in the occupation in the United States and details typical work settings.

Getting a Job provides advice on how to land a job through employment and association websites, career service offices, networking, career fairs, and other methods.

The **Advancement** section provides an overview of typical ways to move up at one's employer or via other means (such as opening a consulting firm or entering academia).

Earnings provides information on starting, median, and top salaries for workers. Information on salaries in particular industries is also provided for many careers.

The **Employment Outlook** section provides an overview of the outlook for the career through 2024. It lists the factors that are fueling employment growth and details career specialties in which there will be especially strong growth. Outlook information is obtained from the U.S. Department of Labor and is augmented by information gathered from professional trade associations. Job growth terms follow those used in the *Occupational Outlook Handbook* (http://stats.bls.gov/search/ooh.htm). Growth described as "much faster than the average" means that employment will increase by 14 percent or more through 2024. Growth described as "faster than the average" means an increase of 9 to 13 percent. Growth described as "about as fast as the average" means an increase of 5 to 8 percent.

Each article ends with **For More Information.** This section provides contact information for professional associations that offer details on educational programs, career paths, scholarships, publications, youth programs, membership, and other resources.

Additionally, many articles in *Hot Health Care Careers* feature one or more interviews with professionals and educators, who provide useful advice on what it takes to land a job and be successful. Other features include:

✔ More than 40 health care scholarships with awards ranging from $500 to $20,000

✔ More than 40 health care-related college summer exploration programs

✔ Nearly 70 informative sidebars such as Cool Career: Perfusionist; Demand Grows for Dementia Care Workers; Genetic Counselors in Demand; Emerging Health Care Careers; What is Public Health?; Demand Strong for Information Technology Health Workers; Interesting Career: Medical Flight Worker; A Closer Look: Alternative and Complementary Medicine; and The Best Places to Work in Health Care.

✔ A career title and association index.

We hope that *Hot Health Care Careers* provides you with some great ideas for possible career paths. But this book is just the beginning. Contact the professional associations listed at the end of each article to obtain more information; perhaps they can even help arrange an information interview with a worker in a field that interests you. Check out associations and potential employers on social networking sites such as LinkedIn. Attend one or more of the college summer exploration programs listed on pages 262 to 273. Follow the suggestions in the Exploring section of each article to get hands-on experience. That way, you will be able to try out each field before making the big decision of choosing a career. Learning about health care careers can be fun, and we hope this book is useful to you as you begin your search. We wish you the very best during your career exploration!

ADVANCED PRACTICE NURSES

OVERVIEW

Advanced practice nurses (APNs) are registered nurses who provide specialized health care, promote health, prevent and treat disease and injuries, and help patients cope with illness. APNs have earned master's degrees and certifications to become either a *certified nurse-midwife,* a *clinical nurse specialist,* a *certified registered nurse anesthetist,* or a *nurse practitioner.* There are more than 200,000 advanced practice nurses employed in the United States. Employment for APNs is expected to be excellent during the next decade.

THE JOB

What makes nurses unique from other health care professionals? Many agree it is the job of the nurse to treat the individual— not just the presenting health problem. In addition, nurses are often tasked with caring not only for the patient, but for his or her loved ones and family, keeping them comfortable and "in the know" about a health crisis of a loved one. Finally, nurses are stewards in their community, keeping the public informed on ways to get and stay healthy. Advanced practice nursing is an umbrella term given to registered nurses who have completed a master's degree and passed additional clinical practice requirements specific to their chosen career path. Advanced practice nursing specialties are detailed in the following paragraphs:

Certified nurse-midwives (CNMs) provide gynecological wellness checks and consultations on conception and pregnancy, and they assist in childbirth. Approximately 8.3 percent of U.S. births are attended by certified

---

FAST FACTS

High School Subjects
Biology
Chemistry
Mathematics

Personal Skills
Active listening
Communication
Critical thinking
Judgment and decision making

Minimum Education Level
Master's degree

Salary Range
$50,000 to $90,000 to $185,620+

Employment Outlook
Much faster than the average

O*NET-SOC
29-1141.00, 29-1141.02, 29-1141.03, 29-1141.04, 29-1151.00, 29-1161.00, 29-1171.00

NOC
3012, 3124

Calling Dr. Nurse!

The nursing field has added yet another specialty—doctor of nursing practice, or DNP. DNPs are graduates of a two-year doctoral program (that includes a one-year residency), which advocates believe allows them to enter the medical field with the training, skill, and medical experience of a primary care physician. In 2015, there were 289 DNP programs at schools of nursing nationwide, and an additional 128 new DNP programs were in the planning stages (62 post-baccalaureate and 66 post-master's programs), according to the American Association of Colleges of Nursing. Doctor of nursing practice programs are now available in 48 states plus the District of Columbia. States with the most programs (more than five) include Florida, Illinois, Massachusetts, Minnesota, New York, Ohio, Pennsylvania, and Texas. Visit www.aacn.nche.edu/dnp/about-the-dnp for more information.

nurse-midwives. CNMs work in hospitals and birthing centers, and they conduct home visits for women who want to deliver their babies at home. The common misconception is that all these professionals do is deliver babies. In fact, they spend only about 10 percent of their workday assisting in childbirth. The majority of their work involves providing routine annual exams and giving primary, preventive care to women of all ages.

Clinical nurse specialists (CNSs) specialize in a wide range of physical and mental health areas. Their area of clinical expertise may be in a setting such as emergency room nursing, a type of health problem such as stress or wounds, a population such as pediatrics or the elderly, or a type of care such as rehabilitation. In addition to direct care, they may serve as consultants, researchers, educators, and medical administrators. CNSs work in clinics, offices, community centers, hospitals, and other medical facilities.

Nurse anesthesia is the oldest advanced nursing specialty. *Certified registered nurse anesthetists (CRNAs)* administer anesthesia to patients undergoing surgery or other medical treatments. They also provide pain management and emergency services. CRNAs administer approximately 43 million anesthetics to patients annually in the United States. Men make up more than 40 percent of nurse anesthetists, according to the American Association of Nurse Anesthetists. Fewer than 10 percent of workers in all nursing fields are men. CRNAs work alongside surgeons, anesthesiologists, dentists, podiatrists, and other health care professionals in hospitals, in medical offices, and in other settings.

Nurse practitioners (NPs) are qualified to provide some of the direct health care services that are generally performed by physicians. They treat illnesses ranging from the common cold to diabetes. Americans make more than 916 million visits to NPs every year, according to the American Association of Nurse Practitioners. NPs have a variety of duties, including diagnosing and treating minor illnesses or injuries and prescribing medication. They also conduct physical examinations; provide immunizations;

help patients manage high blood pressure, diabetes, depression, and other chronic health problems; prescribe medications; perform certain medical procedures; order and interpret lab results, x-rays, and EKGs; and educate and counsel patients and their families. Nurse practitioners can write prescriptions in all 50 states and practice independently from physicians in nearly 20 states. While many NPs focus on primary care, others—with additional training—become *pediatric, gerontological, oncology, neonatal, acute care, school, occupational health, psychiatric,* and *women's health care nurse practitioners.* NPs work in hospitals, offices of physicians, clinics, nursing homes, pharmacies with health clinics, and other medical facilities.

Work settings for advanced practice nurses vary based on their specialty, but they generally work in medical offices or hospitals. Since there is a 24-hour demand for health care, some of these professionals work nights, weekends, and holidays. Regardless of the shift, APNs find their work rewarding. They enjoy caring for patients and their families and promoting wellness education in the field and in the community.

REQUIREMENTS

HIGH SCHOOL

Take health, mathematics, biology, chemistry, physics, English, speech, business, and sociology classes in high school to prepare for a career in advanced practice nursing.

POSTSECONDARY TRAINING

The first step to become an APN is to complete training to become a registered nurse. Prospective RNs have the option of pursuing one of three training paths: associate's degree, diploma, and bachelor's degree. Associate's degree programs in nursing last two years and are offered by community colleges. Diploma programs in nursing typically last three years and are offered by hospitals and independent schools. Bachelor of science in nursing programs are offered by colleges and universities. They typically take four—and sometimes five—years to complete. Graduates of all three paths are known as graduate nurses and must take a licensing exam in their state to obtain the RN designation. Visit Discover Nursing (www.discovernursing.com) for a database of nursing programs.

Graduates of midwifery education programs must have a master's degree in order to be able to take the national certifying exam, which is offered by the American Midwifery Certification Board (www.amcbmidwife.org). The Accreditation Commission for Midwifery Education has accredited nearly 40 nurse-midwifery education programs in the United States. A list of programs can be accessed at www.midwife.org/Education-Programs-Directory.

Clinical nurse specialists need at least a master's degree to work in the field. The National Association of Clinical Nurse Specialists offers a list of educational programs at its website, www.nacns.org.

Nurse anesthetists must have at least a master's degree to practice. The Council of Accreditation of Nurse Anesthesia Educational Programs has accredited 115 programs. Visit the American Association of Nurse Anesthetists' website, www.aana.com, for a list of programs. Nurse anesthesia programs typically last from 24 to 42 months, depending on the requirements of the college or university.

You will need a master's degree to work as a nurse practitioner. Visit the website (www.aanp.org) of the American Association of Nurse Practitioners for a database of education programs.

Doctorate degrees (such as a Doctor of Nursing Practice) are typically required for those who want to work in top levels of administration, in research, or in education. These degrees normally take four to five years to complete.

CERTIFICATION AND LICENSING

Voluntary certification is available for all four advanced practice nursing specialties. The American Midwifery Certification Board offers certification to midwives. Clinical nurse specialists can become certified by the American Nurses Credentialing Center (ANCC), the American Association of Critical Care Nurses Certification Corporation, the Oncology Nursing Certification Corporation (ONCC), Orthopaedic Nurses Certification Board, and other organizations. Nurse anesthetists can become certified by the Council on Certification of Nurse Anesthetists and the American Society of PeriAnesthesia Nurses. Nurse practitioners can obtain certification from such organizations as the American Academy of Nurse Practitioners, the ANCC, the American Nurses Association, the ONCC, and the Pediatric Nursing Certification Board. Contact these organizations for more information.

Cool Career: Perfusionist

One of the most important medical advances in history was the invention of the heart-lung machine, which takes over the functions of a patient's heart and lungs, pumping oxygenated blood through the body, while the patient is undergoing heart surgery. *Perfusionists,* also known as *cardiovascular perfusionists,* operate this lifesaving machine and are responsible for the management of circulatory and respiratory functions of the patient. They may also operate other life-support devices, and they generally assist the surgical team as necessary. Because of the nature of their work, perfusionists are trained in the biological science of artificial circulation, as well as in the mechanical functioning of the heart-lung machine and any other devices they operate and monitor during medical procedures. Seventeen schools in the United States offer training to become a perfusionist. These schools are accredited by the Commission on Accreditation of Allied Health Education Programs. Perfusionists earned median annual salaries of $122,710 in January 2017, according to Salary.com. Earnings ranged from less than $110,135 to $133,967 or more. For more information, contact the American Academy of Cardiovascular Perfusion (717-867-1485, Office@TheAACP.com, www.theaacp.com) and the American Society of ExtraCorporeal Technology (312-321-5156, amsect@amsect.org, www.amsect.org).

Did You Know?

✔ Certified nurse midwives (CNMs) and certified midwives (CMs) attended 8.3 percent of all births in 2014.

✔ Approximately 82 percent of CNMs have a master's degree; 4.8 percent hold a doctoral degree.

✔ In 2014, 94.2 percent of CNM/CM-attended births occurred in hospitals, 3 percent occurred in freestanding birth centers, and 2.7 percent occurred in homes.

Source: American College of Nurse-Midwives

Nurses must be licensed to practice nursing in all states and the District of Columbia. Licensure requirements vary by state, but they typically include graduating from an approved nursing school and passing a national examination. Visit the National Council of State Boards of Nursing's website, www.ncsbn.org, for details on licensing requirements by state.

OTHER REQUIREMENTS

Successful APNs are detail oriented, caring, sympathetic, responsible, and emotionally stable. They need excellent communication skills in order to interact well with patients and coworkers. They have good judgment, are able to remain calm and decisive under pressure, have good leadership abilities, and are willing to continue to learn and upgrade their skills throughout their careers.

EXPLORING

Read books about nursing, talk with your counselor or teacher about setting up a presentation by a nurse and take a tour of a hospital or other health care setting, or volunteer at one of these facilities. Nursing-related websites, including those of professional associations, can also be a good source of information. Here are a two suggestions: Discover Nursing (www.discovernursing.com) and Nurse.com (www.nurse.com).

EMPLOYERS

There are more than 200,000 advanced practice nurses employed in the United States. The following paragraphs provide information on work settings for the four advanced practice nursing specialties.

Certified nurse-midwives work in hospitals and birthing centers, and they conduct home visits for women who want to deliver their babies at home.

Clinical nurse specialists are employed in clinics, offices, community centers, hospitals, and other medical facilities.

Certified registered nurse anesthetists work in hospitals; outpatient surgery centers; and offices of dentists, ophthalmologists, plastic surgeons, podiatrists, and pain management specialists.

FOR MORE INFORMATION

For information on opportunities for men in nursing, contact
**American Assembly
for Men in Nursing**
www.aamn.org

For information on accredited nursing programs, contact
**American Association
of Colleges of Nursing**
www.aacn.nche.edu

For certification information, contact
**American Nurses
Credentialing Center**
www.nursecredentialing.org

For information on gerontological advanced practice nursing, contact
**Gerontological Advanced
Practice Nurses Association**
www.gapna.org

For information about nursing, contact
National League for Nursing
www.nln.org

For information on membership, contact
National Student Nurses' Association
www.nsna.org

For resources for aspiring and current nurses with disabilities, visit
ExceptionalNurse.com
www.exceptionalnurse.com

To learn more about opportunities in Canada, contact
**Canadian Association of
Advanced Practice Nurses**
http://caapn-aciipa.org

NURSE-MIDWIVES
For info on education, careers, and certification for certified nurse-midwives, contact the following organizations

**American College
of Nurse-Midwives**
www.midwife.org

**American Midwifery
Certification Board**
www.amcbmidwife.org

**Midwives Alliance
of North America**
844-626-2674
www.mana.org

CLINICAL NURSE SPECIALISTS
For information on education and careers, contact
**National Association
of Clinical Nurse Specialists**
www.nacns.org

NURSE ANESTHETISTS
For information on education, careers, and certification, contact the following organizations
**American Association
of Nurse Anesthetists**
www.aana.com

**American Society of
PeriAnesthesia Nurses**
www.aspan.org

NURSE PRACTITIONERS
For more info on education and careers, contact the following organizations
**American Academy of Nurse
Practitioners Certification Board**
www.aanpcert.org

**American Association
of Nurse Practitioners**
www.aanp.org

**National Association
of Pediatric Nurse Practitioners**
www.napnap.org

Nurse practitioners are employed in hospitals, clinics, nursing homes, mental health centers, colleges and universities, student health centers, home health agencies, hospices, offices of physicians, community health centers, rural health clinics, prisons, and industrial organizations.

Advanced practice nurses also work for government agencies, including the U.S. Department of Veterans Affairs, the U.S. Public Health Service, and the U.S. military. Some teach at colleges and universities.

GETTING A JOB

Many APNs obtain their first jobs as a result of contacts made through college internships or networking events. Others seek assistance in obtaining job leads from college career services offices, nursing registries, nurse employment agencies, state employment offices, newspaper want ads, and employment websites. Additionally, professional nursing associations (such as the National Association of Clinical Nurse Specialists and the American Association of Nurse Practitioners) provide job listings at their websites. See For More Information for a list of organizations.

ADVANCEMENT

The position of advanced practice nurse is not entry-level. Most APNs enter the field after working as registered nurses and obtaining several years of experience and advanced education and certification. APNs can eventually advance to managerial or senior-level administrative roles. These positions often require APNs to earn a doctorate degree in nursing or management. Some APNs are hired by hospitals, pharmaceutical manufacturers, insurance companies, and managed care organizations to provide health planning and development, policy development, marketing, consulting, and quality assurance consulting. Other APNs work as teachers at colleges, universities, and teaching hospitals.

EARNINGS

Salaries for APNs vary by type of employer, geographic region, and the worker's experience, education, and skill level. Median annual salaries for registered nurses were $67,490 in May 2015, according to the U.S. Department of Labor (USDL). Salaries ranged from less than $46,360 to $101,630 or more. Salaries for APNs are typically higher. The USDL provides the following salary ranges for APNS:

✔ nurse anesthetists: $105,410 to $185,620+
✔ nurse-midwives: $50,310 to $132,270+
✔ nurse practitioners: $70,540 to $135,830+.

In 2017, clinical nurse specialists had earnings that ranged from $89,349 to $108,218 or more, according to Salary.com.

APNs usually receive benefits such as health and life insurance, vacation days, sick leave, and a savings and pension plan. Self-employed workers must provide their own benefits.

EMPLOYMENT OUTLOOK

Employment for registered nurses is expected to be excellent, according to the U.S. Department of Labor (USDL). The USDL reports that these professionals "will be in high demand, particularly in medically under-served areas such as inner cities and rural areas. As states change their laws governing APRN practice authority, APRNs are being allowed to per-form more services. They are also becoming more widely recognized by the public as a source for primary healthcare." APNs with doctoral degrees and certification will have the best employment prospects.

Interview: Diane   Padden

Diane Padden, PhD, CRNP, FAANP, Vice President of Professional Practice and Partnerships at the American Association of Nurse Practitioners

Q. How long have you been a nurse practitioner? What made you want to enter this career?

A. I have been a nurse practitioner (NP) for 18 years. When I graduated from my basic nursing program over 30 years ago I knew I wanted to become a nurse practitioner. The NP role was new at that time, but I saw it as an opportunity to make a difference in patients' lives. Being a registered nurse working in a hospital I saw sick patients for a limited period of time but as an NP I would be able to develop a relationship with my patients over time. I wanted to provide patients with holistic care, not just treating an illness or disease, but rather to better understand them and their specific needs. It was also important to me to practice in primary care, where I could focus on health promotion and disease prevention.

Q. What is one thing that young people may not know about a career in the field?

A. Nurse practitioners can own their own practices (this may involve some caveats/restrictions, see below under "cons").

Q. What are some of the pros and cons of your job?

A. Pros:

✔ It's a privilege to be able to care for patients and hopefully make a dif-ference in their overall health.

✔ Feeling connected with patients and their families as their health care provider. They share so much of their lives and circumstances which many times are both happy and sad, but yet so important to fully understand who they are and how best to care for them.

✔ Multiple opportunities in terms of work settings: outpatient clinics, community centers, private practice, hospitals, rural/underserved areas, correctional institutions, etc.

Cons:

✔ Limited practice authority in some states requiring practice or collab-oration agreements

Demand Grows for Dementia Care Workers

Nearly 15 percent of people age 71 or older (approximately 3.8 million people) have dementia, according to a study by the RAND Corporation. By 2040, this number will skyrocket to 9.1 million. Yet, while direct health care expenses (including nursing home care) for dementia care treatment now exceed those for heart disease and cancer, the *New York Times* reports that America is "unprepared for the coming surge in the cost and cases of dementia." This unpreparedness will result in a shortage of caregivers for patients with dementia.

This shortage will translate into a wealth of employment opportunities in the field. Career options include:

✔ **Geriatric nurses** and **nurse aides,** who provide direct patient care to patients in their homes, or in nursing homes, hospitals, and clinics;

✔ **Geriatric care managers,** who coordinate the many aspects of the short- and long-term care of the elderly;

✔ **Geriatric social workers,** who help elderly people adjust to the challenges of growing older; and

✔ **Geriatricians,** specialized physicians who treat patients with dementia and other diseases of aging.

Educational requirements vary for dementia care workers—from a high school diploma for nurse aides, to a bachelor's degree for geriatric care managers and nurses, to a medical degree for geriatric physicians.

Contact the following organizations to learn more:

✔ **Aging Life Care Association:** www.aginglifecare.org

✔ **American Geriatrics Society:** www.americangeriatrics.org

✔ **American Medical Association:** www.ama-assn.org

✔ **Association for Gerontology in Higher Education:** www.aghe.org

✔ **Gerontological Advanced Practice Nurses Association:** gapna.org

✔ **National Academy of Certified Care Managers:** www.naccm.net

✔ **National Gerontological Nursing Association:** www.ngna.org.

✔ Misunderstanding of what a nurse practitioner is and scope of their practice

✔ At times, not recognized as being part of the health care team or being allowed to lead the team, if appropriate

Q. What is the employment outlook for nurse practitioners?

A. The outlook for employment for nurse practitioners is very good. In 2015, *U.S. News and World Report* ranked the career of nurse practitioner as the second-best job (out of a total of 100 jobs). See http://money.usnews.com/careers/best-jobs/rankings/the-100-best-jobs. Additionally, data shows there is a shortage of primary care physicians. Nurse practitioners—who are educated to evaluate patients; diagnose, order, and interpret diagnostic tests; and initiate and manage treatments (including prescribe medications)—are well positioned to provide health care and improve health outcomes for millions of Americans.

Q. **What advice would you give to high school and college students who are considering a career as a nurse practitioner?**

A. My advice to individuals who are considering a career as a nurse practitioner would be to talk to several nurse practitioners and ask them about their practices and, if possible, shadow them for a day. This really gives a sense of what a day in the life of a nurse practitioner would entail. A decision to pursue a career as a NP would involve attending nursing school and obtaining a BSN. Upon completion of a bachelor's degree, one would apply to an NP program. I'd recommend careful review of program options in terms of the population focus (i.e., family, adult/gerontology, pediatrics, women) and select a program that is accredited. It is also important to review NP program length, curriculum, and delivery methods (in person versus distance) to ensure that it is a good fit. Finally, NP education is vigorous so it's very important that students ask themselves if this is the right time to pursue this advanced education given their individual life circumstances.

Q. **Can you tell us about the American Association of Nurse Practitioners? What are the benefits of membership? What opportunities are available for student members?**

A. The American Association of Nurse Practitioners (AANP) is a nonprofit national professional membership organization for nurse practitioners of all specialties with a mission to lead NPs in transforming patient-centered health care. With more than 65,000 individual members and more than 200 group members, AANP represents the interests of more than 205,000 NPs practicing in the United States and is a recognized leader in public policy and advocacy, promoting access to quality care, collecting and analyzing workforce data, and delivering continuing education. The top priorities at AANP include promoting excellence in NP practice, education, and research; advancing health policy to shape the future of health care; and building a positive image of the nurse practitioner as a leader in the national and global health care community.

AANP professional membership provides free continuing education activities, up-to-date news on health care topics, advocacy at the national and state levels, and the resources needed for nurse practitioners' professional growth. Opportunities for students include scholarships and grants that support NPs and the advancement of the NP profession; a marketplace for student loan refinancing; and advanced notice of jobs and premium résumé placement in the AANP JobCenter, a career service center for NP job seekers and employers.

Genetic Counselors in Demand

Families with genetic disorders such as Down Syndrome, PKU deficiency, hemophilia, or a history of physical defects such as cleft palate or short stature often seek medical advice to help them understand these anomalies and determine the chance of recurrence in future generations. Professionals who specialize in this field are known as *genetic counselors*. They work as part of a medical team to provide testing and give informational support to families at risk for these genetic disorders or inherited birth defects. Genetic counselors investigate genetic issues by conducting extensive interviews with families and researching the medical histories of past generations. They conduct genetic testing in order to interpret and analyze inheritance patterns and risks of recurrence. They present different options and scenarios based upon their findings. Genetic counselors provide education to help families better understand their risks, give advice on how to best live with these conditions, or refer them to government agencies or nonprofit organizations that focus on a particular disorder.

Due to evolving technology used to detect diseases, medical advances in treatment, and increased public awareness, employment opportunities for genetic counselors will continue to grow. Their expertise will be in demand in clinical, educational, and administrative settings. Jobs will also be plentiful for those interested in working in private genetic counseling practices or consulting agencies. Overall, the U.S. Department of Labor predicts that employment for genetic counselors will grow by 29 percent during the next decade. Genetic counselors earned average salaries of $81,377 in 2016, according to the NSGC. Salaries can range as high as $250,000.

The American Board of Genetic Counseling mandates the following prerequisites before granting certification: a master's degree in genetic counseling or related field, clinical experience with a minimum of 50 supervised cases, and successful completion of a certification exam.

In order to be successful in the field, genetic counselors should have compassion when counseling families, be excellent communicators and good listeners, and be able to effectively analyze complex scientific information.

Genetic counselors are employed at hospitals, universities, laboratories, nonprofit organizations, government research agencies, and in private practice. According to the National Society of Genetic Counselors (NSGC), genetic counselors can work in the following areas: Assisted Reproductive Technology/Infertility Genetics, Cancer Genetics, Cardiovascular Genetics, Cystic Fibrosis Genetics, Fetal Intervention and Therapy Genetics, Hematology Genetics, Metabolic Genetics, Neurogenetics, Pediatric Genetics, Personalized Medicine Genetics, and Prenatal Genetics.

For more information, visit the following websites: **American Board of Genetic Counseling** (www.abgc.net), **American Society of Human Genetics** (www.ashg.org), **National Society of Genetic Counselors** (www.nsgc.org), **Careers in Human Genetics** (www.ashg.org/education/careers.shtml).

BIOMEDICAL ENGINEERS

OVERVIEW

Biomedical engineers use their knowledge of engineering principles and medical and biological science to improve medical instrumentation, equipment, and products; health management and care delivery systems; and medical information systems. Their work has led to important medical developments such as artificial limbs, magnetic imaging equipment, and pharmaceuticals. A minimum of a bachelor's degree in biomedical engineering, along with secondary study in another engineering discipline (such as mechanical engineering), is needed to enter the field. Approximately 20,890 biomedical engineers are employed in the United States. Job opportunities for biomedical engineers are expected to be excellent during the next decade.

FAST FACTS

High School Subjects
Biology
Chemistry

Personal Skills
Complex problem solving
Critical thinking
Judgment and decision making

Minimum Education Level
Bachelor's degree

Salary Range
$51,000 to $86,000 to $139,000+

Employment Outlook
Much faster than the average

O*NET-SOC
17-2031.00

NOC
2148

THE JOB

If you have certain vision problems, you can wear disposable contact lenses to correct your vision. If you suffer from heart failure, you may be a candidate to receive an artificial heart transplant. If you recently lost a tooth, your dentist may recommend a dental implant. If you are injured during a football game, an x-ray may be ordered to rule out any fractures. As a child, you received important immunizations to guard against potentially deadly childhood diseases. What do all these situations have in common? These procedures and treatments were made possible through the work of biomedical engineers.

Biomedical engineering is a field that combines the problem-solving techniques and analytical principles of engineering with medical and biological sciences in order to help improve the diagnosis and delivery of health care.

Many biomedical engineers are involved in the research and development of medical devices that help diagnose diseases or conditions, and they develop technology that can cure, treat, or prevent diseases. Many patients owe their quality of life, if not their actual lives, to the implantation of artificial organs such as hearts, pacemakers, and cochlear implants. These devices are self supporting, and they function without a stationary power supply. Other devices currently in various stages of research and development include a bio-artificial liver and an artificial lung.

Biomedical engineers are also responsible for many devices, which, while needing continuous power supply, filtering, or chemical processing, are critically important in providing life support. An example of such a device is a dialysis machine, which improves the quality of life for people with diabetes.

Biomedical engineers also design various prostheses—artificial body parts that replace real ones. Artificial hip and knee implants help many elderly patients escape the pain caused by age or chronic diseases such as arthritis. People who have lost arms and legs due to injury or disease can increase their mobility with robotic prostheses.

Delivery of health care treatment is also improved due to the work of biomedical engineers. Tools developed by engineers range from the familiar—latex gloves, wheelchairs, tongue depressors, bedpans, and adhesive bandages—to the highly specialized, such as laser surgical tools and instruments. Think of what your next hospital procedure or doctor's visit would be like without these items!

Some biomedical engineers specialize in the design and development of biotherapies and biotechnologies. These projects include pharmaceuticals and immunizations. Biotechnology improvements include tissue engineering in the form of artificial skin embedded in collagen, which is used for skin grafts; human-made insulin, to help regulate diabetes; and the development of laboratory-generated bone substitute, to replace human bones lost due to injury or disease.

Biomedical engineers also adapt computer software or hardware to create various health care applications. Medical imaging equipment includes 2D or 3D x-rays, magnetic resonance imaging instruments, and nuclear imaging equipment, such as positron emission tomography. These systems allow physicians to diagnose an injury or disease or to identify the location of tumors or other abnormalities. Computer applications can also help guide medical procedures such as angioplasty.

Some biomedical engineers develop computerized models to help teach students about bodily functions and systems. For example, a model of the human circulatory system is often used for teaching purposes in classrooms and museums.

Biomedical engineers do not come up with these advancements and technologies overnight. Rather, they are the result of years of research, testing, and more testing—regardless of the size or scope of the project. First the need for the application or project is identified. For example, when developing the artificial heart, the medical community expressed the need for such a device in order to lower the number of heart transplant procedures, considering the demand far exceeded the supply. Working with the design and functions of available heart-lung machines at the time, biomedical engineers along with physicians went through several drafts of artificial heart designs. The first few hearts were implanted in many test animals before the first clinical trial could be conducted on a human. Throughout the testing, approval was sought in the United States, and it was finally granted by the Food and Drug Administration. Much additional research, more redesigning, and more testing were done to the prototype before the artificial heart reached the type used in surgical procedures today. Biomedical engineers are constantly improving the design, quality, and durability of artificial hearts due to changing research and technology.

In addition to their laboratory duties, some biomedical engineers supervise technicians and laboratory assistants. They present their research to the medical community, government agencies, or private companies. Some biomedical engineers teach at the university level.

Biomedical engineers have a variety of work environments depending on their employer. However, they typically work indoors in comfortable, well-lit offices and laboratories. Full-time biomedical engineers typically work 40 hours a week, but they often work longer hours as deadlines approach or if assigned an urgent project. They often travel from laboratory to laboratory or to meet with other specialists working on a project.

REQUIREMENTS

HIGH SCHOOL

In high school, take as many courses as possible in the life sciences, such as biology, anatomy and physiology, and chemistry. Other useful classes include English, mathematics, (especially algebra, advanced algebra, geometry, trigonometry, and pre-calculus), drafting, physics, shop, computer science, computer programming, speech, and health.

POSTSECONDARY TRAINING

You will need a minimum of a bachelor's degree in biomedical engineering, along with secondary study in another engineering discipline (such as electronics or mechanical engineering), to enter the field. Another option is to earn a bachelor's degree in electrical, chemical, or mechanical engineering with a specialty in biomedical engineering. Engineers who work in research laboratories typically need a graduate degree. ABET accredits biomedical engineering programs. Visit its website, www.abet.org, to access a database of accredited programs in the United States.

Typical college courses include biology, physiology, biochemistry, general physics, electronic circuits and instrumentation design, inorganic and organic chemistry, statics and dynamics, signals and systems, biomaterials, thermodynamics and transport phenomenon, and engineering design. Students also take advanced science and engineering courses related to their biomedical engineering specialty (such as bioelectronics, virtual reality, or rehabilitation engineering).

IEEE Engineering in Medicine & Biology reports that many biomedical engineers go on to medical or dental school, and a few even attend law school with an end goal of working in patent and intellectual property law. Others earn a master's degree in business administration and enter managerial positions.

Did You Know?

Only 20 percent of engineering degrees were awarded to women in 2015, despite the fact that women comprised 47 percent of the workforce. Yet, several engineering specialties boast a much-higher percentage of female graduates. In 2015, 49.7 percent of environmental engineering graduates were women. Other popular engineering specialties for women were biomedical (40.9 percent of graduates), biological and agricultural (34.4 percent), and chemical (32.4 percent).

Sources: American Society for Engineering Education, U.S. Department of Labor

CERTIFICATION AND LICENSING

Engineers whose work affects property, health, or life must be licensed as professional engineers. According to the U.S. Department of Labor, "this licensure generally requires a degree from an ABET-accredited engineering program, four years of relevant work experience, and completion of a state examination. Recent graduates can start the licensing process by taking the examination in two stages. The initial Fundamentals of Engineering examination can be taken upon graduation. Engineers who pass this examination commonly are called engineers in training (EITs) or engineer interns. After acquiring suitable work experience, EITs can take the second examination, called the Principles and Practice of Engineering exam." Visit the National Council of Examiners for Engineering and Surveying website, www.ncees.org, for more information on licensure.

OTHER REQUIREMENTS

Communication skills are important, since biomedical engineers often meet with other members of a design team or with other health care professionals. They must be able to explain the goals and scientific framework of their project to other engineers, technicians, medical professionals, and laypeople. At times the job is quite stressful and demanding, especially when working with an extremely complicated design or system, or when faced with tedious testing and retesting of a product. Successful biomedical engineers are calm and focused, even during the most demanding of situations. Other important traits include an analytical personality, the ability to solve problems, and scientific ability.

Cool Career: Biomedical Equipment Technologist

Students who are mechanically inclined may enjoy working in the field of biomedical equipment technology. *Biomedical equipment technicians* maintain and repair key medical equipment such as lasers, x-ray equipment, and machines used to perform tests such as EKGs, CT scans, and MRIs. They also modify or operate some medical instruments or equipment. Biomedical equipment technicians work in laboratories and hospitals, for medical equipment manufacturers, and for other employers that use medical equipment. They must be able to think quickly and work effectively under pressure because they may be called to repair lifesaving equipment in time-sensitive situations. In addition to being mechanically inclined, workers in the field of biomedical equipment technology should also have good computer skills, be organized, and be excellent communicators. Demand for biomedical equipment technicians is expected to grow about as fast as the average for all careers during the next decade, according to the U.S. Department of Labor, which reports that "employment growth will stem from both greater demand for health care services and the increasing types and complexity of the equipment these workers maintain and repair." A minimum of an associate's degree in biomedical technology or engineering is required to enter the field.

Contact the following organizations for more information: **American Society for Healthcare Engineering** (312-422-3800, ashe@aha.org, www.ashe.org), **Association for the Advancement of Medical Instrumentation** (703-525-4890, www.aami.org), and the **Medical Equipment and Technology Association** (www.mymeta.org).

EXPLORING

There are many ways to learn more about a career as a biomedical engineer. You can read books and magazines about the field, attend an after-school or summer engineering program (see www.careercornerstone.org/pcsumcamps.htm for more information), and join the Technology Student Association (www.tsaweb.org), which will provide you with a chance to explore career opportunities in science, technology, engineering, and mathematics, allow you to participate in summer exploration programs at colleges and universities, and enter academic competitions. Ask your teacher or school counselor to arrange an information interview with a biomedical engineer. If you're a college student, you can join the Biomedical Engineering Society and other organizations. Visit the websites of college biomedical engineering programs to learn about typical classes and possible career paths. Professional associations can also provide information about the field. IEEE Engineering in Medicine & Biology offers a useful brochure, Designing a Career in Biomedical Engineering, at www.embs.org/docs/careerguide.pdf. Another useful resource is the American Institute for Medical and Biological Engineering's Navigating the Circuit website, www.navigate.aimbe.org.

EMPLOYERS

Approximately 20,890 biomedical engineers are employed in the United States. They work for colleges and universities, hospitals, laboratories, research facilities, pharmaceutical companies, manufacturing facilities, and government agencies.

GETTING A JOB

Many biomedical engineers obtain their first jobs as a result of contacts made through college internships, career fairs, or networking events. Others seek assistance in obtaining job leads from college career services offices, newspaper want ads, and employment and social media websites. Additionally, professional associations, such as the Biomedical Engineering Society (http://jobboard.bmes.org/jobseekers), provide job listings at their websites. See For More Information for a list of organizations. There are many opportunities available with federal agencies. Those interested in positions with the federal government should visit the U.S. Office of Personnel Management's website, www.usajobs.gov.

ADVANCEMENT

Biomedical engineers who are employed in nonacademic settings advance by receiving pay raises and supervisory duties, by working on more prestigious projects, and by receiving additional grant money to work on research projects. Those who work at colleges and universities as educators advance from the position of instructor, to assistant professor, to associate professor, and finally to professor—with an overall goal of attaining tenure. According to the U.S. Department of Labor, "tenured professors cannot be fired without just cause and due process." Once a professor is tenured, he or she might advance by serving as department head or becoming a dean or even college president.

Some biomedical engineers use their bachelor's degree in biomedical engineering as a first step toward attending graduate or medical school and pursuing careers in law, business, medicine, dentistry, or veterinary science.

EARNINGS

Median annual salaries for biomedical engineers were $86,220 in May 2015, according to the U.S. Department of Labor (USDL). Salaries ranged from less than $51,480 to $139,520 or more. The USDL reports the following mean annual earnings for biomedical engineers by employer: scientific research and development services, $104,490; medical equipment and supplies manufacturing, $96,870; navigational, measuring, electromedical, and control instruments manufacturing, $88,950; pharmaceutical and medicine manufacturing, $85,130; and general medical and surgical hospitals, $75,530.

Employers offer a variety of benefits, including the following: medical, dental, and life insurance; paid holidays, vacations, and sick and personal days; 401(k) plans; profit-sharing plans; retirement and pension plans; and educational-assistance programs. Self-employed workers must provide their own benefits.

EMPLOYMENT OUTLOOK

Employment for biomedical engineers is expected to be excellent during the next decade, according to the U.S. Department of Labor (USDL). The growing and aging U.S. population and demand for new medical devices and equipment are creating many opportunities for biomedical engineers. The USDL says that "smartphone technology and three-dimensional printing are examples of technology being applied to biomedical advances." Opportunities will be particularly good in pharmaceutical manufacturing and related industries.

Interview: Sara Beck

Sara Beck is a senior mechanical design engineer at Medtronic (www.medtronic.com), a premier medical technology and services company.

Q. **How long have you worked in the field? What made you want to enter this career?**

A. I have worked as an engineer in the medical devices industry for more than 10 years. I entered this career because I wanted to truly impact the lives of people by using my analytical, organizational, and critical-thinking skills.

Q. **What are some typical projects that you work on as a mechanical design engineer?**

A. I currently support a released implantable drug pump. My primary job is to take complaints/concerns from our customers and investigate them technically. I work with a team of specialists (customer service, quality, physicians, and other engineers). As I dig into these concerns, I try to test the product in the simulated condition to understand if the device could have contributed to the issue. In the past, I have also worked on developing products such as orthopedic shoulder replacements, orthopedic instruments, a handheld device that receives heart-rate information from an internal monitoring device, and an external blood pressure measurement system. In product development, a project would consist of defining design specifications to meet customer requirements, designing a product to meet these specifications, testing the product to ensure it meets the demands, and then verifying it meets the customers' needs. This, of course, involves working with a team of electrical engineers, system engineers, reliability/quality engineers, project managers, etc.

Q. **What are some of the pros and cons of your job?**

A. The best part of my job is knowing my work improves the quality of life of

FOR MORE INFORMATION

Visit the Institute's website for a glossary of biomedical engineering terms.
American Institute for Medical and Biological Engineering
www.aimbe.org

To learn more about engineering education and publications, contact
American Society for Engineering Education
www.asee.org

For information on careers, visit
Biomedical Engineering Society
www.bmes.org

For career information, contact
Biotechnology Innovation Organization
www.bio.org

For information on careers and membership, visit
IEEE Engineering in Medicine & Biology
www.embs.org

many patients. The drug pump allows children with severe spasticity to walk or run by releasing a drug at the right dosage to relax their muscles; it allows people with chronic pain to enjoy active lives with their family and friends. Medtronic improves a life every three seconds. I love working for a company that cares so deeply about improving people's lives. Day to day, I enjoy working in a team to solve very complex problems.

One con of my job is that a biomedical engineer cannot design medical devices in every state, nor in every city. My husband and I are both biomedical engineers; the rest of our family lives in Ohio but there are not many job opportunities there for us.

Q. What advice would you give to young people who are considering a career in biomedical design engineering?

A. Work to obtain a co-op/internship in the field before you graduate. The University of Akron's biomedical engineering (BME) program (which I attended) highly encouraged a one-year co-op before graduation. While it meant it would take me five years to finish my undergraduate degree, the one year of experience I gained at DePuy Orthopaedics was extremely valuable for giving me confidence that this was truly the right field for me and obtaining my first job. While the coursework ensures you can solve problems, your career the next 40 to 50 years will be slightly different day in and out than school. It's important that you experience the environment and type of work you will be doing. At minimum, make sure you can do some job shadowing.

Also, once you know what kind of products (implantables, biologicals, electrical instruments) you want to work on, focus your BME degree on what you want to do. My BME degree focused on mechanical engineering. Because of my coursework focus, co-op/internship and first job, I have the title "mechanical design engineer."

Q. What's the future employment outlook for biomedical design engineers?

A.   The medical devices industry will likely have a continued demand for engineers due to the aging population and need for better medical devices that reduce overall health care costs. In my professional opinion, there are very few medical device jobs with the title "biomedical engineer," which is why I stress the value of a co-op/internship and solid engineering coursework.

CREATIVE ARTS THERAPISTS

OVERVIEW

Creative arts therapy is a health care profession that is built on the fundamental principle that the creative process can enhance a person's physical, mental, and emotional well-being. Therapists use art, music, dance/movement, writing/poetry, drama, and other artistic disciplines to assist patients. Creative arts therapy can be a satisfying career for individuals with strong artistic backgrounds who are also interested in a career in health care. In recent years, creative arts therapies have gained wider acceptance from the public, which is fueling demand for therapists.

FAST FACTS

High School Subjects
Art
Music
Psychology
Speech

Personal Skills
Artistic
Helping

Minimum Education Level
Varies by specialty

Salary Range
$20,000 to $50,000 to $200,000

Employment Outlook
Much faster than the average

O*NET-SOC
29-1125.00, 29-1125.01,
29-1125.02, 29-1129.00

NOC
3144

THE JOB

Major creative arts therapy practice specialties include art, music, drama, dance/movement, and poetry. Creative arts therapists work with people of all ages, although some may specialize to provide therapy to members of a specific age group—such as young children or senior citizens. Therapists work with patients in individual, group, or family sessions. The following paragraphs provide more information on creative arts therapy specialties.

Visual artists have been using creative self-expression as an outlet to express their feelings and emotions since the beginning of time. But you don't have to be a famous painter or sculptor to understand the basic premise behind the discipline of art therapy—expressing oneself can be an emotional, healing, and therapeutic process. *Art therapists* guide clients through the process of resolving conflicts and problems, developing interpersonal skills, reducing stress, increasing self-esteem, and coming to a sense of self-understanding—by means of personal artistic expression. Those who enter the field have a strong commitment to working with people in one-on-one situations. They believe in the nurturing and healing power of art and its importance in helping people resolve personal issues resulting from a variety of life challenges such as physical or mental illness, grief, or trauma. Art therapists use a variety of mediums—from paint and sculpture, to collage and computer art—when working with patients.

Although music has been used for centuries as an informal way of trying to achieve therapeutic goals, it was not until World War I, when professional and amateur musicians visited veteran's hospitals to play music for injured veterans, that the medical community realized the healing power of music and began to consistently incorporate this philosophy into health care regimens. Music therapy involves the use of music to accomplish a variety of therapeutic aims, including the restoration, maintenance, and improvement of physical, emotional, cognitive, and social functioning. Treatment options include creating, singing, moving to, and/or listening to music. A *music therapist* may work with individuals of all ages. For example, a music therapist might help older adults with dementia-related challenges, military veterans with traumatic brain injuries, children with special needs, or teenagers with substance abuse disorders.

Drama therapy is "the intentional use of drama and/or theater processes to achieve therapeutic goals," according to the North American Drama Therapy Association. Therapy methods include pantomime, role playing, puppetry, theater games, storytelling, improvisation, and original scripted dramatization.

Dance/movement therapists create and conduct dance/movement sessions to assist physically, emotionally, and mentally ill people. Therapists also use these sessions to help doctors and rehabilitation specialists measure patients' progress in rehabilitation.

Poetry therapists use poems and what the International Federation for Biblio/Poetry Therapy (IFBPT) calls the "poetic in all literature" to assist people with mental and physical illnesses and disabilities. Treatment methods include the reading, writing, and discussion of poetry; storytelling; and journal writing. The IFBPT says that "it is not necessary to be a poet in order to be a practitioner of poetry therapy, but it is essential to be a reader, to have a thirst for knowledge and a hunger for the interactive wonder of words."

REQUIREMENTS

HIGH SCHOOL

If you've already chosen a career path in the creative arts (such as music therapy), it's important to take as many classes in that area as possible (and, in the case of music therapy, learn how to play at least one musical instrument). If you're not sure what career path to pursue, take courses in all the arts (music, visual art, drama, writing) to learn more about each field, develop your creativity, and identify your talents. Take psychology classes to learn more about human behavior. English and speech classes will help you to develop your communication skills (which are key to success as a creative arts therapist). Other recommended classes include business (especially if you plan to start your own practice), social studies, computer science, biology, philosophy, and sociology.

POSTSECONDARY TRAINING

A master's degree in art therapy is required for professional certification in art therapy. Students entering master's degree programs have undergraduate degrees in areas such as art, education, or psychology. Approximately 35 postsecondary art therapy programs in the United States and Canada are approved/accredited by the American Art Therapy Association

Did You Know?

According to the Music Therapy Program at California State University at Northridge, some of the benefits of music therapy include:

✔ "Development of fine and gross motor skills

✔ Improvement in acquisition and application of academic fundamentals

✔ Development of practical life skills

✔ Increase in socialization

✔ Enhancement of self-esteem

✔ Expansion of the quality of life through musical enjoyment and creative self-expression."

(http://arttherapy.org/aata-educational-programs). Typical classes in an art therapy program include History and Theory of Art Therapy; Studio/Technique of Art Therapy; Marital and Family Art Therapy Counseling; Child Art Therapy; Adolescent Art Therapy; Research Methods; Counseling/Art Therapy Process; Psychopathology/Art and Diagnosis; Social/Cultural Diversity and Art Therapy; Ethics and Professionalism; Group Art Therapy; Human Development and Art Therapy; Trauma I and II; Substance Abuse and Art Therapy; Assessment Procedures; Practicum in Art Therapy; and Advanced Issues in Psychotherapy and Art Therapy.

A bachelor's degree in music therapy and the completion of 1,200 hours of required fieldwork are necessary for employment in the field. More than 70 degree programs in 30 states, the District of Columbia, and Canada are approved by the American Music Therapy Association. For a list of schools, visit www.musictherapy.org/careers.

Students become drama therapists by attending drama therapy master's or doctoral degree programs that are approved by the North American Drama Therapy Association (www.nadta.org/education-and-credentialing/resources-for-students-and-bcts/accredited-schools.html). There are only five such programs in the United States and Canada—Antioch

University, California Institute of Integral Studies, Concordia University, Lesley University, and New York University. Others who have advanced degrees in theater or mental health fields prepare for the field by receiving drama therapy training via the NADTA's alternative training program.

Students become dance/movement therapists by completing a master's degree program in dance/movement therapy that is approved by the American Dance Therapy Association (https://adta.org/approved-graduate-programs). There are only six such programs in the United States—Antioch University, Columbia College, Drexel University, Lesley University, Naropa University, Pratt University, and Sarah Lawrence College. Others who have advanced degrees in theater or mental health fields prepare for the field by receiving drama therapy training via the ADTA's alternative training program, https://adta.org/alternate-route-training. Undergraduate course work in dance/movement therapy is also available.

There are no-university-based training programs in poetry therapy. Most aspiring poetry therapists prepare for the field by participating in an independent study program with an approved mentor/poetry therapist. Such a program can last two to five years.

Typical Classes in a Dance/Movement Therapy Program

✔ Introduction to Expressive Arts Therapy
✔ Dance/Movement Therapy Theory
✔ Clinical Assessment and Treatment Planning
✔ Addiction Counseling
✔ Family Counseling
✔ Social and Cultural Foundations
✔ Introduction to the Body-Mind Experience in Movement
✔ Human Development
✔ Psychopathology Theories and Principles of Counseling
✔ Clinical Techniques of Counseling
✔ Neuroanatomy/Neurophysiology
✔ Methods of Group Therapy
✔ Special Topics: Performance as Therapy
✔ Anatomy and Kinesiology
✔ Laban Movement Analysis

CERTIFICATION AND LICENSING

The following associations provide voluntary certification:

✔ Art Therapy Credentials Board (art therapist registered, art therapist-board certified)

✔ Certification Board for Music Therapists (music therapist-board certified)

✔ American Board of Examiners in Psychodrama, Sociometry and Group Psychotherapy (certified practitioner, certified practitioner-registered practitioner applicant for trainer)

✔ North American Drama Therapy Association (registered drama therapist)

✔ American Dance Therapy Association (registered-dance/movement therapist, board certified dance/movement therapist)

✔ International Federation for Biblio/Poetry Therapy (certified applied poetry facilitator, certified poetry therapist, registered poetry therapist).

Contact these organizations for more information on certification requirements.

Many creative arts therapists are also licensed by their state as counselors, social workers, or marriage and family therapists. In some states, creative arts therapists must be licensed. For example, music therapists are required to be licensed in Oregon.

OTHER REQUIREMENTS

Creative arts therapists must have a strong desire to help others. They must be compassionate, empathetic, caring, and good listeners to effectively assist patients. Because they work so closely with patients, as well as with

Cool Career: Recreation Therapist

Certified therapeutic recreation therapists use leisure and recreation-based activities to improve the physical, cognitive, and emotional well-being of those who are ill or disabled. Recreation therapy interventions include adapted aquatics, adapted fitness activity, adventure programming, animal-assisted therapy, aquatic therapy, creative arts, horticulture, journaling, leisure education, music, social skills training, stress management, t'ai chi chuan, therapeutic horseback riding, wheelchair sports, and yoga. Recreation therapy is sometimes referred to as therapeutic recreation. Recreation therapists typically need a bachelor's degree to work in the field. Some programs offer recreation therapy in the department of education as an option in secondary education, while other programs focus primarily on a health sciences curriculum and/or a parks and recreation curriculum. Approximately 17,880 recreational therapists (RTs) are employed in the United States. Job opportunities for RTs are expected to grow by 12 percent during the next decade, according to the U.S. Department of Labor. Recreational therapists will enjoy good employment prospects because the baby boom generation is aging and will need recreational therapists to help treat age-related injuries and illnesses. RTs will also be needed as the number of Americans who are obese or who have chronic medical conditions increases, legislation goes into effect that requires more federally funded services for students with disabilities, and health maintenance organizations rely on therapists to treat patients in outpatient settings rather than in more-expensive hospitals. Contact the American Therapeutic Recreation Association (601-450-2872, www.atra-online.com) for more information.

other members of the health care team, creative arts therapists need excellent communication, teamwork, and interpersonal skills. Other important traits include flexibility, creativity, the ability to multitask, patience, imagination, tact, and a sense of humor.

EXPLORING

Check out the following journals to learn more about the work of creative arts therapists: *Art Therapy: Journal of the American Art Therapy Association*; *Journal of Music Therapy*; *Journal of Psychodrama, Sociometry, and Group Psychotherapy*; *Drama Therapy Review*; *American Journal of Dance Therapy*; and *Journal of Poetry Therapy*.

Talk to creative arts therapists about their work, and try to set up an appointment to job shadow one. Your art, drama, or music teacher, school counselor, and creative art therapy associations can help arrange opportunities for exploration. Try to land a part-time or summer job or internship at a health care facility that offers creative arts therapy. Finally, check out the following resources to learn about the various specialties:

✔ **What is Art Therapy?:**
www.arttherapy.org/upload/whatisarttherapy.pdf

✔ **A Career in Music Therapy:**
www.musictherapy.org/careers/employment

✔ **Drama Therapy brochure:**
www.nadta.org/assets/documents/nadt-brochure.pdf

✔ **What is Dance/Movement Therapy?:** https://adta.org/faqs.

EMPLOYERS

Creative arts therapists are employed by hospitals (medical and psychiatric), clinics, nursing homes, wellness centers, outpatient counseling clinics, residential treatment facilities, programs for persons with disabilities, hospice programs, public and community agencies, school settings (special education, therapeutic classrooms), businesses, private practice, halfway houses, prisons, domestic violence and homeless shelters, and correctional facilities.

GETTING A JOB

Participating in an internship during college is an excellent way to learn more about the field and get your foot in the door for full-time employment. Many companies use their internship programs to identify candidates for full-time positions. Talk with your professors and career counselors, as well as visit the websites of creative arts therapy associations, to learn about internship opportunities. Use the resources of your college's career services office to learn more about job fairs and develop a strong resume and effective interviewing skills. Network online at social media

FOR MORE INFORMATION

Contact the following organizations for information about education, membership, certification, and careers.

American Art Therapy Association
888-290-0878
info@arttherapy.org
www.arttherapy.org

**American Dance
Therapy Association**
www.adta.org

**American Music
Therapy Association**
301-589-3300
info@musictherapy.org
www.musictherapy.org

**American Society for Group
Psychotherapy and Psychodrama**
609-737-8500
asgpp@asgpp.org
www.asgpp.org

**International Federation
for Biblio/Poetry Therapy**
admin@ifbpt.org
www.ifbpt.org

**National Association
for Poetry Therapy**
naptadmin@poetrytherapy.org
www.poetrytherapy.org

**National Coalition of Creative
Arts Therapies Associations**
www.nccata.org

**North American Drama
Therapy Association**
888-416-7167
office@nadta.org
www.nadta.org

For information on job opportunities in Canada, contact
**Canadian Counselling and
Psychotherapy Association**
Creative Arts in Counselling Chapter
www.ccpa-accp.ca/chapters/creative-arts-counselling

sites such as LinkedIn, at events held by professional associations, and at job fairs. Finally, check out job listings at the following websites:

✔ Art therapy: http://careercenter.americanarttherapyassociation.org

✔ Dance therapy: https://adta.org/forum

✔ Music therapy: www.indeed.com/q-Music-Therapist-jobs.html.

ADVANCEMENT

Creative arts therapists advance by receiving pay raises, by working for larger or more well-known employers, and by taking on managerial duties. Some therapists start their own companies. Others become college professors.

EARNINGS

In 2016, art therapists earned median salaries of $41,486, according to PayScale.com. Earnings ranged from $30,377 to $58,461 or more.

In 2014, music therapists earned average salaries of $50,808, according to a member survey by the American Music Therapy Association. Salaries ranged from $20,000 to $200,000.

Health Care Careers That Require an Associate's Degree or Postsecondary Award That Will Add the Most New Jobs, 2014-24

Career	# of New Jobs	Median Salary
Licensed Practical Nurses	+117,300	$42,490
Emergency Medical Technicians	+58,500	$31,700
Dental Hygienists	+37,400	$71,520
Massage Therapists	+36,500	$37,180
Physical Therapist Assistants	+31,900	$54,410
Medical Records and Health Information Technicians	+29,000	$35,900
Medical and Clinical Laboratory Technologists and Technicians	+29,000	$38,370
Phlebotomists	+28,100	$30,670

Source: U.S. Department of Labor

Median annual salaries of recreational therapists (a career that includes some types of creative arts therapists) were $45,890 in May 2015, according to the U.S. Department of Labor. Ten percent earned less than $28,020, and 10 percent earned $71,790 or more.

Employers offer a variety of benefits, including the following: medical, dental, and life insurance; paid holidays, vacations, and sick and personal days; 401(k) plans; profit-sharing plans; retirement and pension plans; and educational-assistance programs. Part-time and self-employed therapists must provide their own benefits.

EMPLOYMENT OUTLOOK

Employment for recreational therapists (an occupation that includes some types of creative arts therapists) who work in health care and social assistance is expected to grow much faster than the average for all careers during the next decade, according to the U.S. Department of Labor. There is a strong need for therapists—especially those in art and music therapy—to help those with physical, mental, and emotional challenges. Therapists who are certified and who are willing to relocate for job opportunities will have the best job prospects.

DENTAL ASSISTANTS

OVERVIEW

Dental assistants help dentists and other members of the dental team work more efficiently. They are responsible for some patient care, laboratory duties, and administrative duties such as assisting dentists during patient examinations and procedures, preparing casts, handing tools to dentists, and billing. Aspiring dental assistants prepare for the field by receiving on-the-job training or by earning a certificate or diploma in dental assisting at a postsecondary academic institution. Approximately 323,110 dental assistants are employed in the United States. Employment for dental assistants is expected to be good during the next decade.

FAST FACTS

High School Subjects
Business
Health

Personal Skills
Helping
Technical

Minimum Education Level
High school diploma

Salary Range
$24,000 to $35,000 to $50,000+

Employment Outlook
Much faster than the average

O*NET-SOC
31-9091.00

NOC
3411

THE JOB

A good dental assistant can increase the efficiency of an entire dental team, allowing its members to see more patients in a timely manner. Depending on the size of the practice, the dental assistant's role can encompass patient care and administrative and laboratory duties.

Dental assistants prepare the examination room prior to a patient's visit. They clean and sterilize equipment and tools and set up instrument trays, making sure all necessary tools and supplies are in place for the dentist and dental hygienist. When a new patient visits the office, dental assistants record his or her personal information and medical history and enter it in a computer database. They then direct the patient to the exam room and settle him or her into the chair. During the examination or procedure, dental assistants work alongside the dentist, handing him or her tools, providing suction, or wiping water, paste, or saliva from the patient's mouth.

After the examination, dental assistants instruct patients regarding necessary post-operative care of the mouth or any wounds. Some dental assis-

Emerging Health Care Careers

Clinician shortages, an aging population that requires more and different types of medical care, pressure to reduce health care costs, emerging models of person-centered care, and other factors are prompting the creation of a variety of new health care careers, according to AMN Healthcare and The Center for Professional Advancement. Here are some emerging careers:

1. Navigator. Typically a licensed clinical professional who facilitates patient and family health treatment activities in cooperation with the health care facility and insurance providers.

2. Chief Experience Officer. Develops company-wide strategies to enhance patient satisfaction as they interact with medical staff. Already popular in the corporate world.

3. Tele-Health Professional. Physicians, nurses, nurse practitioners, and other health care professionals who are trained to consult, diagnose, and treat patients through virtual means.

4. Medical Scribe. Trained health assistants who shadow physicians as they make patient rounds. They record a patient's medical history and treatment plans, transcribe test and laboratory results, and document procedures and treatments done by physicians and nurses.

tants are trained to remove sutures or apply local anesthetics. They give patients general oral care tips, including describing the proper way to brush and floss teeth. They often assemble and hand out oral care kits to patients after each dental visit.

Dental assistants also have laboratory duties. They may be trained to take x-rays (radiographs) of the patients' gums and teeth as well as process the x-ray films. They also prepare materials for impressions or fillings.

Depending on state regulations, dental assistants can be trained to make casts of teeth from impressions created by dentists. They clean and polish removable appliances or make temporary crowns. If the dental office offers cosmetic procedures such as ultrasonic bleaching treatments, dental assistants can be trained to prepare the patient's mouth and gums with protective wax or other substances.

Administrative duties encompass a large portion of the dental assistant's workday. Dental assistants oversee the front office, including fielding phone calls, scheduling and confirming patients' appointments, and greeting patients as they arrive. They keep careful records of patients and the treatments performed during the appointment. They may be asked to make copies of x-rays, test results, or other paperwork for patients or other dentists.

Depending on the size of the office, dental assistants may be responsible for the billing. They often consult with insurance companies or government agencies such as Medicare regarding procedure costs or patient deductibles. Dental assistants keep track of payments made, either through insurance checks or private methods. Most dental offices now bill insurance companies electronically, so dental assistants are specially trained in the ins and outs of electronic billing, including proper procedural codes.

Dental assistants also keep track of and order supplies and equipment. Some dental assistants, especially those employed at pediatric dental offices, take photographs of children after a no-cavity dental visit. In general, many dental assistants act as the dental practice's office manager.

Dental assistants work in well-lighted, clean, and comfortable offices. They often sit in the front office when conducting administrative duties. When working with patients or assisting the dental team, they often maintain a work area near the dentist's chair. Nearly 33 percent of dental assistants work part-time. Some evening and Saturday hours are typically required.

Dental assistants are required to wear gloves, masks, eyewear, and other protective clothing, especially when working with patients. Some dental assistants wear a uniform of smock and pants. Comfortable shoes are a must, since dental assistants spend much of their day on their feet, moving back and forth between exam rooms and the front office.

REQUIREMENTS

High School

Take chemistry, biology, health, speech, computer science, accounting, and business in high school to prepare for this career.

Postsecondary Training

Some dental assistants still learn their skills on the job, but an increasing number prepare for the field by completing a postsecondary dental-assisting education program that lasts nine to 11 months. Completion of this type of program typically results in a certificate or diploma. Associate's degree programs are also available. It is a good idea to attend a training program that is accredited by the Commission on Dental Accreditation (www.ada.org/en/coda/find-a-program). Nearly 260 programs are accredited by the Commission. Once they are hired, dental assistants also complete on-the-job training to learn the specific procedures and protocols of their employer.

Certification and Licensing

Dental assistants can receive the voluntary certified dental assistant (CDA) credential from the Dental Assisting National Board. The CDA is recognized or required in more than 35 states. The Board also offers the following credentials: national entry-level dental assistant, certified orthodontic assistant, certified preventive functions dental assistant, and certified restorative functions dental assistant. In addition, dental assistants must be certified in cardiopulmonary resuscitation.

In some states, dental assistants must be licensed to perform expanded functions or to perform radiological procedures.

OTHER REQUIREMENTS

Dental assistants should have a polite and calm demeanor, especially when dealing with patients in person or over the phone, or when speaking with insurance company clerks or dental supply vendors. They should be organized and work well under pressure, since a good portion of their work day is spent juggling multiple and varied tasks. Finally, they must have good manual dexterity because they need to prepare and hand a variety of instruments and materials to dentists during dental procedures.

EXPLORING

There are many ways to learn more about a career as a dental assistant. You can read books and magazines about dentistry (such as *Dental Assistant Journal,* www.adaausa.org/Publications/Dental-Assistant-Journal), visit the websites of college dental-assisting programs to learn about typical classes and possible career paths, and you can ask your teacher or school counselor to arrange an information interview with a dental assistant. Professional associations can also provide information about the field. The American Dental Association provides a wealth of information on dental assistants at its website, www.ada.org/en/education-careers/careers-in-dentistry/dental-team-careers/dental-assistant. You should also try to land a part-time job in a dental office. This will give you a chance to interact with dental assistants and see if the career is a good fit for your interests and abilities.

EMPLOYERS

Approximately 323,110 dental assistants are employed in the United States. About 91 percent work in offices of dentists. Other employers include government agencies, the U.S. military, offices of physicians, schools and clinics (public health dentistry), hospitals, insurance companies (processing dental insurance claims), and colleges and universities (as dental educators).

GETTING A JOB

Participation in college internships and attending career fairs and networking events are excellent ways to learn more about job opportunities. Others seek assistance in obtaining job leads from college career services offices, newspaper want ads, and employment websites (such as Dentalworkers.com, www.dentalworkers.com/employment). Some professional dental associations provide job listings at their websites or in their journals. Those interested in positions with federal agencies—such as the Veterans Health Administration or Indian Health Service—should visit the U.S. Office of Personnel Management's website, www.usajobs.gov.

ADVANCEMENT

Dental assistants advance by receiving pay raises and by being assigned more demanding duties—such as handling all billing for their office. With additional training, they can become office managers, dental hygienists, dental educators, or dentists. Others work in dental product sales or as insurance claims processors for dental insurance companies.

EARNINGS

Median annual salaries for dental assistants were $35,980 in May 2015, according to the U.S. Department of Labor (USDL). Salaries ranged from less than $24,950 to $50,660 or more.

Becoming certified often translates into higher earnings. Dental assistants who were certified earned average hourly wages of $19.00 in 2014, according to the Dental Assisting National Board (DANB). Those who did not have certification earned only $17.02 an hour.

Dental assistants usually receive benefits such as health and life insurance, vacation days, sick leave, a savings and pension plan, and an allowance for uniforms. Seventy-five percent of certified dental assistants (CDAs) received paid vacation from their employers in 2014, according to the DANB. Fifty-nine percent received a 401(k) pension plan, and 52 percent received free dental care. Part-time workers must provide their own benefits.

EMPLOYMENT OUTLOOK

Employment for dental assistants is expected to grow much faster than the average during the next decade, according to the U.S. Department of Labor. Job opportunities for dental assistants will be excellent as a result of several factors. The U.S. population is growing, which will create more demand for dental professionals. More middle-aged and elderly people are keeping their natural teeth, which is creating a need for more dental assistants. Finally, the overall focus on preventive dental care for people of all ages will ensure a strong employment outlook for dental professionals in coming years.

FOR MORE INFORMATION

For career information, contact
**American Dental
Assistants Association**
www.adaausa.org

For information on dental assisting education and careers, contact
American Dental Association
www.ada.org

For information on dental education, contact

**American Dental
Education Association**
www.adea.org

For information about certification, contact
Dental Assisting National Board
www.dentalassisting.com

For information on job opportunities in Canada, contact
**Canadian Dental
Assistants' Association**
613-521-5495
www.cdaa.ca/da-promotion

DENTAL HYGIENISTS

OVERVIEW

Dental hygienists perform prophylaxis procedures on patients (preventive care that helps a patient avoid gum disease and cavities), take oral x-rays, administer local anesthetics, and remove sutures and dressings. They perform administrative duties such as charting and/or taking oral and medical histories of patients. Dental hygienists also educate patients about the importance of oral preventive care. A minimum of an associate's degree or certificate is required to work as a dental hygienist. About 200,550 dental hygienists are employed in the United States. Employment in this field is expected to grow much faster than the average for all careers during the next decade.

FAST FACTS

High School Subjects
Biology
Health

Personal Skills
Helping
Technical

Minimum Education Level
Associate's degree

Salary Range
$50,000 to $72,000 to $98,000+

Employment Outlook
Much faster than the average

O*NET-SOC
29-2021.00

NOC
3222

THE JOB

Dental hygienists are licensed dental professionals who are responsible for many of the routine duties once performed by dentists—which leaves dentists free to complete more complicated and invasive procedures.

At the beginning of the appointment, the dental hygienist first assesses the patient. He or she reviews the patient's medical and oral history, takes x-rays, and conducts a clinical exam. Then he or she examines the condition of the patient's teeth as well as the periodontal area. Dental hygienists report their findings to the dentist, who then conducts a follow-up exam for a final diagnosis of any dental problems.

If the patient is there for a routine cleaning, the dental hygienist can perform the prophylaxis. This involves the removal of any tartar (hardened mineralized plaque) and stains from the surface of the teeth. Dental hygienists use various hand instruments and power-driven dental instruments to help them during the process. If the patient suffers from peri-

odontal disease, the dental hygienist may administer a local anesthetic before continuing on with scaling (removing plaque and other stains) or root planing (more involved cleaning that focuses on the roots) to help curb the disease. The dental hygienist may also finish the session with an application of fluoride, which prevents tooth decay.

Dental hygienists may also be specially trained to remove sutures or change dressings for patients who have had oral surgery or other invasive procedures. They also assist the dentist by creating teeth molds in preparation for denture pieces, tooth caps, or implants. They may help the dentist when providing ultrasonic teeth whitening by prepping the gum line with wax or other protective coverings.

Dental hygienists also teach patients about good oral health. They instruct the patient about the proper techniques to use when brushing and flossing their teeth. They may use a model of upper or lower teeth to demonstrate these techniques. If the patient complains of tooth sensitivity, the dental hygienist recommends a special toothpaste or rinse to help alleviate this problem.

Did You Know?

The typical dental hygiene educational program requires 84 credit hours for an associate degree and 118 credit hours for a bachelor's degree. Eighty-eight percent of programs are semester-based, and 34 percent include summer study.

Depending on the size and scope of the dental office, dental hygienists have additional duties such as charting and keeping track of and ordering necessary medical supplies.

Full-time dental hygienists work about 40 hours a week. Some evening and weekend shifts are required to accommodate patients' schedules. Dental hygienists wear professional attire, often a lab coat or smock. Comfortable shoes are a must, since dental hygienists are on their feet for much of the day, or walking from exam room to exam room. They also wear latex gloves, masks, and other protective equipment when working with patients.

Dental hygienists work in clean, comfortable, well-lit offices. They often sit on stools when performing procedures in order to better reach the patient. Dental hygienists are at high risk of developing carpal tunnel syndrome—nerve damage to the hand caused by the use of small tools in repetitive movements. They often use special braces and perform stretching exercises to reduce the risk of developing carpal tunnel syndrome.

At times, dental hygienists' work schedules can be quite hectic, especially when handling a heavy patient load. They can also fall behind schedule due to a difficult case or a patient who is especially nervous or jittery. They may work at more than one office—sometimes even in the course of a single workday. If the dental hygienist is employed at more than one facility, he or she needs a reliable means of transportation in order to travel from one office to another.

REQUIREMENTS

HIGH SCHOOL

Take courses in biology, chemistry, psychology, math, and health. Speech classes will help you develop your communication skills, which you will use often when interacting with patients, dentists, dental assistants, and other hygienists.

POSTSECONDARY TRAINING

A minimum of an associate's degree or certificate is required to work as a dental hygienist. More than 330 dental hygiene programs are accredited by the Commission on Dental Accreditation. Visit www.ada.org/en/coda/find-a-program for a list of accredited programs. Most programs award an associate's degree, but some offer certificates, bachelor's degrees, and master's degrees. According to the American Dental Hygienists' Association (ADHA), a typical associate's degree program offers courses in the basic sciences (anatomy, physiology, pathology, general chemistry, biochemistry, microbiology, pathology, nutrition, and pharmacology), the liberal arts (English, speech, sociology, and psychology), dental science courses (dental anatomy, head and neck anatomy, oral pathology, radiography, oral embryology and histology, periodontology, and pain control and dental materials), and dental hygiene science courses (patient management, clinical dental hygiene, oral health education/preventive counseling, community dental health, and medical and dental emergencies). Students also participate in preclinical and clinical experiences in which they work directly with patients under the close supervision of dental educators. The average associate's degree program requires 86 credit hours, according to the ADHA. Dental hygienists who plan to work in research, clinical practice, or teaching typically have at least a bachelor's degree.

CERTIFICATION AND LICENSING

All states require dental hygienists to be licensed. According to the U.S. Department of Labor, "every state requires dental hygienists to be licensed; requirements vary by state. In most states, a degree from an accredited dental hygiene program and passing grades on written and clinical examinations is required for licensure."

OTHER REQUIREMENTS

To be a successful dental hygienist, you should have excellent communication and interpersonal skills, since you will spend the majority of your workday interacting with patients, dentists, and dental assistants. You should have good manual dexterity in order to skillfully use dental instruments to conduct prophylaxis procedures. Other important traits include attention to detail, punctuality, cleanliness, and patience and compassion to deal with patients who may be fearful of undergoing dental procedures.

EXPLORING

There are many ways to learn more about a career as a dental hygienist and dentistry as a whole. You can read books and magazines about the field, visit the websites of college dental hygiene programs to learn about typical classes and possible career paths, and ask your health teacher or school counselor to arrange an information interview with a dental hygienist. Professional associations can also provide information about the field. Both the American Dental Association (www.ada.org) and the American Dental Hygienists' Association (www.adha.org/professional-roles) provide a wealth of information about dental hygiene education and careers at their websites. You should also try to land a part-time job in a dental office. This will give you a chance to interact with dental hygienists and see if the career is a good fit for your interests and abilities.

What is Public Health?

According to the Association of Schools of Public Health (ASPH), public health is the "science and art of protecting and improving the health of communities through education, promotion of health lifestyles, and research for disease and injury prevention." Career opportunities are found in environmental health, biostatistics, behavioral sciences/health education, epidemiology, health service administration, dentistry, maternal and child health, nutrition, international/global health, and public health laboratory practice. The ASPH predicts that there will be a shortage of 250,000 public health workers by 2020 if more people do not pursue careers in the field. Public health workers have a variety of educational backgrounds and skill sets. Some workers can find employment with a bachelor's degree (majors vary by career path), while other positions require a graduate degree in public health or a related field or a medical degree. Some public health workers have dual degrees in public health and fields such as nursing, public policy, business, medicine, dentistry, law, social work, or veterinary medicine.

EMPLOYERS

Approximately 200,550 dental hygienists are employed in the United States, with nearly all working in dental offices. Others work for employment services and in physicians' offices, hospitals, nursing homes, prisons, schools, and public health clinics. Some dental hygienists work for companies that sell dental-related equipment and supplies. Opportunities are also available in the U.S. military. About 50 percent of dental hygienists work part time.

GETTING A JOB

Many dental hygienists obtain their first jobs as a result of contacts made through college internships or networking events. Others seek assistance in obtaining job leads from college career services offices, newspaper want ads, employment websites, and dental auxiliary placement services (which charge a fee for their services). Additionally, professional dental associations—such as the American Dental Association (http://careercenter.ada.org) and the American Dental Hygienists' Association (www.adha.org/career-center)—provide job listings at their web sites. See For More Information for a list of organizations.

ADVANCEMENT

Dental hygienists advance by receiving salary increases or by working at larger practices. Some hygienists pursue advanced education and become dentists. Others pursue bachelor's or master's degrees in dental hygiene and work as college educators or public health researchers and educators.

FOR MORE INFORMATION

To learn more about education and careers, contact
American Dental Association
www.ada.org

For information on education, contact
American Dental Education Association
www.adea.org

For comprehensive information about a career as a dental hygienist, contact
American Dental Hygienists' Association
312-440-8900
www.adha.org

For information on job opportunities in Canada, contact
Canadian Dental Hygienists Association
www.cdha.ca

EARNINGS

Salaries for dental hygienists vary by type of employer, geographic region, and the worker's experience level and skills. Median annual salaries for dental hygienists were $72,330 in May 2015, according to the U.S. Department of Labor (USDL). Salaries ranged from less than $50,140 to $98,440 or more. The USDL reports the following mean annual earnings for dental hygienists by employer:

✔ offices of dentists, $73,050;
✔ outpatient care centers, $70,370;
✔ employment services, $68,800; and
✔ offices of physicians, $68,300.

Some dental hygienists receive fringe benefits such as paid sick leave and vacation, retirement plans, and free or discounted dental care.

EMPLOYMENT OUTLOOK

Employment for dental hygienists is expected to grow much faster than the average for all careers during the next decade, according to the U.S. Department of Labor. Demand will increase for dental hygienists as a result of the growth of the U.S. population, the increasing focus on preventive dental care, and a growing reliance on hygienists to perform duties that were previously handled by dentists. Competition for jobs will vary by geographic region. In some areas, there is an overabundance of hygienists, which will make finding a job more difficult.

Interview: Betty Kabel

Betty Kabel, RDH, BS, President of the American Dental Hygienists Association

Q. **What made you want to enter this career?**
A. I knew from middle school that I wanted to be a dental hygienist. It was a career that my grandmother had wanted to pursue but didn't have the opportunity. The inspiration from my grandmother combined with my personal enthusiasm to visit my own dental hygienist made this career my first and only choice.

Q. **What is one thing that young people may not know about the field?**
A. While working in a private dental office continues to be the primary place of employment for dental hygienists, the women and men who comprise today's dental hygiene professionals have many different career pathways to explore. With opportunities in clinical, corporate, public health, research, education, and many other areas, there has never been so many options for professional growth. To begin a career in dental hygiene you need to earn a college degree and secure your license. The college curriculum is packed with high standards, heavy science, clinical research, and hands-on training.

Q. **What are the most important personal and professional skills for dental hygienists to have?**
A. It is critical for dental hygienists to have good communication skills combined with a compassion and understanding for the patients they serve. This is definitely a career for a self-motivator who has good conflict management skills, is organized, and can work collaboratively to be successful. Also, having a strong desire to improve and not settle for the status quo is key to success.

Q. **What are some of the pros and cons of your job?**
A. There are many positive aspects to being a dental hygienist, but the biggest one is the flexibility of the job and the ability to take it in so many different directions.

   The dental hygiene practice is regulated at the state level, and so there can be variations in the scope of practice from state to state that can restrict how we can access and treat the public. As a result, we cannot always provide care to those who need it most.

Q. **Can you tell us about ADHA? How important is association membership to career success?**
A. Membership in ADHA is extremely important for career success. ADHA membership provides opportunities for dental hygienists to network with colleagues locally and nationally. ADHA also gives us many opportunities to advance our own careers through continued education and networking. Plus, through our collective public policy support, we can increase access to care for the public and advocate for the changes we desire in the ways we can practice. Most of all, ADHA offers a place for dental hygiene professionals to call their own. This is our association—built by and lead by dental hygienists.

DENTISTS

OVERVIEW

Dentists provide dental care to patients of all ages. They diagnose and treat problems with teeth and surrounding tissues and administer care to prevent future dental problems. They use lasers, digital scanners, and other types of technology to do their jobs. Some dentists specialize in a particular dental field, such as orthodontics or pediatric dentistry. A doctoral degree in dentistry is required to work as a dentist. Approximately 116,750 dentists are employed in the United States. Employment opportunities for dentists should be strong during the next decade.

THE JOB

While many people dread a visit to the dentist, a twice-yearly visit to the dentist is important to maintain your oral health. Good dental care is becoming even more important, as medical studies have linked dental health to overall health. Dentists diagnose and treat patients of all ages with any problems dealing with teeth and surrounding tissues.

When seeing a new patient, dentists may ask about the patient's medical history, including any pre-existing conditions or any medications he or she is taking. The dentist may also ask the patient if he or she is experiencing any oral pain or discomfort. The next phase of the assessment can involve an oral examination and x-rays. In some dental offices, dental hygienists and assistants handle these duties. The dentist then reviews the x-ray and double-checks the patient's mouth for cavities or other dental issues.

If the patient is there for a routine visit, the dentist may proceed with the prophylaxis, or teeth cleaning, or ask the dental hygienist to complete the procedure. Dentists can also apply fluoride treatments or sealants to protect teeth from decay.

Many times, patients see dentists for pain or discomfort due to dental caries (cavities), cracked teeth, or other oral problems. For example, when

FAST FACTS

High School Subjects
Chemistry
Health

Personal Skills
Critical thinking
Helping
Technical

Minimum Education Level
Dental degree

Salary Range
68,000 to $152,000 to $304,000+

Employment Outlook
Much faster than the average

O*NET-SOC
29-1021.00, 29-1022.00, 29-1023.00, 29-1024.00, 29-1029.00

NOC
3113

treating a patient with a cavity, the dentist will first use tools such as a sickle probe (also known as a dental explorer) to locate the cavity. Once found, the dentist uses a variety of tools—picks, probes, and drills—to remove the decay. The next step involves filling the cavity with medicine to retard decay, and finally filling the cavity with a dental restoration—usually composite resin, porcelain, or even gold. Once the filling is in place, the dentist uses a file and other tools to create a natural finish. If the decay is extensive, the dentist may be forced to file the tooth down and cover it with a crown or cap made of porcelain or gold. In these instances, dentists take measurements and make a temporary model of the crown.

A Truly Unique Career

To encourage more people to become dentists, the American Dental Association (ADA) has created the following list of reasons why dentistry is "truly a unique career."

✔ **Provides the Opportunity to Provide Service to Others.** There is great personal satisfaction helping people attain better oral health. Conducting research and teaching future dentists also are rewarding.

✔ **Offers Good Balance of Professional and Personal Goals.** Approximately 75 percent of dentists are solo practitioners, which allows them to establish their own work schedules that work well with their personal lives. Most experienced dentists work a standard week of 35-40 hours—far less than the 50+ hours worked by physicians. New dentists may work longer hours as they attempt to build their practices.

✔ **Offers Strong Earning Potential.** In 2015, general dentists earned average salaries of $152,700, according to the U.S. Department of Labor. The career ranked as the 14th highest-paying job in the United States.

✔ **Prestige/Social Status.** Dentists often have strong reputations in their communities and have a "distinguished history of leadership in improving world health."

✔ **Provides Opportunities to Be Creative.** This might be surprising to some, but the ADA calls dentists "artists," who "combine keen visual memory, excellent judgment of space and shape, and a high degree of manual dexterity in the delivery of patient services."

✔ **Variety.** There are nine dental specialties available in addition to general dentistry and a variety of employment settings that will take dentists from small towns and big cities in the United States to countries throughout the world.

Sometimes teeth are so damaged that they cannot be saved. In this case, they must be extracted before infection sets in (or gets worse) or more damage is done. When conducting an extraction, dentists may need to administer a form of local anesthetic or even nitrous oxide to prevent the patient from feeling pain. They may also prescribe antibiotics if infection is detected.

In order to maintain optimum dental health, dentists counsel their patients on the proper way to care for their teeth. They demonstrate the correct way to brush and floss teeth and suggest special toothpastes to address issues such as tooth or gum sensitivity.

Dentists can also change the appearance of teeth through cosmetic procedures. Many patients wishing for straighter, whiter, or bigger teeth can opt for veneers, tooth bridges, bleaching, tooth reshaping, or gum lifts.

In addition to patient care, some dentists perform administrative duties. They maintain the financial records of their practice (including billing) and supervise dental hygienists, dental assistants, and other office staff.

Some dentists specialize in a particular area of dentistry. The American Dental Association recognizes nine professional specialties, which are detailed in the following paragraphs.

Dental public health specialists promote good dental health and prevent dental diseases within the community. They study the oral health needs of a community, then develop plans and policies that help community members attain better dental health.

Endodontists specialize in treating the tooth pulp and the tissues surrounding the tooth root. Endodontic procedures include root canals, endodontic retreatments, and repairing cracked teeth or other dental trauma.

Oral and maxillofacial pathologists focus on the identification and management of diseases affecting the oral and maxillofacial region—the jaws and face.

Oral and maxillofacial radiologists focus on the production and interpretation of radiological images of the oral and maxillofacial region. X-rays, MRIs, subtraction radiography, arthrography, and dental panoramic radiographs are some procedures used by these dentists.

Oral and maxillofacial surgeons operate on the mouth, jaws, teeth, gums, neck, and head, as well as the soft tissues in these regions. Some procedures done by these dental specialists include facial implants, treatments for temporomandibular joint disorder, and corrective jaw surgery.

Orthodontics is the dental specialty dealing with malocclusions of the teeth due to tooth irregularity, disproportionate jaw relationships, or both. *Orthodontists* correct these malformations using procedures and techniques including expansion appliances, retainers, or fixed multi-bracket therapy—otherwise known as braces.

Pediatric dentists specialize in the comprehensive preventive and therapeutic oral health of infants and young children, as well as those with special needs. Pediatric dentists tailor their dental surroundings and approach to suit and soothe young children.

Periodontists specialize in the supporting and surrounding tissues of the teeth including the gums, aveola bone, cementum, and periodontal ligaments, and the diseases and conditions affecting them.

Prosthodontists replace missing teeth with permanent fixtures, such as crowns and bridges, or with removable fixtures such as dentures.

Dentists work in comfortable, well-lit offices. Many offices equip each examining room with overhead music or a video screen to keep patients occupied during examinations. All equipment and tools are sanitized and

New Dental Specialties

Most of us are familiar with the typical paths in dental care—such as dentist, dental hygienist, dental assistant, and dental laboratory technician—but now the American Dental Association (ADA) has created two new dental team members to "assist dentists in increasing care for all." Here are summaries of the new positions, courtesy of the ADA:

Community dental health coordinators (CDHCs) are community health workers who focus on oral health awareness and prevention (fluoride treatments, sealants, etc.). They work in underserved, rural, urban, and Native American communities where residents have limited or no access to dental care. The ADA reports that CDHCs now serve in more than 25 communities in eight states: Arizona, California, Montana, Minnesota, Oklahoma, Pennsylvania, Texas, and Wisconsin.

Oral preventive assistants "support the dental profession by providing a variety of preventive services as well as patient oral health care education." Preventive services within the dental office include "collection of diagnostic data such as medical histories, vital signs, charting, radiographs; preventive services for all types of patients, including preventive and oral hygiene instruction, application of fluoride and sealants, coronal polishing for all patients, scaling for plaque induced gingivitis patients; and general office duties including facilitate basic legal and regulatory compliance, e.g., HIPAA compliance, maintain patient treatment records, managing a recall system." Oral preventive assistants also work in community health centers, schools, and other settings to teach people about proper oral health.

organized, and made ready for the dentists' use by trained office staff. Full-time dentists work about 36 hours a week, the majority of which are spent on patient care. Office hours may vary depending on the size of practice, and they often include Saturday and evening hours. Office attire for dentists varies from office to office but generally consists of scrubs or a medical gown. Dentists also wear gloves and masks when treating patients. Many dentists are susceptible to carpal tunnel syndrome due to repetitive movements during examinations and treatments, and continued manipulation of dental tools.

EDUCATION AND CERTIFICATION

HIGH SCHOOL

To prepare for college, take courses in biology, organic and inorganic chemistry, mathematics, physics, computer science, and health. English and speech classes will also be useful.

POSTSECONDARY TRAINING

A doctoral degree in dentistry is required to work as a dentist. Dental students typically enter dental school after earning a bachelor's degree. Some students earn a bachelor's degree in a science-oriented field such as biology or chemistry, while others take the required science coursework while pursuing a major in a nonscientific field. Admissions requirements include strong undergraduate grades, successful completion of the Dental Admissions Test, and participation in personal interviews with dental school admissions officials. More than 65 dental schools in the United States are accredited by the American Dental Association's Commission on Dental Accreditation. Visit www.ada.org/en/coda/find-a-program for a list of programs.

In recent years, the ADA has placed a strong emphasis on improving diversity among dental students. The good news: women now make up nearly 48 percent of dental students. The bad news: African Americans, Hispanic Americans, and Native Americans are still underrepresented in dental schools as compared to their representation in the general population, but the ADA is working hard to ensure that admission rates reflect diversity.

CERTIFICATION AND LICENSING

Dentists may obtain certification from the various dental specialty boards such as the American Board of Pediatric Dentistry and the American Board of Oral and Maxillofacial Surgery. Certification, while voluntary, is highly recommended. It is an excellent way to stand out from other dentists and demonstrate your abilities to prospective patients.

All 50 states and the District of Columbia require dentists to be licensed. Licensing requirements typically involve graduating from an accredited dental school and passing practical and written examinations. Dental specialists must also receive special licensing. Those seeking specialty licensure must complete two to four years of postgraduate education. In some instances, applicants must also take and pass a state-level examination and complete a postgraduate residency term of up to two years.

OTHER REQUIREMENTS

Dentists need to be calm and perform well under pressure, especially when working on a difficult case or with a fearful patient. Strong communication skills are also very important. Pediatric dentists often use a gentle speaking voice or rename certain tools or procedures to help calm younger patients. Other key traits for dentists include excellent manual dexterity, attentiveness to detail, diagnostic ability, and good business acumen.

EXPLORING

There are many ways to learn more about a career in dentistry. You can read books and magazines about the field, visit the websites of dental schools to learn about typical classes and possible career paths, and ask your teacher or school counselor to arrange an information interview with a dentist (or talk to your own). Professional associations can also provide information about the field. The American Dental Association (ADA) provides a wealth of information on education and careers at its website, www.ada.org. The ADA offers membership options for high school and college students who plan to pursue a career in dentistry. Try to land a part-time job in a dental office. This will give you a chance to interact with dentists and see if the career is a good fit for your interests and abilities.

EMPLOYERS

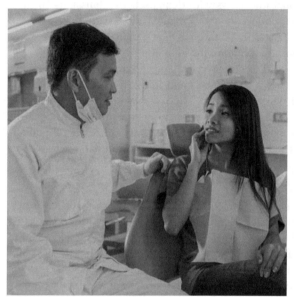

A dentist discusses treatment options with a patient.
(Adobe Stock)

Approximately 116,750 dentists are employed in the United States. About 75 percent of dentists who work in private practice are sole proprietors, and nearly 15 percent belong to a partnership. Dentists also work in many other employment settings, including those in academics as teachers, at public health facilities and hospitals, in research, and in international health care (with the World Health Organization, the Food and Agricultural Organization of the United Nations, and the United Nations Educational, Scientific and Cultural Organization). Additionally, about 15 percent of dentists practice in dental specialties. The three largest specialties are:

✔ orthodontists: 5,410 people employed in this field,
✔ oral and maxillofacial surgeons: 5,000, and
✔ prosthodontists: 710.

GETTING A JOB

After graduation, most dental school graduates purchase an established practice or open a new practice. Dentists who do not purchase a practice or start their own business can obtain their first jobs as a result of contacts made through college internships, career fairs, or networking events. Others seek assistance in obtaining job leads from college career services offices, newspaper want ads, and employment websites (such as Dentalworkers.com, www.dentalworkers.com/employment). Professional associations, such as the American Dental Association (http://career-

FOR MORE INFORMATION

For a wealth of information on dental education and careers, contact
American Dental Association
publicinfo@ada.org
www.ada.org

For information on educational programs in the United States and Canada, contact
American Dental Education Association
202-289-7201
www.adea.org

Contact the following organizations to learn more about on education and careers in dentistry:
Academy of General Dentistry
888/AGD-DENT
www.agd.org

American Academy of Oral & Maxillofacial Pathology
888-552-2667
info@aaomp.org
www.aaomp.org

American Academy of Oral & Maxillofacial Radiology
admin@aaomr.org
www.aaomr.org

American Academy of Pediatric Dentistry
312-337-2169
www.aapd.org

American Association of Endodontists
info@aae.org
www.aae.org

American Association of Orthodontists
www.aaoinfo.org

American Association of Public Health Dentistry
217-529-6941
info@aaphd.org
www.aaphd.org

American Association of Women Dentists
800-920-2293
info@aawd.org
www.aawd.org

American Student Dental Association
800-621-8099, ext. 2795
www.asdanet.org

For information on job opportunities in Canada, contact
Canadian Dental Association
613-523-1770
www.cda-adc.ca

center.ada.org) provide job listings at their websites. Information on job opportunities at federal agencies is available at www.usajobs.gov.

ADVANCEMENT

Dentists advance by earning higher salaries or by developing a successful practice that attracts more patients. Dentists who work as associates for established dentists may eventually start their own practice or purchase an existing practice from a dentist who is retiring or leaving the field for other reasons. Dentists also conduct research for private organizations or government agencies. Others teach dentistry at dental colleges.

EARNINGS

Salaries for general dentists vary by type of employer, geographic region, and the worker's experience. Median annual salaries for general dentists were $152,700 in May 2015, according to the U.S. Department of Labor (USDL). Ten percent earned less than $68,310. The USDL reports the following mean annual earnings for general dentists by employer:

✔ state government, $163,070;

✔ offices of physicians, $151,380;

✔ outpatient care centers, $150,570; and

✔ general medical and surgical hospitals, $133,880.

The American Dental Association reports that dental specialists average more than $304,000 per year.

Dentists who are salaried employees receive a variety of benefits, including the following: medical and life insurance; paid holidays, vacations, and sick and personal days; 401(k) plans; profit-sharing plans; retirement and pension plans; and reimbursement for continuing education. Self-employed dentists must provide their own benefits. About 23 percent of dentists are self-employed.

EMPLOYMENT OUTLOOK

Employment for general dentists, orthodontists, prosthodontists, and oral and maxillofacial surgeons is expected to grow by 18 percent during the next decade, according to the U.S. Department of Labor, or much faster than the average for all careers. Job opportunities for dentists in all other specialties are expected to grow by 9 percent (faster than the average). More opportunities are emerging for dentists as a result of the growing U.S. population and the increasing number of people age 65 and older, who often need more dental care than other demographic groups. Other factors that are fueling growth include the increasing number of people who have dental insurance, advances in technology that are expanding treatment options, and the growing popularity of cosmetic dental procedures.

Interview: Steve Morris

Dr. Steve Morris is a dentist in Chicago, Illinois.

Q. What made you want to become a dentist?

A. I decided to become a dentist for several reasons. I worked in a pharmacy all through high school and got a chance to become acquainted with people in many areas of medicine—physicians, dentists, pharmacists, optometrists, and so on. I found of the various professions that dentistry piqued my curiosity the most. And frankly, as a child I spent quite a bit of time in the dental office, so I was very familiar with the procedures and environment. There was a kind of fascination with all the instruments and machinery. The instrumentation these days is a lot more high-tech, and it's been interesting to be able to advance as the profession does. Dentistry is a nice blend of medicine, art, and microtechnology, and it is basically all hands-on. Dentistry is also nice in that you can work in whatever setting is most appealing to you—a large group practice or small solo practice—with whatever hours work best for you.

Q. What is one thing that young people may not know about a career in dentistry?

A. People don't always realize the many areas of dentistry that are available. There are areas to appeal to just about everyone. If you're surgically inclined, there are opportunities to do surgical reconstruction, cancer treatment, and implant dentistry. For those more artistically inclined, one can specialize in cosmetic dentistry with veneers, bonding, and orthodontics. You can work with children only with developing faces, or with the other side of the spectrum, geriatric patients with implants, dentures, or other methods of restoring lost function and esthetics. If you enjoy a little more variety, general dentists delve a bit into all the specialties and work with a wide range of age groups. There is also research and technical development, which is less patient oriented.

Q. What are the most important personal and professional qualities for dentists?

A. There are several important qualities for dentists that will help make them happy and successful in the profession. It helps to be very patient, as some procedures can be rather time consuming and tedious, and if things don't go according to plan you have to be able to shift gears and make treatment modifications. Having good tactile sense and hand-to-eye coordination is very helpful as well. Many times procedures are accomplished by feel as much as sight, and sometimes they have to be visualized in reverse on a mirror. Practice and repetition improve these qualities, but good inherent ability makes it much easier. You have to be able to work in a small area and still be able to be pretty precise about what you're doing. Being mechanically inclined is also helpful, as many times you have to get creative and be able to use available materials for a problem you weren't expecting. You can't always prepare for what a patient will come in with, or have things go according to plan, so it pays to be flexible. You have to be even tempered enough to be able to handle the pressure of a busy schedule, and you have to be able to not get discouraged if things don't always work out as planned. Inevitably there will be times when treatment won't work well, or patients won't be satisfied no matter what you do, so you have to be able to work with that. Having a pleasant disposition helps when dealing with patients, especially if they happen to be in pain and not in the best mood. A good disposition and a "we're all on the same team" approach works well with staff, too.

Q. What are some of the pros and cons of your job?

A. The pros of the job are extreme satisfaction when patients are thrilled about improved esthetics, or are out of intense pain due to something you've done for them. They are usually very, very appreciative. Your hours can be very flexible: you can work four long days and have three off, or work short days for six days, whatever suits you. You can work in any setting you'd like, a large, high-tech, group practice with specialists on site, or you can

Demand Strong for Information Technology Health Workers

Dentists, nurses, primary care physicians, and some technician and therapist jobs are not the only careers that are enjoying strong growth in the health care industry. The expanding U.S. population and federal laws such as the HITECH Act and the American Recovery and Reinvestment Act are fueling demand for information technology (IT) workers in the health care industry. For example, job opportunities for network and computer systems administrators in the health care industry are expected to grow by 22.3 percent from 2014 to 2024, according to the U.S. Department of Labor, or much faster than the average for all careers. Employment for software applications developers in the health care industry is expected to grow by 17.3 percent during this same time span. Skills that are in the strongest demand (in descending order) include project management, Structure Query Language, troubleshooting, oral and written communication skills, and problem solving.

have a lower-key solo practice. You can specialize if a certain area interests you more, or have a general practice with more variety. Some of the cons are that although you work pretty much whatever hours you set, you do get emergencies at inopportune times. Usually you don't get many, but they are inevitable. In a larger practice this isn't as big a problem, as doctors cover for each other, but in a solo practice you're obligated to cover your emergencies whenever they occur. Sometimes money is an issue for patients, and you have to be able to compromise treatment to get the best result you can with what they can afford. There are patients even today with a tremendous fear of the dentist, so you have to be able to deal with people who are fearful, in pain, and not happy at all to see you.

Q. What advice would you give to young people who are interested in the field?

A. I would advise anyone interested in the field to visit a dental office and observe for a day, talk to the staff and especially the dentist, and get a feel for an average day. You might even want to work part-time in an office for a summer. If there is a dental school in your area, it might be good to visit that as well. I would also check out related fields if you're medically inclined, to see if any of them seem more appealing. It is also a good idea to evaluate your situation, your strengths and weaknesses. All medical fields require some strength in science, so if that isn't your interest, dentistry is probably not for you. You'll need a certain grade point average, especially in science, as admission is very competitive. A certain amount of manual dexterity is also very helpful in dentistry.

DIAGNOSTIC MEDICAL SONOGRAPHERS

OVERVIEW

While many of us instinctively think of ultrasound as a means of determining the sex of a fetus, the technology of sonography is also used to diagnose a variety of medical problems associated with the female and male reproductive systems, liver, kidneys, gallbladder, spleen, pancreas, brain, and eyes. *Diagnostic medical sonographers* are the professionals who explain the procedure to patients, take medical histories, and operate the transducer which transmits high-frequency sound waves that hit a boundary between tissues (e.g., between fluid and soft tissue, soft tissue and bone) and bounce back to create images that are captured for review by physicians. While physicians make the medical diagnosis, sonographers must possess the knowledge of which images to take and which angles best show healthy versus unhealthy organs and tissues. Approximately 61,250 diagnostic medical sonographers are employed in the United States.

FAST FACTS

High School Subjects
Biology
Health
Mathematics

Personal Skills
Helping
Technical

Minimum Education Level
Associate's degree

Salary Range
$48,000 to $68,000 to $97,000+

Employment Outlook
Much faster than the average

O*NET-SOC
29-2032.00

NOC
3216

THE JOB

Diagnostic medical sonographers use ultrasound equipment to obtain images of organs, tissues, and blood vessels in the body, or in the case of pregnancy, to assess the health, development, and gender of a fetus. Ultrasound technology is increasingly being used to detect heart attacks and heart and vascular disease.

To begin the procedure, the sonographer applies a thin layer of gel to the skin on the area of the patient's body that is to be imaged. The gel helps the ultrasound waves to be transmitted from the transducer (i.e., the probe that sends and receives the sound waves) into the body. The sonographer places the transducer directly on the skin or inside a body opening to record echoes of high-frequency sound waves as they bounce from the patient's organs or tissues, or the fetus back to the equipment in real time. These echoes are generated into a real-time image, which is saved for later review by physicians. Doppler ultrasound technology is used to detect levels of blood flow in a patient; this technology also provides audible signals that can be recorded and analyzed. Sonographers use their knowledge of sonographic technology and the human body to determine if the images they have recorded are sufficient for analysis by a physician, or if more comprehensive tests are necessary. When the procedure is complete, sonographers provide an oral or written summary of their findings, and are available for follow-up with the physician, if necessary.

Specialties in the field include abdominal (abdominal cavity and nearby organs, such as the kidney, liver, gallbladder, pancreas, or spleen), breast, echocardiography (anatomy of the heart, including its valves and blood flow), neurosonography (brain and nervous system), obstetrics (fetus and womb), gynecology (female reproductive system), vascular (blood vessels and blood flow), musculoskeletal (joints, tendons, ligaments, and muscles), and ophthalmology (eyes). Some sonographers specialize in conducting procedures on people in specific age groups, such as children or the elderly.

Most sonographers are employed full time. Many work a standard Monday-Friday, 9-to-5 workweek, while others work at nights and on weekends.

EDUCATION AND CERTIFICATION

HIGH SCHOOL

In high school, take classes in health, biology, mathematics, and computer science. English and speech classes will help develop your communication skills, which you'll use frequently when interacting with coworkers, physicians, and patients.

POSTSECONDARY TRAINING

A minimum of an associate's degree in diagnostic medical sonography is required to enter the field. The Commission on Accreditation of Allied Health Education Programs (www.caahep.org/Find-An-Accredited-Program) and the Joint Review Committee on Education in Diagnostic Medical Sonography (www.jrcdms.org) accredit programs in diagnostic medical sonography. In addition, certificates offer professionals the opportunity to obtain advanced certifications (e.g., abdominal ultrasound), but are not alone a path to a job.

Typical classes in a sonography program include Introduction to Sonography; Anatomy and Physiology; Medical Terminology; Sonographic Physics; Sonographic Instrumentation; Sonographic Cross Sectional Anatomy; Obstetric and Gynecologic Sonography; and Clinical Experience.

Debunking Common Misconceptions About Health Care Careers

Health care is the largest industry in the United States, according to the U.S. Department of Labor. It employs more than 18 million people, features 19 of the top 25 fastest-growing occupations, and offers great opportunities to those with less than a four-year college education, as well as those, such as physicians and nurse practitioners, with advanced education. And the industry continues to grow: about 39 percent (or nearly 3.8 million) of all new jobs created between 2014 and 2024 will be in health care.

Despite this rapid growth and the large number of people employed in the field, many people have misconceptions about the health care industry that keep them from reaching their career potential. Here are a few of the most common health care career myths and the facts about them.

Myth #1: All health care professionals work in hospitals and medical centers.
The Facts. Employment in these settings was the norm for years, but, today, health care professionals—especially registered nurses, physicians, and therapists—work in a variety of nontraditional settings. These include staffing or recruitment agencies, managed care companies, professional associations, insurance companies, publishing companies, occupational health companies, research facilities, law firms, private corporations, and colleges and universities.

Myth #2: The nursing shortage means that you will get any job that you want.
The Facts. Yes, you will definitely get a job at some point, but your job search may take longer than you expect—especially if you have not received specialized training. Additionally, some hospitals do not hire new graduates to work in demanding specialties such as critical care nursing.

Myth #3: Medical technicians, nurses, and other health care positions require a four-year degree.
The Facts. Not true for many careers. Many employers—especially due to the nursing shortage—are hiring nurses with two-year associate degrees from community colleges. Other rewarding careers that only require an associate degree include occupational therapy assistant, physical therapist assistant, respiratory therapist, and radiologic technologist.

CERTIFICATION AND LICENSING

The American Registry for Diagnostic Medical Sonography, the American Registry of Radiologic Technologists, Cardiovascular Credentialing International, American Society of Echocardiography, and Sonography Canada offer certification to diagnostic medical sonographers.

Currently, only Oregon, New Mexico, New Hampshire, and North Dakota mandate the licensure of sonographers, but more states may adopt licensure requirements in coming years. Contact your state's department of regulation for information on requirements in your state.

OTHER REQUIREMENTS

Patient contact is a major part of this job, so you'll need to have excellent communication and interpersonal skills, as well as an empathetic and caring personality. You should also be detail-oriented to effectively scan a patient's body (and differentiate between healthy and unhealthy areas) and follow the instructions of the physician to record an accurate image. Other important traits include good hand-eye coordination, physical stamina (because you will be on your feet often during your workday and may have to help move or reposition patients), intelligence, and excellent critical thinking skills.

EXPLORING

There are many ways to learn more about sonography and a career in the field. First, learn the lingo of sonography by checking out a glossary of commonly-used terms at www.aace.com/ecnu_resources/ECNU_RESOURCES/Glossary-of-Ultrasound-Terminology.pdf. Then read industry journals such as the *Journal for Vascular Ultrasound,* the *Journal of the American Society of Echocardiography,* and *ECHO.* While some of the technical terms may be a bit over your head, these journals can provide a good introduction to the types of issues sonographers face daily. Talk to sonographers about their careers, and join health care career explorations clubs in high school and college. Finally, check out the following web resources to learn more:

✔ **American Institute of Ultrasound in Medicine-Diagnostic Medical Sonography Career Information:**
http://files.aium.org/DMS/handout.pdf

✔ **Society of Diagnostic Medical Sonography-What is Sonography:**
www.sdms.org/resources/what-is-sonography

✔ **Society of Diagnostic Medical Sonography-Careers:**
www.sdms.org/resources/careers

✔ **Ultrasound Imaging:** www.fda.gov/Radiation-Emitting Products/RadiationEmittingProductsandProcedures/Medical Imaging/ucm115357.htm.

EMPLOYERS

Approximately 61,250 diagnostic medical sonographers are employed in the United States. They work at hospitals, physicians' offices, clinics, diagnostic imaging centers, public health facilities, laboratories, and in other medical settings. The U.S. Department of Labor reports that the states with the largest number of sonographers are (in descending order): California, Florida, New York, Texas, and Pennsylvania.

GETTING A JOB

Many people land their first jobs in sonography through contacts made during college internships or practicums. Sonography professors and career services counselors can also provide job leads. The Society of Diagnostic Medical Sonography (SDMS) is a strong proponent of using networking to land a job. It suggests that new members access its membership directory, attend its annual conference, volunteer with the association, and check out SDMS social media resources to begin building their networks. Finally, the SDMS and other associations provide job listings at their websites:

✔ **SDMS:** www.sdms.org/resources/careers/job-board

✔ **Society for Vascular Ultrasound:** http://careers.svunet.org

✔ **National Healthcare Career Network:** www.nhcnnetwork.org.

ADVANCEMENT

Sonographers advance by receiving higher pay, better benefits, and managerial duties. Some become college professors.

EARNINGS

Salaries for sonographers vary by type of employer, geographic region, and the worker's experience, education, and skill level. Diagnostic medical sonographers earned median annual salaries of $68,970 in May 2015, according to the U.S. Department of Labor (USDL). Ten percent earned less than $48,720, and 10 percent earned $97,390 or more. The USDL reports the following mean annual earnings for sonographers by employer: outpatient care centers, $83,600; medical and diagnostic laboratories, $74,360; general medical and surgical hospitals, $70,500; and offices of physicians, $68,460.

Employers offer a variety of benefits, including the following: medical, dental, and life insurance; paid holidays, vacations, and sick and personal days; 401(k) plans; profit-sharing plans; retirement and pension plans; and educational-assistance programs. Part-time workers must provide their own benefits.

EMPLOYMENT OUTLOOK

Employment in the field is expected to grow much faster than the average for all careers during the next decade, according to the U.S. Department of Labor. The field of sonography is experiencing growth due to an aging population and the increased popularity of sonography over more invasive, costly radiologic diagnostic procedures. Sonographers with certification (ideally in more than one area) will have the best job prospects.

Interview: Joy Guthrie

Dr. Joy Guthrie, RDMS, RDCS, RVT is a practicing sonographer and the Past-President of the Society of Diagnostic Medical Sonography.

Q. What made you want to enter this career?

A. I started in the medical field as a medical assistant/EMT. I was introduced to sonography by an obstetrician who I worked for during my training as a medical assistant. The first time I saw an echocardiogram (sonogram of the heart) I was hooked for life. The ability to see the inside of the heart using a non-invasive technology (sonography) was just amazing to me. My first employer advised me to go back to school and become a radiology technologist since that was what was required to practice sonography in a hospital setting in the 1980s. Now, we have more than 200 programmatically accredited and dedicated sonography education programs throughout the country.

Q. What do you like most and least about your job?

A. Sonography is a great combination of art and science. The technical challenge of obtaining accurate images, as well as the knowledge base needed to determine the preliminary diagnosis for the interpreting physician, makes our field very exciting. I believe we can all share stories where our timely diagnosis made a great difference in a patient's life. You get to work very closely with the patients and your physician partners. I love doing sonography research and actively participating in both entry-level and advanced sonography education.

What I like least is, depending on the specific demands of your job, is that the position may require long hours or "on-call" hours, which can become a struggle over time.

Q. What are the key qualities for sonographers?

A. Integrity, caring, and dependability are personal qualities that are needed to succeed in sonography. Professional qualities include intelligence, good hand-eye coordination, excellent critical thinking skills, and good communication skills.

Q. Any career advice for students?

A. Do your research before committing to a sonography education program.
Look for programs that have exhibited a sustained record of good outcomes
for their graduates for both full-time sonography job placement and national registry pass rates. Make sure that the program provides students with a
pathway to take their national sonography credentialing exams immediately
upon graduation. The entry to practice standard applied by most health
care organizations are graduates from a CAAHEP-accredited program and
either ARDMS, CCI, or ARRT sonography certification. It is really important for students to understand the difference between sonography education programs that have programmatic accreditation (the CAAHEP pathway), and those that may lack programmatic accreditation but who may say
that their institution is accredited—either institutionally, regionally, or
through one of the proprietary accreditation options. Only those students
who graduate from a CAAHEP-accredited sonography education program
are qualified to sit for their national credentialing exams immediately upon
graduation. Otherwise, they will have to acquire experience working full-
time as a sonographer for a year before they are allowed to take the national
credentialing exams. The problem is that most employers, and for good reason, only want to hire sonographers who are already certified. It can be a
Catch-22 for students who can spend thousands of dollars going through a
sonography education program only to find they are not qualified to sit for
the national credentialing exams after they graduate and cannot find an
employer willing to hire them so that they can get their full year of work as
a sonographer to qualify for the national exams. It can be a very frustrating
and discouraging experience for students who find themselves in this situation, and it all can be avoided by making sure that you find a CAAHEP-
accredited sonography education program.

**Q. What is the future employment outlook in diagnostic medical sonogra-
phy? How is the field changing?**

A. The U.S. Department of Labor is predicting a 24 percent increase in sonography jobs by 2024. Additionally, not only are the prospects for sonography
jobs on a tremendous growth curve, the salaries for sonographers are quite
attractive. Based on a large and recent salary and benefits survey for sonography, the median total annual compensation for sonographers is $78,520*.

With the rapid evolution of ultrasound technology, sonographers are
finding additional avenues for employment including education, research,
application specialists, and advanced practice working within a physician-
extender role. The future of sonography appears to be bright, and career
options and job security are growing exponentially. As healthcare focuses
more on patient safety, quality outcomes, and expense control, it is likely
that sonography will continue to be an attractive source for medical imaging services because of the non-invasive nature of the technology, the ability to produce high-quality imaging results for the patients we serve, and the
lower cost of sonography compared to many of the other medical imaging
modalities.

*Source: *SDMS Sonographer Salary & Benefit Survey Report,* copyright 2013, Society
of Diagnostic Medical Sonography. All rights reserved.

EMERGENCY MEDICAL TECHNICIANS

OVERVIEW

Emergency medical technicians (EMTs) are the first medical respondents at the scene of an accident, injury, crime, fire, or other emergency. They provide medical care to victims, including stopping bleeding, applying splints or braces to broken bones, or administering cardiopulmonary resuscitation, often while in transit to hospitals or medical facilities. EMTs also transfer patients between hospitals and other medical facilities for specialized treatment. Most work in ambulances, but some travel to accident scenes in special medically equipped helicopters. Duties of EMTs vary according to their level of training. Approximately 236,890 EMTs are employed in the United States. There will be excellent employment opportunities for EMTs during the next decade.

FAST FACTS

High School Subjects
Biology
Health

Personal Skills
Critical thinking
Helping
Judgment and decision making
Technical

Minimum Education Level
Some postsecondary training

Salary Range
$20,000 to $31,000 to $55,000+

Employment Outlook
Much faster than the average

O*NET-SOC
29-2041.00

NOC
3234

THE JOB

A horrible car-versus-semi crash. A four-alarm fire. A man suddenly collapses on a city street clutching his chest. Seconds after an emergency 911 call is placed, an emergency medical team is dispatched to provide help to victims in need. The work done by emergency medical technicians (EMTs) often means the difference between life and death. EMTs treat a wide spectrum of patients and their injuries including accidents, heart attacks, strokes, untimely birth deliveries, severe burns, and gunshot and stab wounds.

EMTs have different job titles based on their level of training. EMTs at the basic level (*EMT-Basic*) provide emergency assistance to assess, stabilize, and manage respiratory, cardiac, and trauma emergencies. They are trained to administer non-invasive emergency care. EMTs at the intermediate level (*EMT-*

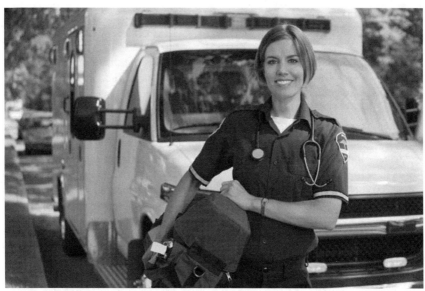

Approximately 35 percent of emergency medical technicians are women. (Thinkstock)

Intermediate) provide more advanced emergency care, including some invasive procedures, cardiac monitoring, intubations, and IVs. *Paramedics* have the highest level of training and are able to administer drug IVs, give defibrillation, and interpret electrocardiograms (EKGs). EMTs perform their duties under direct orders from doctors and nurses at a hospital or other health care facility.

EMTs are known for their quick thinking and immediate response to any situation, whether it is minor or critical. Dispatchers from a 911 center alert them to an emergency situation and its location. EMTs often arrive at the scene in a matter of minutes—usually in an ambulance, but sometimes in a helicopter or other mode of transportation. Once there, they determine the nature of the accident or illness. For example, if dispatched to a multi-car accident, EMTs determine the priority of injuries sustained. Sometimes, victims trapped in their vehicle must be freed before emergency care can be given. EMTs often work alongside police and firefighters to rescue victims, sometimes using rescue tools such as cutters, spreaders and rams that are frequently referred to as the "Jaws of Life." Once they have access to the victims, EMTs may ask victims to identify pain or discomfort if they are conscious; if not, EMTs take vital signs and visually assess the patient (including looking for medical alert bracelets or other identification to signal certain medical conditions).

EMTs administer emergency care, depending on the condition of the victim and the extent of injuries sustained. They use bandages and gauze to control bleeding. They apply splints to set broken bones. A neck brace or backboard may be used if a neck or back injury is suspected. If the victim is short of breath, EMTs treat the individual with oxygen to help him or her regain a normal breathing pattern. If the victim is unconscious and does not appear to be breathing, EMTs administer CPR.

Useful Website: ExploreHealthCareers.org

ExploreHealthCareers.com has been created to inspire minority students to pursue careers in the health care industry and encourage students to consider working in medically underserved communities. The site has several useful sections. Career Explorer helps students assess whether a career in health care is right for them, provides an overview of the wide range of health careers (and the educational requirements to enter them), and offers a health careers database that allows users to search for careers based on the salary they desire and the number of years they want to attend school. The Your Education section provides information on applying to and paying for college, planning your studies, and achieving academic success. Finally, there is a health careers blog and links to national and state health career organizations and their websites, diversity-oriented medical websites, and student health care organizations. This is a comprehensive resource not just for minorities, but all students who are interested in learning about educational and career options in health care.

Once the victim is stabilized, EMTs use boards or stretchers to move him or her from the scene of the accident and into the ambulance for transportation. They make sure the victim is comfortable and securely strapped onto the stretcher. They monitor the victim en route to the hospital or other medical facility and administer medical care as needed. EMTs maintain communication with emergency department doctors and nurses regarding the condition of the patient. If the patient's condition or vital signs worsen during transport, doctors may advise EMT-Intermediates or paramedics to administer additional emergency care. EMT-Intermediates may start intravenous fluids or open airway passages by intubation. Paramedics may draw an IV line to administer drugs or use a defibrillator to shock a patient's stopped heart back into action. EMT-Intermediates and paramedics may also be asked by doctors to perform an EKG, interpret its results, and relay the information for review.

When the ambulance reaches the hospital, EMTs transfer the patient to the emergency room. They update doctors and nurses about the treatment they gave the patient at the scene and en-route.

EMTs also treat people suffering from injuries, accidents, or illness happening in their homes. For example, relatives of someone suffering from a heart attack or seriously injured from a fall may call 911 for emergency care. EMTs arrive at the scene and assess the situation. For a suspected heart attack, they take the patient's vital signs, including blood pressure and heart rate. EMTs may take an EKG reading or use bag-valve mask resuscitators for critical cases. They make sure the patient is stabilized before transferring him or her to the hospital.

After each run, EMTs clean and decontaminate their vehicle. This is especially important if they have treated patients with infectious diseases such as Hepatitis B and AIDS/HIV. They make sure instruments and equipment are maintained and medical supplies are replenished.

At the scene of a traffic accident, EMTs not traveling to the hospital with the victim may often help firefighters and police create a safe traffic environment. They light flares or use flashing signals to detour cars and pedestrians. If hazardous materials are present on the street, they use fire extinguishers or other equipment to absorb oil or harmful chemicals.

EMTs and paramedics also work with public agencies, schools, and community centers to educate the public about safety, or to teach first-aid programs.

EMTs usually work in teams of two or more; many times EMTs and paramedics work together as a pair, with the paramedic acting as team leader. A full-time EMT can expect to work 40 hours a week. Since accidents and illnesses occur 24 hours a day, EMTs work weekends and holidays.

EMTs work indoors and outdoors in all kinds of weather. This is an especially strenuous job. EMTs perform a considerable amount of kneeling, bending, and lifting. EMTs train to keep physically fit, yet despite this, they are often at risk for injuries. They are also at risk of catching communicable or infectious diseases, especially when dealing with high-risk patients such as those with HIV/AIDS or Hepatitis B.

EMTs face many stressful and traumatic situations. Patients sometimes die no matter how intense the efforts to save them. Others are injured so badly that they will have difficulty living productive lives. EMTs also risk injury when treating violent patients or those under the influence of drugs or alcohol. Most consider these challenges to be part of their job and enjoy helping people in need.

REQUIREMENTS

High School

You will need a high school diploma to enter an EMT training program. In high school, take classes in health, psychology, mathematics, biology, anatomy and physiology, and speech. Taking a foreign language such as Spanish will come in handy if you work in an area that has a large population that does not speak English as a first language.

Postsecondary Training

Training for EMTs is offered at several levels: Emergency Medical Technician (EMT), Advanced Emergency Medical Technician (AEMT), and Paramedic.

At the EMT level, students study the basics of emergency caregiving. They learn how to react to and manage medical emergencies such as respiratory distress, obstructed airways, heart attacks, emergency childbirth, or broken bones, wounds, or other injuries caused by accidents, physical assaults, or other events. Their education includes about 150 hours of both classroom time and experience out in the field with experienced EMTs.

Training requirements for those at the AEMT level vary by state, but students learn advanced skills such as the use of advanced airway devices, intravenous fluids, and some medications. Programs at this level require about 400 hours of instruction.

Paramedics receive the most advanced training (including how to stitch wounds and administer intravenous medications), which often culminates in the awarding of an associate's or bachelor's degree. Programs at this level require about 1,200 hours of instruction.

The Commission on Accreditation of Allied Health Education Programs accredits paramedic education programs. Visit its website, www.caahep.org/Find-An-Accredited-Program, for a list of accredited programs. The National Association of Emergency Medical Technicians offers a list of baccalaureate and graduate degrees in emergency medical services at www.naemt.org/EMS_Careers/degreeprograms.aspx.

Programs at the Advanced EMT level typically require about 400 hours of instruction. At this level, candidates learn EMT-level skills as well as more advanced ones, such as using complex airway devices, intravenous fluids, and some medications. Paramedics have the most advanced level of education. They must complete EMT and Advanced EMT levels of instruction, along with courses in advanced medical skills. Community colleges and technical schools may offer these programs, which require about 1,200 hours of instruction and may lead to an associate's degree. Paramedics' broader scope of practice may include stitching wounds or administering intravenous medications.

CERTIFICATION AND LICENSING

The National Registry of Emergency Medical Technicians (NREMT) offers certification to emergency medical service providers at four levels: emergency medical responder (a designation that is typically held by police officers and firefighters); emergency medical technician, advanced emergency medical technician, and paramedic. Additionally, some states have their own certification programs.

All 50 states and the District of Columbia require EMTs to be licensed. Licensing requirements vary by state. Some states have their own licensing examinations and also require EMTs to be certified by NREMT.

OTHER REQUIREMENTS

To be a successful EMT, you should be calm under pressure, decisive, and emotionally stable, since you will occasionally encounter heartbreaking or stressful situations. Other important traits include good overall physical condition (including dexterity, good eyesight and accurate color vision, and endurance to lift heavy loads), the ability to work as a member of a team, and strong communication skills.

EXPLORING

There are many ways to learn more about a career as an EMT. You can read books and magazines about the field, take first-aid and CPR classes offered by the Red Cross or other organizations, visit the websites of college EMT programs to learn about typical classes and possible career paths, and ask your teacher or school counselor to arrange an information interview with an EMT.

Interesting Career:
Medical Flight Worker

Medical flight workers (MFWs) transport critically injured or ill patients from accident scenes and outlying hospitals. The Association of Air Medical Services (AAMS) estimates that the air medical community conducts 550,000 air medical transports in the U.S. each year. The medical flight crew consists of a pilot; specially trained nurses, emergency medical technicians, and respiratory therapists; and, in some instances, emergency medicine-trained physicians. Medical flights may also be staffed by organ transplant specialists, who rush human organs to people who desperately need a transplant. MFWs fly in specially equipped helicopters or fixed-wing aircraft—sometimes called "emergency rooms with wings." They are on call 24-hours a day and are only grounded in the instance of bad weather that might put their own lives in danger. Successful medical flight workers are extremely calm under pressure, organized, able to work as members of a team, and committed to providing top-flight care to injured or ill people. For more information on these exciting careers, contact the following organizations:

✔ **AAMS:** 703-836-8732, www.aams.org

✔ **National Association of EMS Physicians:** 800-228-3677, info-NAEMSP@NAEMSP.org, www.naemsp.org

Check out emergency services blogs to learn about the issues EMTs face every day. Visit www.naemt.org/members_audience/blogsandpodcasts.aspx for a list of popular blogs.

EMPLOYERS

Approximately 236,890 EMTs are employed in the United States. EMTs work for private ambulance companies, fire departments, police departments, public emergency service agencies, and hospitals. While the majority of EMTs work in paid positions in urban areas, some work in volunteer positions in small, rural communities.

GETTING A JOB

Many EMTs obtain their first jobs as a result of contacts made through college internships, career fairs, or networking events. Others seek assistance in obtaining job leads from college career services offices, newspaper want ads, and employment and social media websites.

ADVANCEMENT

EMTs advance by receiving higher pay and by gaining additional training to move from EMT, to Advanced EMT, to paramedic. Paramedics can also advance to supervisory positions. With additional training, some EMTs become teachers, dispatchers, physician assistants, registered nurses, physicians, or sales or marketing professionals for emergency medical equipment manufacturers.

EARNINGS

Salaries for emergency medical technicians vary by type of employer, geographic region, and the worker's experience, education, and skill level. Median annual salaries for EMTs were $31,980 in May 2015, according to the U.S. Department of Labor (USDL). Salaries ranged from less than $20,860 to $55,110 or more. The USDL reports the following mean annual earnings for EMTs by employer: state government, $59,890; local government, $39,000; general medical and surgical hospitals, $36,700; and other ambulatory health care services, $32,550.

Emergency medical technicians usually receive benefits such as health and life insurance, vacation days, sick leave, and a savings and pension plan. Part-time workers must provide their own benefits.

EMPLOYMENT OUTLOOK

Employment for EMTs is expected to grow much faster than the average for all careers during the next decade, according to the U.S. Department of Labor (USDL). Growth is occurring as a result of an increase in the U.S. population—especially among the elderly, who typically require more medical care than other age groups. The USDL reports that "demand for part-time, volunteer EMTs and paramedics in rural areas and smaller metropolitan areas will also continue." EMTs who receive advanced certifications and education will have the best job prospects.

HEALTH AIDES

OVERVIEW

Health aides help patients who are elderly, sick, or physically or mentally disabled with their daily living activities. These activities are conducted in the patients' homes, though aides often accompany patients to medical appointments and other activities. Some aides are certified to provide medical assessment or help with therapy exercises. Health aides learn their skills via on-the-job training. About 820,630 health aides are employed in the United States. Employment opportunities for health aides are expected to be excellent during the next decade.

FAST FACTS

High School Subjects
Family and consumer science
Health

Personal Skills
Communication
Following instructions
Helping

Minimum Education Level
High school diploma

Salary Range
$16,000 to $21,000 to $29,000+

Employment Outlook
Much faster than the average

O*NET-SOC
31-1011.00, 39-9021.00

NOC
3413, 3414

THE JOB

Many people who are ill, injured, or infirm want to stay in their own homes instead of living in a residential, long-term care facility or nursing home. However, they require a degree of care that their family or friends are incapable of providing. In these cases, many people turn to the services of *home health aides* or *personal care aides* (also known as *homemakers, caregivers, companions,* and *personal attendants)* for assistance.

Home health aides and personal-care aides share many of the same duties, with some differences, especially in regards to their employer. Home health aides work for certified home health agencies or hospice agencies. These agencies receive government funding, and so they must comply with state regulations. Personal-care aides work for public or private agencies supplying health care services.

Home health aides travel from site to site, providing skilled care to people of all ages. They complete medical and/or psychological assessments, maintain records, and note any changes in their client's condition. They work alongside other health care professionals such as nurses or therapists. Their duties include cleaning and dressing wounds, administering medications, and educating patients and their families about

Emerging Career: Medical Scribe

The digitalization of health care records has created extra duties for physicians, who must take their attention away from treating patients to record medical data. Many doctors frustrated by these digital demands are looking to a new worker called a *medical scribe* to take notes in real time during medical examinations at clinics and in emergency rooms. ScribeAmerica, a company that provides scribes to assist physicians, estimates that there are nearly 10,000 scribes employed in the United States. This number is expected to grow as more hospital and doctors' offices use digital health records—especially as a result of government incentives to use such programs.

It typically takes between 15 and 21 days to become a medical scribe, with training provided by companies such as ScribeAmerica. Some scribes have college degrees. Scribes earned between $8 to $16 an hour in 2017, according to Salary.com. Considering the short training involved, a job as a scribe might be a good option for college students who are training for high-paying health care careers or for those simply trying to break into the industry.

The American College of Medical Scribe Specialists (https://theacmss.org) is the leading professional organization for medical scribes. It offers membership, certification, and other resources.

patients' particular diseases or conditions. Some home health aides are trained to assist patients with daily physical, speech, or occupational therapy exercises as prescribed by health care professionals.

Some home health aides also provide nonmedical care to patients, as do personal and home care aides. Their duties include helping patients with the many activities of daily living. Aides help patients take baths and showers, or perform daily grooming, such as brushing patients' teeth or combing their hair. They also help patients get dressed or undressed. Other daily responsibilities include bringing patients to the toilet throughout the day, transferring them in and out of wheelchairs, and assisting them in walking or climbing and descending stairs. Aides also help patients during mealtimes by preparing their food and helping them eat, if needed. They make sure that patients eat to maintain their strength, as well as take their medications at the appropriate times.

Depending on the time spent with a patient, aides may do light housework, laundry, or other tasks around the house. At times, they may accompany patients to the grocery store, the doctor's office, or on another appointments or errands. Patients sometimes ask their aides to help them use the telephone or even manage their finances.

Aside from the many tasks done by home health aides and home care aides, equally important is the sense of psychological support and well-being they give to their patients. Patients, as well their concerned families, feel comforted knowing a reliable person is available to help with daily tasks and provide companionship.

Most aides work full time, about 40 hours a week. They often work evenings or weekends to accommodate patients' needs. The work is demanding, both physically and emotionally.

Some tasks done by health aides are unpleasant—emptying bedpans or Foley catheter bags, changing soiled bed linens or clothing, or cleaning patients when they become incontinent. Patients can sometimes become irritable, stubborn, angry, or disoriented and can be quite difficult to handle. Regardless of the challenges they face, health aides perform their duties with compassion for their patients.

Oftentimes, health aides care for multiple patients—up to five a day—working with each for a few hours before moving on to the next client. Health aides should be able to shift gears easily, adapting for a variety of patient personalities, situations, and work environments.

Most aides work independently, with occasional visits from health professionals, their supervisor, or manager. They must have a reliable vehicle, or access to another mode of transportation, in order to travel from patient to patient.

REQUIREMENTS

HIGH SCHOOL

Take health, psychology, and family and consumer science courses in high school. Since you will need strong communication skills to interact effectively with your clients and coworkers, it is a good idea to take as many speech and English classes as possible. Taking a foreign language such as Spanish will come in handy if you work in an area that has a large population that does not speak English as a first language.

POSTSECONDARY TRAINING

Health aides typically do not need to have a high school diploma, but it is always a good idea to graduate from high school since you will need at least a high school education, and at least some college training, to work in most careers. Aides learn their skills via on-the-job training from licensed practical nurses, registered nurses, experienced aides, and managers. They learn how to cook and clean, feed patients, recognize health issues, and react effectively during emergencies.

CERTIFICATION AND LICENSING

Health aides can receive national certification from the National Association for Home Care and Hospice (NAHC). Certification, while voluntary, is highly recommended. It is an excellent way to stand out from other job applicants and demonstrate your abilities to prospective employers.

Health aides who are employed by agencies that receive reimbursement from Medicaid or Medicare must complete a minimum 75-hour

Emerging Career: Dementia Care Nurse

More than 5 million people in the United States have been diagnosed with Alzheimer's disease (one of many types of dementia)—more than twice the number in 1980. By 2050, the number of people age 65 and older with Alzheimer's disease may nearly triple, to a projected 13.8 million. As a result, nurses who care for dementia patients will be in strong demand in the coming decades. The National Council of Certified Dementia Practitioners offers certification in the field. Dementia care nurses need a strong love of others, patience to deal with patients who are sometimes confused or even violent, and familiarity with the special care that is necessary for those with dementia.

training program and a competency evaluation or state certification program. Many employers require aides to complete the NAHC's certification program as proof of competency. Requirements vary by state. Contact your state's department of licensing for more information on requirements in your state.

OTHER REQUIREMENTS

Health aides must be in excellent physical condition. They frequently move patients in and out of beds or wheelchairs, or support them as they descend stairs, cross streets, or get in and out of vehicles. Aides should be strong and physically fit, especially when working with obese patients or those with limited mobility. Since lift apparatus are not often found in patient's homes, aides must lift and shift patients, following procedures to prevent injury to themselves. Other important traits for health aides include compassion for people who are suffering from illness, injury, or old age; excellent communication skills; patience; an upbeat personality; and strong ethics, since you will be working in patients' homes and trusted with their well-being.

EXPLORING

There are many ways to learn more about a career as a health aide. You can read books and magazines (such as *Caring*, www.nahc.org/caringmagazine) about the field. You can ask your health teacher or school counselor to arrange an information interview with a health aide. If you are in high school, you could try to land a job as a health aide with a home health care service or at a nursing home. This will give you a chance to see if the duties of a health aide are a good fit for your interests and abilities.

EMPLOYERS

Approximately 820,630 health aides are employed in the United States. Most work for home health care services or hospice agencies, residential care facilities, individual and family services, and private households. A few operate their own businesses.

GETTING A JOB

Many health aides obtain job leads from newspaper want ads and employment websites. Additionally, national- and state-level professional associations, such as the National Association for Home Care and Hospice (NAHCH), provide job listings at their websites. The NAHCH career website can be found at www.homecarecareers.com.

ADVANCEMENT

Other than salary increases, health aides have few ways of advancing unless they continue their education. Those who go back to school can become nursing aides, licensed practical nurses, registered nurses, or health care managers. Self-employed aides may start their own businesses.

FOR MORE INFORMATION

For information on certification and statistics about home health care, visit the following Web site.
National Association for Home Care and Hospice
202-547-7424
www.nahc.org

For information on career opportunities in Canada, contact
Canadian Home Care Association
www.cdnhomecare.ca

EARNINGS

Salaries for home health aides vary by type of employer, geographic region, and the worker's experience, education, and skill level. Median annual salaries for home health aides were $21,920 in May 2015, according to the U.S. Department of Labor. Salaries ranged from less than $17,480 to $29,950 or more. Earnings for personal care aides ranged from less than $16,910 to $28,620 or more, with a median of $20,980.

Health aides usually receive benefits such as health and life insurance, vacation days, sick leave, and a savings and pension plan. Self-employed workers must provide their own benefits.

EMPLOYMENT OUTLOOK

Employment for health aides is expected to grow much faster than the average for all careers during the next decade, according to the U.S. Department of Labor. In fact, the careers of home health aide and personal-care aide are expected to grow by 38 percent through 2024—adding 348,400 new jobs during this time span. Several factors are fueling growth. The U.S. population is continuing to grow, and the number of people—especially elderly people—needing care is increasing rapidly. Health care costs in hospitals and other nonresidential settings are rising, which is prompting more people to seek care in their own homes. There is also high turnover in this career because the pay is low and work responsibilities are demanding. Many young people view this career as a stepping-stone to other health care careers in nursing, therapy, or health care management.

HEALTH CARE MANAGERS

OVERVIEW

Health care managers, also known as *health care executives, health care administrators,* and *medical and health services managers,* plan, direct, coordinate, and supervise the delivery of health care services. They work at hospitals, clinics, nursing homes, home health agencies, private offices, and other health care facilities. A master's degree in health care management or a related field is required for employment at large facilities; a bachelor's degree may be sufficient for entry-level positions at small facilities. Approximately 314,950 medical and health services managers are employed in the United States. Employment is expected to be good during the next decade.

THE JOB

Health care managers are responsible for the operations of a health care facility, including its clinical health services, financial office, human resources department, educational programs (some facilities offer training to health care students), security, janitorial services, information technology department, and other departments.

A large part of a manager's job involves managing the daily fiscal operations of the facility. Managers look for ways to reduce costs without sacrificing quality health care for patients. This entails keeping up to date on insurance policies, changes in Medicare or Medicaid reimbursements, and federal laws or regulations regarding health care reform.

Health care managers oversee improvements to equipment and medical technology, building repairs and additions, and the procurement of medications, equipment, and supplies. At least once a year, state health inspectors visit the facility to make sure it meets health regulations. Violations may result in fines or, in severe cases, a forced shut-down. Health care managers ensure their facilities are safe and up to standards as mandated by the state.

Supervision of personnel is another duty. Health care managers often interview potential employees and have final say in employee hiring and firing. They are in charge of training and continuing education offered to staff members. They establish pay scales and sometimes are asked for input regarding benefits packages offered to staff members. Health care managers also mediate disputes between employees or address complaints made by patients or family members.

Security is another important duty. Health care managers ensure that employees and patients at their facilities are physically safe while on the hospital's premises. Health care managers also ensure patient privacy and confidentiality by protecting the security of all patient records, whether in paper or electronic format. Recent government regulations mandate that all health care facilities and providers maintain patient records in secure electronic format. Health care managers, as well as select staff and department members, must participate in service training to keep up to date on changing computer and software technology.

Health care managers meet regularly with department heads, such as the director of nursing or the medical director. These meetings provide department heads with an opportunity to update the administrator regarding current or future projects and to address any issues that are affecting the smooth operation of the facility.

Health care managers often act as their facilities' representative for community functions and events. They participate in community outreach programs and health fairs that educate the public on health issues.

Duties and responsibilities of health care managers vary by facility. Large facilities such as hospitals may have several assistant administrators who manage clinical departments such as therapy, nursing, surgery, and medical records and health information. For example, the nursing department is managed by the director of nursing, and the medical records department or therapy departments are supervised by separate managers. These managers typically have experience in their department's specialty. For example, a director of physical therapy is typically a practicing physical therapist. A director of nursing typically is a nurse with advanced education. There are managers who supervise security, information technology, janitorial services, billing, and other departments. All departmental managers report to the head hospital administrator. At facilities that are smaller in size, such as a nursing home, administrators may handle all daily activities as well as issues regarding personnel, faculty operations, admissions, and resident care. Some medical practices employ medical administrators to manage the business aspect of the practice, including staff, billing, budgeting, equipment procurement, and overall patient flow.

Full-time health care managers work five days a week for about 40 hours a week. However, since many health care facilities operate 24 hours a day, health care managers often work long hours, including those at night and on weekends, to manage any crisis or emergency situations that arise. They carry pagers or dedicated cell phones for such emergencies. Health care managers and administrators work in comfortable, well-lit offices.

Many health care managers have limited patient contact, instead spending much of their time dealing with policy issues or other changes needed to make their institutions or departments run smoothly. This in turn serves the patient population. They deal with insurance companies, Medicare or Medicaid, government health service agencies, medical contractors, and medical supply companies to ensure the efficient operation of their facilities.

Health care managers supervise the work of assistant administrators or managers. Some travel may be necessary to attend meetings and community events, or to inspect satellite facilities.

Other Career Options in Health Care

✔ Biomedical Equipment Technicians
✔ Chiropractors
✔ Dental Laboratory Technicians
✔ Dietitians and Nutritionists
✔ Clinical Laboratory Technologists and Technicians
✔ Health Advocates
✔ Histologic Technicians
✔ Holistic Physicians

✔ Kinesiologists
✔ Medical Ethicists
✔ Nursing Home Administrators
✔ Ophthalmologists
✔ Optometrists
✔ Orthotists and Prosthetists
✔ Perfusionists
✔ Respiratory Therapists and Technicians
✔ Transplant Coordinators

REQUIREMENTS

HIGH SCHOOL

High school classes that will be useful for aspiring health care managers include business, computer science, health, mathematics, English, and speech.

POSTSECONDARY TRAINING

A master's degree is required for employment at large health care facilities; a bachelor's degree may be sufficient for entry-level positions at small facilities. Most people earn a graduate degree in health services administration, long-term care administration, health sciences, or public health. Others pursue graduate degrees in business or public administration, with a concentration in health care management, or seek joint degrees in business administration and public health. The Commission on Accreditation of Healthcare Management Education (www.cahme.org) accredits graduate-level health care management programs. The

Association of University Programs in Health Administration offers a list of baccalaureate, master's, and doctoral health care management programs at its website, www.aupha.org/resourcecenter/auphaprogramdirectory. Offices of physicians and other health care facilities sometimes hire managers with extensive on-the-job experience but no college degree.

CERTIFICATION AND LICENSING

Voluntary certification is offered by several professional associations including the American Health Information Management Association, the American College of Health Care Administrators, AMDA-The Society for Post-Acute and Long-Term Care Medicine, the Professional Association of Health Care Office Management, and the Medical Group Management Association. Certification, while voluntary, is highly recommended. It is an excellent way to stand out from other job applicants and demonstrate your abilities to prospective employers.

All states require nursing home administrators to be licensed, but requirements vary by state. The U.S. Department of Labor reports that "in most states, these administrators must have a bachelor's degree, complete a state-approved training program, and pass a national licensing exam. Some states also require applicants to pass a state-specific exam; others may require applicants to have previous work experience in a health care facility. Some states also require licensure for administrators in assisted-living facilities. A license is not required in other areas of medical and health services management." The National Association of Long Term Care Administrator Boards offers information on state licensing at its website, www.nabweb.org.

OTHER REQUIREMENTS

Health care managers must have strong leadership abilities to effectively lead staff members and inspire them to provide excellent health care services to patients. They should be decisive, organized, diplomatic, flexible, and good at solving problems. Strong communication skills are important because they frequently interact with other managers, staff members, inspectors, and others. Health care managers must have excellent financial management skills and strong ethics, since they are tasked with managing multimillion dollar budgets and making financial decisions that will affect the future of the facility and the quality of the health care services provided to patients.

EXPLORING

There are many ways to learn more about a career as a health care manager. You can read books [such as *The Emerging Healthcare Leader: A Field Guide,* by Laurie K. Baedke and Natalie D. Lamberton (Health Administration Press, 2015)] and journals about the field, and visit the websites of college health care management programs to learn about typical classes and possible career paths. Professional associations can also provide information about the field. The American College of Healthcare Executives provides a wealth of information on health care managers and careers at its website, Make a Difference: Discover a Career in Healthcare Management! (www.healthmanagementcareers.org). You should also try to land a part-time job in a medical office. This will give you a chance to interact with health care managers and see if the career is a good fit for your interests and abilities.

Ask your teacher or school counselor to arrange an information interview with a health care manager. Here are some sample questions to ask:

✔ What do you like best and least about your job?

✔ What's the work environment like at your company?

✔ What are the most important personal and professional qualities for people in your career?

✔ What's the best way to network in the health care industry?

✔ What are the best job-search strategies?

✔ What advice would you give to job seekers in terms of applying to and interviewing for jobs?

Useful Resources

Aldrich, Jim. *Climbing the Healthcare Management Ladder: Career Advice From the Top on How to Succeed.* Baltimore, Md.: Health Professions Press, 2013.

McConnell, Charles R. U*miker's Management Skills for the New Health Care Supervisor.* 7th ed. Burlington, Mass.: Jones & Bartlett Learning, 2016.

White, Kenneth R., and J. Stephen Lindsey. *Take Charge of Your Healthcare Management Career: 50 Lessons That Drive Success.* Chicago: Health Administration Press, 2015.

EMPLOYERS

Approximately 314,950 medical and health services managers are employed in the United States. Medical and health services managers are employed by hospitals; HMOs; centers for cardiac rehabilitation, urgent care, and diagnostic imaging; group medical practices; offices of health practitioners; nursing homes; adult day care programs; home health care agencies; and other residential facilities.

GETTING A JOB

Participating in an internship during college is an excellent way to get your "foot in the door" at an employer. Many companies offer high-performing interns full-time positions. Other job-search strategies include attending career fairs and networking events, using the resources of one's college career services offices, and checking out newspaper want ads and employment and social media websites.

Many companies provide useful resources for job applicants at their websites. Here are two examples of job-search resources provided by health care employers:

✔ Kaiser Permanente offers information on its interview process, internships, and career paths, as well as details about its more than 35 hospitals, at www.kaiserpermanentejobs.org/university-connection.

✔ Providence Health and Services provides an overview of potential career paths, the application process, and job listings at www.providence-executive.jobs

Additionally, professional associations, such as the American College of Health Care Administrators and the American College of Healthcare Executives (ACHE), provide job listings at their websites, as well as offer networking and job-search resources. For example, the ACHE provides the following networking resources:

✔ The Leadership Mentoring Network, which matches college-level and young members with senior-level executives, who provide advice on career development and developing one's network.

✔ The Career Management Network, which is a group of member volunteers who provide advice about career transitions and names of key contacts in your chosen health care specialty or geographic region.

✔ The Early Careerist Network, which is available to full members or fellows of ACHE who are under the age of 40. Resources include the *Early Careerist Newsletter,* networking and mentoring opportunities, educational programs, and The Early Careerist Message Board, which allows users to interact via e-forums.

✔ Networking Profile, a self-assessment tool that allows users to assess their networking skills.

ADVANCEMENT

Health care managers advance by receiving increases in pay or promotions to higher positions, by moving to larger facilities, and by working as consultants or college professors.

EARNINGS

Salaries for health care managers vary by type of employer, geographic region, and the worker's experience, education, and skill level. Median annual salaries for health care managers were $94,500 in May 2015, according to the U.S. Department of Labor (USDL). Salaries ranged from less than $56,230 to $165,380 or more. The USDL reports the following mean annual earnings for health care managers by employer:

✔ general medical and surgical hospitals, $114,180;

✔ offices of physicians, $102,080;

✔ outpatient care centers, $100,470;

✔ home health care services, $95,260; and

✔ nursing care facilities, $87,970.

Employers offer a variety of benefits, including the following: medical, dental, and life insurance; paid holidays, vacations, and sick and personal days; 401(k) plans; profit-sharing plans; retirement and pension plans; and educational-assistance programs. Health care managers who work as freelance consultants must provide their own benefits.

EMPLOYMENT OUTLOOK

The U.S. Department of Labor predicts that employment for health care managers will grow much faster than the average for all careers during the next decade. Opportunities will be best in home health care services, outpatient care centers, and offices of health practitioners (as services traditionally provided by hospitals shift to these settings, especially as medical technologies improve). There will also be increasing opportunities at health care management companies that provide management services to health care facilities on a contract basis. Health care managers who oversee care for the elderly (from independent assisted-living facilities to supervised 24-hour care) will have strong job prospects. Health care managers with master's degrees in health care administration and related fields and knowledge of health information technology and informatics systems will have the best job prospects.

FOR MORE INFORMATION

Contact the AMDA for information about medical directors who work in long-term care.
AMDA-The Society for Post-Acute and Long-Term Care Medicine
800-876-2632
info@paltc.org
www.amda.com

To learn more about certification and state licensing, contact
American College of Health Care Administrators
202-536-5120
info@achca.org
www.achca.org

For information on education, careers, and certification, contact
American College of Healthcare Executives
contact@ache.org
www.ache.org

For information on accredited programs and careers, contact
Association of University Programs in Health Administration
aupha@aupha.org
www.aupha.org

To learn more about certification, contact
Medical Group Management Association
877-275-6462
www.mgma.org

To learn more about careers in health care office management and certification, contact
Professional Association of Health Care Office Management
800-451-9311
www.pahcom.com

For information on career opportunities in Canada, contact
Canadian College of Health Leaders
613-235-7218
www.cchl-ccls.ca

HEALTH INFORMATION MANAGEMENT SPECIALISTS

OVERVIEW

Health information management specialists, also known as *health information management technicians,* capture, analyze, and protect patients' medical information. This information is stored in paper or digital format. Information they coordinate includes patients' medical history, diagnoses, laboratory tests, x-ray and other diagnostic procedure reports, and treatment plans. An associate's degree or apprenticeship is typically required to enter the field. Approximately 247,760 medical records and health information management technicians are employed in the United States. Employment opportunities are expected to be very good during the next decade.

THE JOB

Every time a patient goes to the emergency room, is admitted to the hospital, visits a primary care physician for an annual physical, or undergoes laboratory tests, a record is made of that visit or procedure, as well as every referral or second-opinion consultation. The notes taken during an actual examination or procedure are considered the "primary patient record." It includes patient data, which physicians use to get a better idea of a patient's medical condition. Primary patient records also include any documentation, observations, or instructions made by the physician. A "secondary patient record" is created from information taken from the primary record and includes data pertinent to nonclinical people such as administration, regulation, and billing/payment history. The collection of information documenting a patient's health care services is considered the "patient health record." It includes all clinical or office records, all care, tests, and procedures done in health care or home care settings, as well as patient evaluations, and any participation in research or clinical databases. It's important that all medical records are organized and can be accessed by physicians, nurses, and other health care workers. A complete record gives a clear picture of a patient's medical condition as well as saves time and money by preventing duplication of laboratory tests and other procedures. It also allows medical billing workers to send appropriate bills to the patient or request reimbursement from insurance companies.

Great efforts have been made to organize and streamline the methods used by hospitals, clinics, and physicians' offices to gather and store patient records. At the center of this system are health information management specialists, who are key to the day-to-day operations of medical records departments.

At the start of every workday, health information management (HIM) specialists receive a request list from different physicians or departments of, say, a hospital or clinic. This list names every patient who will be seen that day—whether for an examination or follow-up, or perhaps for a blood test or x-ray. Other physicians may submit a list of patients needed for charting purposes or further research. Using this list, HIM specialists "pull" or electronically retrieve patients' records and deliver them to the appropriate physician or department.

Throughout the day, the medical records department will receive additional patient information from various sources, including off-site laboratories, hospitals, and physician's offices. This information could contain test results, physician consults, or a variety of other medical information. HIM specialists are responsible for coding any new diagnoses and incorporating new information into the patient's existing medical records.

As recently as 10 years ago, most medical records were in paper form, and a great deal of time was spent filing these papers into a patient's medical chart. Unfortunately medical records were sometimes misfiled due to human error. Today, most hospitals and clinics, and the majority of physician's offices, keep their medical records in digital format. Not only do digital medical records reduce the chance for human error, they make it easier to quickly enter and obtain information. HIM specialists often attend training sessions to keep abreast of any new computer software applications or techniques to manage electronic medical records.

Some technicians are specially trained to work with medical coding. *Medical coders*, also known as *coding specialists*, transform medical diagnoses and procedures into a universally accepted set of numeral codes known as ICD-10-CM, which helps providers and insurance companies in their diagnosis and treatment of a disease, reimbursement, and surveillance of potential disease outbreaks. This coded information is used by insurance companies or programs such as Medicare in the processing of claims.

Other technicians are specially trained to keep track of patients as they manage their illnesses. *Cancer registrars*, also known as *tumor registrars*, are needed to track information regarding patients and their fight against cancer. This information is used by researchers, health care professionals, and public policymakers to identify cancer groups, track treatment success, create cancer education programs, and support funding for additional treatment centers. Cancer registrars begin their work by creating a case file for every newly diagnosed patient in their assigned workplace, usually a hospital or cancer clinic. Information compiled includes the diagnosis of a cancerous or benign tumor, pathology reports, and medical reports. This first step will determine the patient's eligibility in the cancer registry. Next, cancer registrars abstract the case, or summarize the patient's medical records into standard coding used by the medical and research community. Specific coding is assigned to different data such as the patient's demographic, the type of cancer and its location, the stage of disease, and prescribed treatment details. Cancer registrars need to locate information and results from different locations, as patients are often sent to various physicians, clinics, and hospitals for various tests and procedures. Cancer registrars also conduct a yearly follow-up with each case, detailing any hospital admissions or changes in treatment as well as surveys from all attending physicians. Also important is the written follow-up with patients on how they have fared in the past year. All registry data is submitted to state

Books to Read

Abdelhak, Mervat, and Mary Alice Hanken. *Health Information: Management of a Strategic Resource.* 5th ed. Philadelphia: W. B. Saunders, 2015.

Gartee, Richard. *Electronic Health Records: Understanding and Using Computerized Medical Records.* 3rd ed. New York: Pearson Education, 2016.

Green, Michelle A., and Mary Jo Bowie. *The Essentials of Health Information Management: Principles and Practices.* 3rd ed. Farmington Hills, Mich.: Delmar Cengage Learning, 2015.

cancer registries to identify high-risk groups, implement screening procedures, and give an estimated prognosis for many types of cancer.

Other HIM specialists work as *medical transcriptionists*. This is the process of taking handwritten notes or recorded evaluations and transforming them into an electronic format. Some hospitals and health care settings often outsource this duty, while others may keep it in-house. Transcription could mean simply keyboarding the physicians' notes, or finding and including the appropriate diagnosis or procedural code.

Health information administrators supervise health information management workers. They develop and implement policies that assure the appropriate storage and dissemination of health information.

Health information management specialists have other duties, including speaking with physicians or representatives from insurance companies, creating monthly work schedules, and ordering office supplies.

Full-time health information management specialists work about 40 hours a week, with opportunity for overtime. Those employed at hospitals or other health care facilities that offer round-the-clock care will have shift work.

HIM specialists work indoors in comfortable offices with cutting-edge computer technology. There may be separate areas for specific tasks such as file retrieval, transcription, coding, or quality review. Much of the work is detail oriented and done using a computer.

While they work in health care, HIM specialists (except cancer registrars) do not have any patient contact. However, they do interact with people from many different professions in order to clarify diagnoses or to obtain additional data.

REQUIREMENTS

HIGH SCHOOL

In high school, take courses in anatomy and physiology, biology, chemistry, mathematics (especially algebra), health, and computer science to prepare for the field.

POSTSECONDARY TRAINING

An associate's degree is typically required to enter the field, though some move into this field with work experience and on-the-job training. Health information administrators need at least a bachelor's degree.

The Commission on Accreditation for Health Informatics and Information Management Education accredits health information management programs. Visit its website, www.cahiim.org, for a list of accredited programs. More than 200 programs are accredited by the Commission. Typical classes in a health information management program include Medical Terminology; Human Anatomy, Physiology, and Pathology; Health Data Management; Introduction to Pharmacology; Clinical Classification Systems; Clinical Data Analysis; Legal and Qualitative Aspects of Health Information; Principles of Health Information Management; Medical Reimbursement; Medical Transcription Practicum; Medical Coding Practicum; Medical Ethics; and Database Security and Management.

The American Health Information Management Association approves certificate programs in medical coding. Visit www.ahima.org for a list of accredited programs. Sixty-nine percent of coders have some postsecondary training, according to a member survey from the AAPC; 18 percent have a bachelor's degree or higher.

An emerging pathway in this career field is the registered apprenticeship. "Registered apprenticeships are a customizable work-and-learn program that combines on-the-job training with job related technical instruction that meets national standards for registration with the Department of Labor or state apprenticeship agencies," according to Bill Rudman, the executive director of the AHIMA Foundation and the vice president of education visioning at AHIMA. "AHIMA Foundation's Managing the Talent Pipeline in Health Information Management Registered Apprenticeship program provides individuals skills training and experiential learning for our four registered roles (coding professional/hospital coder, coding documentation improvement specialist, business analyst, data analyst) through an intense immersion program and on-the-job training of the apprentice at no cost to the employer or to the employee."

CERTIFICATION AND LICENSING

Certification is offered by several professional associations, including the American Health Information Management Association, the AAPC, the Board of Medical Specialty Coding, the Association for Healthcare Documentation Integrity, the Professional Association of Healthcare Coding Specialists, the Practice Management Institute, the Institute of Certified Records Managers, and the National Cancer Registrars Association. Certification, while voluntary, is highly recommended. It is an excellent way to stand out from other job applicants and demonstrate your abilities to prospective employers. A few states and health care facilities require cancer registrars to be licensed.

OTHER REQUIREMENTS

Although the work is administrative in nature, HIM specialists must have a background in the health sciences, since accuracy and understanding of medical terminology are exceptionally important in these careers. They must translate physician notes, spot any inconsistencies, and avoid errors at all costs. Being detail oriented is a must for a career in health information management. Other important traits for HIM specialists include strong communication skills, the ability to work as a member of a team, and a willingness to continue to learn throughout one's career.

EXPLORING

There are many ways to learn more about a career as a health information management specialist. You can read books and journals (*Advance for Health Information Professionals*, http://health-information.advanceweb.com) about the field, visit the websites of college health information management programs to learn about typical classes and possible career paths, and ask your teacher or school counselor to arrange an information interview with a HIM specialist. Professional associations can also provide information about the field. The American Health Information Management Association provides information on education and careers at its website, www.ahima.org/careers. If you're in college, consider becoming a member of the association. Membership benefits include access to scholarships, networking events, career prep webinars, a mentor program, and other resources. You should also try to land a part-time job in a medical office. This will give you a chance to interact with HIM specialists and see if the career is a good fit for your abilities and interests.

EMPLOYERS

Approximately 247,760 medical records and health information technicians are employed in the United States. Approximately 35 percent work in hospitals. Other employers of HIM specialists include offices of physicians and other health care practitioners, outpatient clinics, surgical centers, nursing homes, managed-care facilities, home health agencies, pharmaceutical companies, long-term care facilities, state and federal government agencies that collect and disseminate health care information, and other health care facilities. Some HIM specialists are self-employed.

GETTING A JOB

Many health information management specialists obtain their first jobs as a result of contacts made through college internships, career fairs, or networking events. Others seek assistance in obtaining job leads from college career services offices, newspaper want ads, and employment websites. Additionally, professional associations, such as the American Health Information Management Association, the Association for Healthcare Documentation Integrity, the National Cancer Registrars Association, and the AAPC, provide job listings at their websites. See For More Information for contact information. *Advance for Health Information Professionals* also offers job listings for HIM specialists at its website, www.advanceweb.com/jobs/healthcare. Medical transcriptionists can access job listings at MTJOBS (www.mtjobs.com). Those interested in positions with the federal government should visit the U.S. Office of Personnel Management's website, www.usajobs.gov.

ADVANCEMENT

Health information management specialists advance by receiving pay raises and by earning bachelor's or master's degrees, which qualifies them to become health information managers. Those who obtain specialty certifications can become specialists such as medical transcriptionists.

EARNINGS

Median annual salaries for HIM specialists were $37,110 in May 2015, according to the U.S. Department of Labor (USDL). Salaries ranged from less than $24,190 to $61,400 or more. The USDL reports the following mean annual earnings for HIM specialists by employer: federal agencies, $47,520; general medical and surgical hospitals, $43,080; nursing care facilities, $37,550; outpatient care centers, $37,370; and offices of physicians, $34,940.

Medical transcriptionists earned salaries that ranged from less than $34,192 to $52,664 or more in 2017, according to Salary.com.

Employers offer a variety of benefits, including the following: medical, dental, and life insurance; paid holidays, vacations, and sick and personal days; 401(k) plans; profit-sharing plans; retirement and pension plans; and educational-assistance programs. Self-employed and part-time workers must provide their own benefits. Approximately 14 percent of HIM specialists are self-employed.

EMPLOYMENT OUTLOOK

Employment for health information management specialists is expected to grow much faster than average for all careers during the next decade, according to the U.S. Department of Labor (USDL). More opportunities are becoming available because of the increasing number of medical tests, procedures, and treatments that are being conducted and the federally mandated transition of paper medical records to electronic format. HIM specialists with a good knowledge of computer software and other technology will have the best job prospects.

Demand is expected to continue to be strong for cancer registrars. "As the population ages," according to the USDL, "there will likely be more types of special purpose registries because many illnesses are detected and treated later in life."

FOR MORE INFORMATION

For information on certification, contact the following organizations

AAPC
800-626-2633
info@aapc.com
www.aapc.com

ARMA International
800-422-2762
headquarters@armaintl.org
www.arma.org

Association for Healthcare Documentation Integrity
ahdi@ahdionline.org
www.ahdionline.org

Practice Management Institute
800-259-5562
info@pmimd.com
www.pmimd.com

Professional Association of Healthcare Coding Specialists
888-708-4707
www.pahcs.org

For information on careers in health information management and accredited programs, contact
American Health Information Management Association
info@ahima.org
www.ahima.org

For a list of schools offering accredited programs, contact
Commission on Accreditation for Health Informatics and Information Management Education
info@cahiim.org
www.cahiim.org

To learn more about a career as a cancer registrar, contact
National Cancer Registrars Association
703-299-6640
www.ncra-usa.org

For information on career opportunities in Canada, contact
Canadian Health Information Management Association
519-438-6700
www.echima.ca

Interview: Bill Rudman

The American Health Information Management Association (AHIMA)
has created an interactive Health Information Management (HIM)
Career Map© to help students and HIM professionals chart their career
paths. The editors of *Hot Health Care Careers* spoke with Bill Rudman,
the Vice President of Education Visioning at AHIMA and Executive
Director of the AHIMA Foundation, about the HIM Career Map© and
opportunities in health information management.

Q. **Can you tell us about the HIM Career Map©?**

A. The Health Information Management (HIM) Career Map© is an interactive
visual representation of the job titles and roles that make up the scope of
HIM and associated career pathways. The map contains both current and
emerging roles in HIM, and promotional and transitional career pathways.
The map is based on data collected from volunteer subject matter experts,
AHIMA staff, and a member survey. The HIM Career Map© illustrates the
full breadth and depth of the profession, and it serves as an educational
tool for those inside and outside the field. To view the HIM Career Map©,
visit http://hicareers.com/CareerMap.

Q. **What are some of the most popular careers in HIM?**

A. The HIM Career Map© is divided into six job families within the HIM profes-
sion: Compliance/Risk Management; Education/Communication; Informatics/
Data Analysis; Information Technology and Infrastructure; Operations: Medical
Records Administration; and Revenue Cycle Management/Coding and Billing.
Currently, the most popular careers for HIM professionals are in Operations:
Medical Records and Revenue Cycle Management/Coding and Billing.

   HIM careers are shifting from traditional roles in coding to roles that are
more focused on data governance, integrity, and analytics. Coding auditors,
chief knowledge officers, documentation specialists, registry specialists,
professors, revenue cycle, and risk/compliance are among the most-popular
emerging career titles.

Q. **What are the key skills for HIM professionals?**

A. By studying health information management, students will acquire a versa-
tile, yet focused, skill set incorporating clinical, analytical, information
technology, leadership, legal, and management skills. Health information
professionals use their knowledge of information technology and records
management to form the link between clinicians, administrators, technology designers, and information technology professionals. Health information
programs incorporate the disciplines of medicine, management, finance,
information technology, and law into one curriculum. Because of this
unique mixture, health information graduates can choose from a variety of
work settings across an array of health care environments. As for personal
skills, HIM professionals must be detail-oriented, hard-working, and passionate about their field. They must also have strong interpersonal skills.

Q. **What advice would you give to those seeking jobs in HIM?**

A. Health information is a rapidly growing field. Finding the right entry-level
position, however, can be a challenge. The difficulty often lies not in acquiring the necessary skills or credentials, but rather integrating yourself into the
professional community. To become an HIM or health informatics profession-

al, you'll have to think like one, and work with the collaborative nature of the industry. One helpful tip is to volunteer at a hospital, physician's office, or other facility where you'd like to work. Think of volunteering as a way to help patients and demonstrate your commitment to health information in a low-pressure environment. By volunteering, you'll build your network from within, and will increase your chances of being notified about job vacancies.

Also, consider job shadowing. Once you've established a professional relationship with someone in health information, ask to shadow them for a day. You will gain a perspective that can't be taught in a classroom or through intern experience. As a natural next step after an informational interview, job shadowing can be a great way to observe intangibles, like culture.

In the HIM field, it is also important to join a professional association. Joining AHIMA as a student or new graduate member automatically extends your potential network by thousands. Associations like AHIMA offer students the resources to turn knowledge and connections into real opportunities. AHIMA also offers job search resources like the top industry-specific job board, Career Assist: Job Bank.

Lastly, make sure to network. Estimates reveal that 70 to 80 percent of jobs are obtained through networking. Networking does not involve directly asking for a job, but rather developing a broad list of contacts and professional relationships within a given occupation. In most areas, health information is a tight-knit field. Ask your professors, friends, or mentors if they can introduce you to someone in your area of interest. Most are happy to oblige and genuinely want to see students succeed. You can also use social media for networking. Find others with similar career goals online through AHIMA's Engage Communities, LinkedIn, Facebook, and Twitter.

The Best Places to Work in Health Care

Earning a good salary is not the only thing you should consider when choosing a health care employer. A supportive work environment, good benefits, and other criteria should also be considered. Each year, *Modern Healthcare* selects the top 100 health care employers that offer a rewarding work environment for their employees. Criteria included work environment, job satisfaction, benefits, and training and development programs. Here were the 10 best places to work in 2016:

1. Texas Health Presbyterian Hospital Flower Mound (Flower Mound, TX)

2. CQuence Health Group (Omaha, NE)

3. Impact Advisors (Naperville, IL)

4. Black River Memorial Hospital (Black River Falls, WI)

5. Pantherx Specialty Pharmacy (Pittsburgh, PA)

6. CompHealth (Salt Lake City, UT)

7. The Women's Hospital (Newburgh, IN)

8. Louisiana Organ Procurement Agency (Metairie, LA)

9. Pivot Point Consulting (Brentwood, TN)

10. Weatherby Healthcare (Fort Lauderdale, FL)

Some companies have locations throughout the United States. Visit modernhealthcare.com/community/best-places/2016 to read the complete list.

LICENSED PRACTICAL NURSES

OVERVIEW

Licensed practical nurses (LPNs), also known as licensed vocational nurses in Texas and California, provide general health care to patients under the supervision of registered nurses and physicians. Their job duties depend largely on their work setting. To prepare for the field, LPNs must complete at least one year of postsecondary nursing training at a vocational or technical school or a community or junior college. Approximately 697,250 licensed practical nurses are employed in the United States. Employment opportunities are expected to be very good during the next decade.

FAST FACTS

High School Subjects
Biology
Chemistry

Personal Skills
Active listening
Communication
Critical thinking
Judgment and decision making

Minimum Education Level
Some postsecondary training

Salary Range
$32,000 to $43,000 to $59,000+

Employment Outlook
Much faster than the average

O*NET-SOC
29-2061.00

NOC
3233

THE JOB

LPNs care for sick, injured, and disabled people. They handle a large share of the direct patient care in health care facilities today. They observe, record, and report changes in patients' conditions by taking patients' vital signs (blood pressure, pulse, respiration, temperature, height, and weight); administer medications and therapeutic treatments; and assist patients with bathing, dressing, and general personal hygiene. They help patients in and out of bed, dress wounds, and administer medication, taking careful note of the amount of the medication and the time it was administered and entering this information on patients' medical charts. They also note the patient's fluid intake and output. More and more today, these charts are now in digital format.

LPNs must be comfortable using medical equipment such as IV lines, catheters, tracheotomy tubes, and respirators. For patients who need physical assistance, LPNs may help in getting them dressed and move about, or LPNs may assist them during mealtimes.

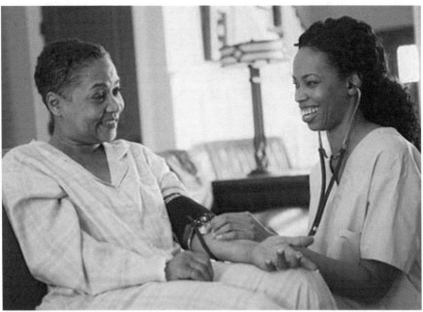

A licensed practical nurse takes a patient's blood pressure.
(Jupiterimages/Thinkstock)

Most LPNs are generalists and are trained to work in any medical office setting, treating patients of all ages. Some specialize in a certain population, such as caring for the elderly in a nursing home or treating babies and young children in a pediatric ward in a hospital. Experienced LPNs supervise nursing assistants and aides.

Regardless of where they work, LPNs play a critical role in gathering information about the patient and communicating it to other members of the patient's health care team. They ask the patient about his or her medical history, current symptoms, and any medications he or she might be taking. They monitor the patient for adverse reactions to newly prescribed medications or treatments and note changes in vital signs that may signal a problem. All this information is vital to help assist physicians and other specialists make diagnoses and prescribe treatments.

In addition to communicating with the patient's doctors and nurses, LPNs also spend time talking to the patient and his or her family about healthy living suggestions or how to care for a healing injury or newly diagnosed illness. They help make everyone more comfortable during a possibly stressful time and try to answer any questions patients or family members may have.

Licensed practical nurses work in medical offices, hospitals, nursing homes, medical clinics, schools, and community health centers. Those who work in 24-hour settings such as hospitals may work evening or overnight shifts, and some LPNs work weekends or holidays. Since much of their work is physically demanding, LPNs must be in good shape. They help patients in and out of bed or move them to gurneys. They often bend, stoop, reach, and otherwise physically exert themselves during their shifts.

Like all health care workers, LPNs must follow standard procedures when caring for sick patients, such as wearing latex gloves or a mask and frequently washing their hands. While this career can be stressful and physically demanding at times, most LPNs view their careers as very rewarding.

REQUIREMENTS

HIGH SCHOOL

Take health, mathematics, biology, chemistry, physics, English, and speech in high school to prepare for a career in nursing.

POSTSECONDARY TRAINING

To become a LPN, you should attend a practical nurse training program at a technical or vocational school or a community college. Training lasts for approximately one year. Typical course work includes basic nursing concepts, anatomy, physiology, nutrition, first aid, nursing specialties

Nursing Informatics Blends Patient Care with Information Science

Modern patient health care is increasingly supported by the use of computers and information science for data management and communication. Such reliance on computers and technology in the field of nursing has created a career specialty for professionals with skills in patient care as well as information science—*nursing informatics specialist.*

Nursing informatics specialists organize a database of patients' medical information in an accessible format. They may customize and test the database according to the needs of different medical departments or specialties. Nursing informatics specialists also train nurses on computer charting, which consists of adding information to or retrieving it from the database. They write and install new programs or software applications to help nursing staff work more efficiently.

Most nursing informatics specialists come to the field with a degree in nursing, though some employers will consider candidates with a degree in information or computer science. The demand for nursing informatics specialists is expected to rise due to increasing regulation of medical practices and stricter standards for the management of patients' records, making this an appealing career choice for those wanting to combine patient care with their interest in information science.

For more information, contact the **American Nursing Informatics Association,** 866-552-6404, ania@ajj.com, www.ania.org.

Emerging Career: Health Care Coach

About 75 percent of health care costs in the United States are spent on the management of chronic diseases, but according to research, only slightly more than half of people with chronic diseases are receiving guidance on preventive care. Health care companies are realizing that to reduce health care costs, patients need to be "coached" on proper care, to monitor blood pressure and blood sugar, to make and keep regular medical appointments, and to otherwise stay healthy. As a result, the career of *health care coach* is growing in popularity. These professionals dispense advice, monitor the well-being of patients, and generally serve as cheerleaders and motivators to help patients with diabetes, hypertension, asthma, and other chronic diseases live better lives. Others help people quit smoking, lose weight, or eliminate other addictive habits. Health insurance companies, hospitals, and other health care providers are employing health care coaches to work with patients. Health care coaching businesses are also being founded by entrepreneurs with little or no health experience, but strong communication and organizational skills. A study led by Eric Coleman, M.D., a professor of medicine and the head of the Division of Health Care Policy and Research at the University of Colorado Anschutz Medical Campus, found that patients who worked with a coach "were less likely to require re-hospitalization, significantly cutting their health care costs."

(such as pediatric, obstetric, or gerontological nursing), and hands-on clinical experience. Visit Discover Nursing (www.discovernursing.com) for a database of nursing programs.

CERTIFICATION AND LICENSING

Certification, while not required, is an excellent way to demonstrate your nursing skills and expertise to potential employers. The National Association for Practical Nurse Education and Service offers specialty certification in pharmacology, IV therapy, and long-term care. Contact the association for more information.

Nursing students need to pass the National Council Licensure Examination, or NCLEX-PN, in order to obtain licensure. The examination is administered by the National Council of State Boards of Nursing.

OTHER REQUIREMENTS

To be a successful LPN, you should have empathy for others, be decisive, enjoy working as a member of a team, be able to follow instructions (but also work independently, when necessary), have strong communication skills, and be willing to continue to learn throughout your career to keep your skills up to date.

EXPLORING

Read books and visit websites about nursing, talk with your counselor or

More Men Pursuing Careers in Nursing

Although their numbers are still relatively small, men are increasingly pursuing careers in nursing. Registered nurses make up the largest occupational group in the health care industry, comprising more than 2.7 million jobs. About 10 percent of this total are men, but this percentage has climbed steadily since 1980, according to the U.S. Census Bureau.

There are many resources for men who are interested in careers in nursing. Discover Nursing (www.discovernursing.com/men-in-nursing#.WHZFavkrK70) offers a section about males in nursing. The American Association of Nurse Anesthetists offers a Men in Nursing DVD. Visit www.aana.com for more information. Other useful resources include American Association for Men in Nursing (www.aamn.org/resources/aamn-resources), MinorityNurse.com, and *Men in Nursing* magazine (www.nursingcenter.com).

teacher about setting up a presentation by a nurse, take a tour of a hospital or other health care setting, or volunteer at one of these facilities. Nursing websites, including those of professional associations, can also be a good source of information. Here are two suggestions: Discover Nursing (www.discovernursing.com) and Nurse.com (www.nurse.com). You should also join Future Nurses organizations or student health clubs at your school.

EMPLOYERS

Approximately 753,600 LPNs are employed in the United States. Twenty-five percent work at hospitals, 28 percent in nursing care facilities, and 12 percent in offices of physicians. Others are employed by rehabilitation centers, home health care services, employment services, residential care facilities, nursing homes, and other health care facilities. Federal, state, and local government agencies employ licensed practical nurses. Opportunities can also be found in the U.S. military.

GETTING A JOB

Many LPNs obtain their first jobs as a result of contacts made through college clinical experiences or networking events. Other job-search resources include college career services offices, newspaper want ads, and employment and social networking websites. Some professional associations, such as the National Association for Practical Nurse Education and Service, provide job listings at their websites. See For More Information for a list of organizations. Those interested in positions at federal agencies—such as the Veterans Health Administration—should visit the U.S. Office of Personnel Management's website, www.usajobs.gov.

ADVANCEMENT

Licensed practical nurses advance by receiving pay raises and becoming *charge nurses,* who supervise the work of other LPNs. Others become registered nurses by attending LPN-to-RN training programs. Some become nurse educators.

EARNINGS

Salaries for licensed practical nurses vary by type of employer, geographic region, and the worker's experience level and skills. Median annual salaries for LPNs were $43,170 in May 2015, according to the U.S. Department of Labor (USDL). Salaries ranged from less than $32,040 to $59,510 or more. The USDL reports the following mean annual earnings for LPNs by employer:

> **FOR MORE INFORMATION**
>
> For information on certification and state boards of nursing, contact
> **National Association for Practical Nurse Education and Service**
> 703-933-1003
> www.napnes.org
>
> For information on licensing, contact
> **National Council of State Boards of Nursing**
> 312-525-3600
> info@ncsbn.org
> www.ncsbn.org

✔ home health care services, $45,460;

✔ continuing care retirement communities and assisted living facilities for the elderly, $45,070;

✔ nursing care facilities, $45,060;

✔ general medical and surgical hospitals, $42,940; and

✔ offices of physicians, $40,950.

Employers offer a variety of benefits, including the following: medical, dental, and life insurance; paid holidays, vacations, and sick days; personal days; 401(k) plans; profit-sharing plans; retirement and pension plans; and educational assistance programs. Self-employed workers must provide their own benefits.

EMPLOYMENT OUTLOOK

Employment for licensed practical nurses is expected to grow much faster than the average for all careers during the next decade, according to the U.S. Department of Labor. The growing population of people age 65 and over and increasing demand for health care services is creating excellent demand for licensed practical nurses. Employment opportunities will be strongest in outpatient care centers; home health care services; residential intellectual and developmental disability, mental health, and substance abuse facilities; and continuing care retirement communities and assisted living facilities for the elderly. There is a shortage of nursing professionals in rural areas, which will create strong opportunities for those who are interested in working in and/or relocating to these and other underserved areas (such as inner cities).

MEDICAL ASSISTANTS

OVERVIEW

Medical assistants perform administrative and clinical duties at medical offices, hospitals, inpatient/outpatient clinics, nursing homes, and long-term care facilities, and in other health care settings. Their duties include taking patients' medical histories, assisting physicians during procedures, conducting simple tests, updating patients' files in databases, and completing paperwork. Some medical assistants have specialized duties based on the size or type of practice. There are no formal education requirements for medical assistants. Some learn their skills via on-the-job training; many train for the field by completing postsecondary programs that last one or two years. Approximately 601,240 medical assistants are employed in the United States. Opportunities for medical assistants are expected to be excellent during the next decade.

THE JOB

Medical assistants work under the supervision of physicians, nurses, and managers. Many of their duties are administrative in nature. These include checking in patients, answering the phone, sorting mail, and scheduling appointments. *Administrative medical assistants* also maintain medical records, file patient records, and complete requests for insurance reimbursement. Some are trained to perform monthly insurance electronic billing for services rendered as well as to send out monthly statements and record payments that are received. Others are specially trained to perform medical transcription (the written or typed transcription of a doctor's recorded notes).

Clinical medical assistants have some administrative duties but largely focus on helping the doctor before, during, and after patient examinations and procedures. Before bringing a patient to the examination room, clinical medical assistants prepare the room, making sure the examination table is clean and supplies and instruments are ready for use. They then take the patient's pulse, blood pressure, and temperature; measure his or her weight; and talk with the patient regarding the nature of his or her visit and any complaints about health or symptoms, writing this information down for review by the physician. They assist the physician during examinations and certain procedures by handing instruments to the physician or readying medications or supplies for use. After each procedure, clinical medical assistants dispose of contaminated supplies and sterilize equipment and instruments. Some clinical medical assistants are trained to remove sutures, change dressings and bandages, administer injections, collect and prepare laboratory specimens, and draw blood. They also operate diagnostic equipment such as electrocardiogram or x-ray machines. As directed by a physician, clinical medical assistants also help patients arrange for hospital admission, give needed orders for laboratory work, pass along physician referrals, and give instruction to patients regarding new prescriptions, special diets, or additional treatments.

Some medical assistants have specialized duties specific to their workplace. For example, *podiatric medical assistants* are trained to make castings of feet, take x-rays of the feet or ankle, and assist the podiatrist during surgeries.

Optometric medical assistants and *ophthalmic medical assistants* have special duties related to care and health of the eyes. They conduct tests such as a lensometry (which measures for proper lens prescription) or tonometry (which determines fluid pressure, a sign of glaucoma). They also conduct other tests to measure visual acuity or eye muscle function. Some administer drops to dilate the eye in preparation for an exam or administer other medicinal drops. Ophthalmic medical assistants also educate patients about the proper care and insertion of contact lenses.

Medical assistants work in well-lit, clean offices. Full-time medical assistants work 40 hours a week, with some evening or weekend hours required. There is no official uniform, but most medical assistants choose to wear medical scrubs or smocks with pants. Comfortable shoes are a must, since medical assistants are on their feet for a good part of the day. Medical assistants often use gloves, masks, or other protective gear, especially when assisting physicians with procedures or handling spent syringes or needles.

REQUIREMENTS

High School

Take health and science classes in high school—especially anatomy, physiology, biology, and chemistry. English and speech classes will help you develop your writing skills, which you will use frequently during your workday. Since medical professionals are increasingly using computers to record and store data about patients, computer science classes (especially those involving database management) will be useful. If you attend a vocational high school, you might be able to take medical-assisting classes or even participate in a formal training program to prepare for the field.

POSTSECONDARY TRAINING

There are no formal education requirements for medical assistants. Some learn their skills via on-the-job training; many train for the field by completing postsecondary programs that last one or two years. Some of the topics covered in medical-assisting classes include anatomy, physiology, medical terminology, clinical and diagnostic procedures, pharmaceutical principles, laboratory techniques, first aid, medical ethics, and office skills (such as keyboarding, recordkeeping, transcription, accounting, and insurance processing). Students also complete an internship at a medical office as part of their studies.

The Accrediting Bureau of Health Education Schools and the Commission on Accreditation of Allied Health Education Programs accredit medical-assisting programs. The Commission on Accreditation of Ophthalmic Medical Programs accredits ophthalmic medical-assisting programs. See the For More Information section for contact information for these organizations.

CERTIFICATION AND LICENSING

Certification is offered by several associations, including the American Association of Medical Assistants, the American Medical Technologists, and the National Healthcareer Association. Specialty certification is available from the American Society of Podiatric Medical Assistants and the Joint Commission on Allied Health Personnel in Ophthalmology. Certification, while voluntary, is highly recommended. It is an excellent way to stand out from other job applicants and demonstrate your abilities to prospective employers.

OTHER REQUIREMENTS

Medical assistants interact with patients, physicians, nurses, and other health care professionals throughout the day, so it's important that you be able to get along with many different types of personalities and work as a member of a team. You should also be organized and work well under pressure, especially when work is busy and you are asked to perform multiple tasks or handle multiple assistants. Other important traits include the ability to follow instructions, compassion, and manual dexterity and good vision.

EXPLORING

There are many ways to learn more about a career as a medical assistant. You can read books and magazines (such as *CMA Today*, www.aama-ntl.org/cma-today), visit the websites of college medical assisting programs to learn about typical classes and possible career paths, and ask your teacher or school counselor to arrange an information interview with a medical assistant. Professional associations also provide valuable resources. The American Association of Medical Assistants provides a wealth of information on medical assistants (MAs) and careers (including a salary survey and profiles of MAs in a wide range of employment settings) at its website, www.aama-ntl.org. Try to land a part-time job in a medical office. This will give you a chance to interact with medical assistants and see if the career is a good fit for your interests and abilities.

Learn More About It

Blesi, Michelle, Barbara A. Wise, and Cathy Kelley-Arney. *Medical Assisting: Administrative and Clinical Competencies.* 8th ed. Farmington Hills, Mich.: Delmar Cengage Learning, 2016.

Booth, Kathryn, Leesa Whicker, and Terri Wyman. *Medical Assisting: Administrative and Clinical Procedures with Anatomy and Physiology.* 6th ed. New York: McGraw-Hill Education, 2016.

French, Linda. *Administrative Medical Assisting.* 8th ed. Farmington Hills, Mich.: Delmar Cengage Learning, 2017.

Kronenberger, Judy, and Julie Ledbetter. *Lippincott Williams & Wilkins' Comprehensive Medical Assisting,* 5th ed. Williams & Wilkins, 2015.

Kronenberger, Judy, and Julie Ledbetter. *Lippincott Williams & Wilkins' Pocket Guide for Medical Assisting.* 5th ed. Philadelphia: Lippincott Williams & Wilkins, 2015.

EMPLOYERS

Approximately 601,240 medical assistants are employed in the United States. About 59 percent work in offices of physicians. Fifteen percent work at public and private hospitals, and 10 percent work in offices of other health practitioners, such as optometrists, podiatrists, and chiropractors. Others are employed at outpatient care centers and residential care facilities.

GETTING A JOB

Many medical assistants obtain their first jobs as a result of contacts made through college internships, career fairs, or networking events. Others seek assistance in obtaining job leads from college career services offices, newspaper want ads, and employment websites. Additionally, professional associations, such as the Association of Technical Personnel in Ophthalmology, provide job listings at their websites. See For More Information for a list of organizations. Those interested in positions with the federal government should visit the U.S. Office of Personnel Management's website, www.usajobs.gov.

ADVANCEMENT

With further education, medical assistants can become nurses, physician assistants, physicians, or health sciences professors. Administrative medical assistants can become office managers or work in other managerial positions.

EARNINGS

Salaries for medical assistants vary by type of employer, geographic region, and the worker's experience, education, and skill level. Median annual salaries for medical assistants were $30,590 in May 2015, according to the U.S. Department of Labor (USDL). Salaries ranged from less than $22,040 to $43,880 or more. The USDL reports the following mean annual earnings for medical assistants by employer:

✔ scientific research and development services, $36,750;
✔ colleges, universities, and professional schools, $36,020;
✔ offices of dentists, $35,710;
✔ outpatient care centers, $33,550;
✔ general medical and surgical hospitals, $33,140;
✔ offices of physicians, $31,960; and
✔ offices of other health practitioners, $28,810.

The American Association of Medical Assistants (AAMA) reports that certified medical assistants earned average annual salaries of $31,089 in 2016. Those who worked in the offices of physicians or clinics earned $31,021, while those who worked for providers of ambulatory surgery services earned $33,487.

Approximately 95 percent of full-time medical assistants receive some type of fringe benefits, according to the AAMA. Eighty-four percent receive paid vacation, 78 percent receive dental insurance, and 75 percent receive major medical insurance. Part-time workers must provide their own benefits.

EMPLOYMENT OUTLOOK

Employment opportunities for medical assistants will be strong during the next decade, according to the U.S. Department of Labor. Factors that are fueling growth include the increasing U.S. population (especially the elderly, who typically need more medical care than other demographic groups), technological advances that are allowing people to live longer, the increasing number of medical facilities that need support staff such as medical assistants, and the increasing prevalence of certain diseases and conditions, such as diabetes and obesity, which will create demand for more support staff to help treat patients. Opportunities will be best for those with formal training, familiarity with digital health records, and certification.

FOR MORE INFORMATION

For information on accreditation, contact
Accrediting Bureau of Health Education Schools
703-917-9503
info@abhes.org
www.abhes.org

For information on careers, earnings, and certification, contact
American Association of Medical Assistants
800-228-2262
www.aama-ntl.org

For certification information, contact
American Medical Technologists
847-823-5169
ail@americanmedtech.org
www.amt1.com

For information on career options for optometric medical assistants, contact
American Optometric Association
800-365-2219
www.aoa.org

To learn more about careers in podiatric medical assisting, contact

American Society of Podiatric Medical Assistants
888-88ASPMA
aspmaex@aol.com
www.aspma.org

For information on careers in ophthalmic medical assisting, contact
Association of Technical Personnel in Ophthalmology
800-482-4858
atpo@atpo.org
www.atpo.org

To learn more about accredited programs, contact
Commission on Accreditation of Allied Health Education Programs
727-210-2350
mail@caahep.org
www.caahep.org

For information on certification, contact the following organizations
Joint Commission on Allied Health Personnel in Ophthalmology
800-284-3937
jcahpo@jcahpo.org
www.jcahpo.org

National Healthcareer Association
www.nhanow.com

Interview: Lisa Lee

Lisa Lee is a certified medical assistant at Tanner Clinic in Layton, Utah. She is also the vice president of the American Association of Medical Assistants.

Q. **Can you tell us about the Tanner Clinic? How long have you worked in the field? What made you want to enter this career?**

A. Tanner Clinic is a large privately owned, multi-specialty clinic with 110+ physicians as well as in-house lab, magnetic resonance imaging, computed tomography, mammography, and radiology. We also have a multiple in-house surgery suites where minor procedures are performed, and we do all our billing in-house as well. I have worked at Tanner Clinic for 23 years, all for the orthopedic department. I worked for the first surgeon for 18 years until his retirement and have been with the second surgeon and his physician's assistant since he started immediately after the retirement of my first doc. I served as

the supervisor of the orthopedic department for 20 years but, due to a restruc-
ture of supervisory roles, I now just work for as a certified medical assistant
for my doctor. Prior to coming to Tanner Clinic, I worked for a plastic surgeon
in his private office for nine years, so I have worked in the field for 32 years.

I entered this field primarily because of the example of my mother. She
was also a certified medical assistant and worked in the field for more than
52 years, all of them at the same clinic, before she finally retired. I watched
her while I was growing up and saw firsthand the compassion she had for
her patients and admired the service she provided for them. After I completed college with a bachelor's degree in sociology I discovered I wasn't
going to enjoy working in that environment, so I thought more about my
mom's example and decided to look into the medical field. I have been
there ever since.

**Q. What is one thing that young people may not know about a career as a
medical assistant?**

A. I think one of the main things that young people may not know is that
medical assisting is hard work, physically as well as emotionally. At least in
our clinic, the job goes way beyond greeting a patient at the reception desk
or walking them back to an exam room. Sometimes we push their
wheelchairs back to the exam rooms, and often we have to assist these
patients up on to the exam tables. We are in constant motion running specimens to the lab, walking patients to radiology or the other ancillary areas,
fitting braces and splints, etc. Emotionally we see patients at their best and
their worst. When someone is in pain or confused, it is not uncommon for
them to lash out at the first available person, which is often the medical
assistant. We have to just know that it is not us they are yelling at. We have
to make decisions constantly as to the priority of the things we are being
asked to do, and those decisions do not always make all parties happy. All
this aside, I will say that there is no greater profession, in my mind. All the
hard work pays off with the satisfaction that I get out of seeing a patient's
smile after helping them or from hearing even one patient say thank you. I
love my job and would not want to trade professions.

Q. Can you please describe a day in your life on the job?

A. No two days are alike, but typically I arrive before my doctor and make
sure the computers are up and ready to go, and then I return any phone
calls that have come in since the last time we were in the office. At our
clinic we are hired to work for just one doctor and do everything that is
required in his/her practice. We are not assigned to just one particular task
such as phlebotomy or loading the patients into an exam room and taking
their vitals and their histories.

A certified medical assistant is described as being highly trained and
multi-skilled, and I use every one of those skills I was trained in almost
every day. During the course of any given day I answer all incoming phone
calls and am responsible for taking care of any actions derived from those
calls. This includes calling in prescription refills and juggling the schedule
sometimes and, of course, documenting all calls in the EMR (electronic
medical record). I obtain prior authorizations from insurance companies for
office procedures as well as for outside surgeries. I also schedule these surgeries at the appropriate facilities. I take care of the hospital billings as well.
All of the above is what I do in between patients or while the doctor is with

the patient. Additionally, I apply and remove all casts, change dressings, remove sutures, apply braces and splints, perform blood draws when directed, and administer all injections other than intra-articular injections. I load the exam rooms and take the histories and record the vitals of the patients. I schedule any radiology exams that the doctor orders and instruct the patients if there are any requirements for their exams. I also give the pre- and post-operative instructions to the patients relative to their specific surgery. When my doctor gives an intra-articular injection or performs minor surgery in our clinic, I do the prep for the procedure as well.

Q. **What are the most important personal and professional qualities for people in your career?**

A. I think you need to honestly like people. It is important to be happy and to smile. Smiles are contagious and can make people feel at ease. If you are not a people person, medical assisting may not be the best career. I think most people are friendly, and I love interacting with our patients and really getting to know them. I try to learn little things about them or their families, and when they come in the next time and I remember those things, the patients really seem to appreciate it. Sometimes this small act makes their day, and I've made a friend for life. I also feel a medical assistant needs to have true compassion for and genuinely care for the patients he or she serves. This makes all the difference in the world for the experience those patients have with the doctor you work for. The medical assistant can make or break the relationship.

It is important to remember that in the medical field we deal with people from all walks of life. No one is offended by professionalism, but many are offended by the lack of it. As a medical assistant, you should remember that you represent the profession as a whole, and it is very important how you look to the public. Wild and crazy hair styles, excessive jewelry or nails, or some of the other fashion trends that are popular are out of place in the physician's office. This sometimes makes the patients feel uncomfortable, and if they are not comfortable they don't very often return. It is also important to make sure we wear uniforms that are clean and pressed. We don't want to look like we woke up and just threw something on. We need to look professional and act professional at all times, and this includes how we speak.

Foul language or slang has no place in a medical office, and even beyond that (which should be obvious), we need to make sure we speak using proper grammar. The public assumes we are professionals in all aspects of the word and that we are well educated, and it only takes one slip to change their perception of that.

Q. **What are some of the pros and cons of your job?**

A. The pros of my job are easy. It is very rewarding to see someone come into the office in pain or scared and have them leave more comfortable and happy and know that I had a part in that outcome, especially when it comes to the kids. I love working with kids. There is nothing false about a child. You know when they are hurting and when they are better, and they always have a true desire to get better. Their smiles are the best. I also love the satisfaction of a job well done. I very much enjoy interacting with the patients and getting to know them. I have some very special friendships that have come about because of my job. I love the smiles, and the pats on the back, and the hugs, and the thank-yous. We have one patient who tells me every time she comes in that I'm a "special person" and she "loves" me, and those kinds of comments make my day even when it's been a bad day. I just love my job and, once again, the feeling of satisfaction I get from a job well done is indescribable.

The cons of my job are much harder to define because I don't know that I really think there are any, other than the occasional grumpy patient and dealing with all the insurance companies and their ever changing rules. About the only things I could come up with that would be considered cons are the wages and the work schedule I have. Taking into account the enormous amount of responsibility and sometimes the liability a medical assistant has, the wages we are paid are not very good, and I believe the pay must improve in order to attract more people to the profession. I think this is slowly beginning to change, as employers are seeing the value of hiring certified medical assistants and are recognizing the asset we are to the offices we work for, but we are not paid very well right now. The work schedule is not very flexible either. I am responsible to be at work when my doctor is at work, and this does not always fit in with the schedule my family may have, or my dentist, or anyone else I may need to schedule an appointment with. If I have sick kids or need a day off for some other reason, I can't just call in sick and figure I can catch up the next day. It is my responsibility to find my own coverage if I am unable to fill my shift. At Tanner Clinic we all help each other out and cover for one another if our doctor is out of the office and we need a day off, but finding coverage can be a problem at times. Another thing about the schedule is that I don't have an 8 to 5 job. I may get to work at 8:00, but I don't leave until the last patient has left and all the paperwork has been completed. This may be 5:00, but most of the time it is more like 7:00 or 8:00. For me, I don't mind the long days because the job is so rewarding and I have a very understanding family, but the schedule can be a con.

Q. What advice would you give to young people who are interested in the field?

A. I would tell them that where they go to school is very important. They should research the schools they are interested in attending and make sure the school they select is accredited by Committee on Accreditation of Allied Health Education Programs (CAAHEP) or Accrediting Bureau of Health Education Schools (ABHES). Young people (or older people, for that matter) should not look for the program they can complete the quickest, they should look for the program that will give them the best education and best prepare them to work with the public and the fast-paced nature of the medical-assisting profession. CAAHEP and ABHES programs provide this training. The programs are more intense and take longer to complete, but upon completion of the program they are eligible to sit for the CMA (AAMA) exam and upon and successfully passing the certification exam they will earn the CMA (AAMA) credential, which is considered by many to be the gold standard of medical-assisting credentials. Some of the other schools will try to convince students the credential they offer is just as good as the CMA (AAMA) credential, but that is not correct. Some credentials are valid only in the states where they were earned, and some credentials are not even recognized by employers. The CMA (AAMA) credential is a national certification and is good in all states and now is even recognized internationally. So, my best advice would be that the education portion of the profession matters a great deal and potential students should make sure that if they are going to invest the time and the money they should get the best bang for their buck, which is the CMA (AAMA) credential.

MEDICAL ILLUSTRATORS AND PHOTOGRAPHERS

OVERVIEW

Medical illustrators use hand-held drawing tools and illustration software to make medical concepts easier to understand. *Medical photographers* use photographs to meet the same end goal. The work of medical illustrators and photographers appears in textbooks and journals, trade and consumer publications, advertisements, continuing medical education resources, patient education materials, museums, and veterinary, dental, and legal markets, as well as on the Internet and television. Together, medical illustrators, photographers, and *multimedia artists* are sometimes known as *biomedical visualization professionals.*

THE JOB

Are you a talented artist with skill in traditional and computer-based drawing, or photography, and an interest in medicine, biology, and related fields? If so, a career as a medical illustrator or photographer may be in your future.

To prepare an illustration, medical illustrators first conduct research on the body part or system, procedure, or other medical-related subjects that need to be illustrated. They may meet with doctors, research, and other medical and scientific experts; observe a surgical procedure or scientists in a laboratory; or read scientific research papers or other documents. Once their research is complete, medical illustrators use hand-held drawing tools or computer design software to create the final product. Examples of the work of medical illustrators include diagrams of the various stages of pancreatic cancer for medical textbooks; illustrations of complex medical

---

FAST FACTS

High School Subjects
Art
Computer science
Health

Personal Skills
Artistic
Creative

Minimum Education Level
Master's degree (illustrators)
Bachelor's degree (photographers)

Salary Range
$19,000 to $67,000 to
$100,000+ (illustrators)
$18,000 to $54,000 to $72,000+
(photographers)

Employment Outlook
Much faster than the average

O*NET-SOC
27-1013.00, 27-1014.00,
27-4021.00

NOC
5221, 5241

information for use in legal settings; and illustrations of the effects of a particular medication on lung disease for consumer publications. Some illustrators have skills in computer animation, interactive development, multimedia, and web and graphic design. Others create three-dimensional physical models, such as anatomical teaching models.

Medical photographers use high-quality cameras to capture images of surgical procedures, human anatomy (such as the eye or the structure of a cell), research studies, and any other health-related subject. They may take photographs during surgery, before and after images of a patient to document his or her medical status before and after treatment, and images of physicians and nurses at work for publication on a hospital's website or in a health maintenance organization's monthly health newsletter. Medical photographers need to be skilled in the use of photo editing software in order to effectively prepare photographs for publication.

Medical illustrators and photographers may specialize in particular subject matter (such as ophthalmology or surgery). Others specialize by focusing on providing illustrations or photographs to specific markets such as pharmaceutical advertising or medical textbook publishing.

REQUIREMENTS

HIGH SCHOOL

In high school, take as many art and science classes as possible—from digital photography and illustration to anatomy/physiology, biology, chemistry, and cell biology. Most illustrators and photographers use computers to either create and/or edit their work, so take classes in graphic design, digital design, and multimedia. Business, mathematics, and accounting classes will be useful to freelance biomedical visualization professionals. Other recommended classes include English, speech, social studies, and health.

POSTSECONDARY TRAINING

A master's degree in medical illustration is required for most positions in medical illustration. Only four graduate medical illustration programs are accredited by the Commission on Accreditation of Allied Health Education Programs: Augusta University (Augusta, Georgia), University of Illinois at Chicago, Johns Hopkins University School of Medicine (Baltimore, Maryland), and the University of Toronto (Mississsauga, Ontario, Canada). The Association of Medical Illustrators reports that a growing number of medical illustrators—particularly those in academic settings—are earning doctorates in science or education.

Typical classes in a master's degree program in illustration include Gross Human Anatomy; Medical Sciences and Human Pathophysiology; Clinical Sciences for Biomedical Visualization; Molecular Pharmacology for Biomedical Visualization; Biochemistry; Molecular Biology; Cell Biology; Foundations of Neuroscience; Visual Learning and Visual Thinking; Anatomical Visualization; Interactive Media Development; 3-D Modeling; and Web Design.

Fast Facts About the Health Care Job Search

Here are some interesting findings from the American Hospital Association's *2016 Health Career Center Job Search Insights Survey:*

✔ The most-popular health care job-search resources were online job boards. They were used by 69 percent of job hunters. Company websites (59 percent) ranked second, followed by family/friend connections (42 percent).

✔ The top three methods of resume distribution included uploading resumes to online job boards/recruitment sites (cited by 33 percent of survey respondents), direct mail/email to organizations (26 percent), and using friends or colleagues (25 percent).

✔ Sixty-four percent of respondents used LinkedIn to search for jobs.

✔ Health care job seekers reported that the most effective networking methods were: keeping in touch with former colleagues (21 percent), engaging with recruiters (18 percent), membership in professional societies and associations (18 percent), and networking through social media (15 percent).

✔ When considering a potential employer, 70 percent of respondents said "competitive compensation" carried the most weight, followed by "great benefits" (61 percent), "flexible hours/scheduling" (41 percent), and "clear long-term growth opportunities" (39 percent).

Most medical photographers have a bachelor's degree in photography. They may also earn certificates or minors in videography or related areas. Students in biomedical photography programs explore the field by learning more about digital and traditional photography and their uses in science, medicine, technology, and industry. Classroom topics include black and white and color photography, close-up and high-magnification photography, lighting, ophthalmic photography, imaging technologies, desktop publishing software, computer graphics, techniques for biomedical news and public relations photography, equipment and techniques for magnified images, and planning, executing, and presenting a professional portfolio. Some colleges offer specialized areas of concentration such as photography of the patient for medical documentation, public relations, standardization of lighting in the studio, close-up photography, photomicrography, digital imaging, and video and audio-visual presentation. The Rochester Institute of Technology offers a bachelor's degree in photographic sciences, with options in biomedical photographic communications AND imaging and photographic technology.

CERTIFICATION AND LICENSING

The Board of Certification of Medical Illustrators awards the certified medical illustrator credential to applicants who pass an examination that covers business practices, ethics, biomedical science, and drawing skills, and has undergone a rigorous portfolio review. The BioCommunications Association awards the total body photography (TBP) certification to applicants who pass a written exam, complete a demonstration of competency in the specialty of TBP, and pass a practical exam (in which he or she completes one complete series of photographs of a patient for TBP). Additionally, the Ophthalmic Photographers' Society Board of Certification awards the certified retinal angiographer credential.

OTHER REQUIREMENTS

Medical illustrators must have artistic talent and be skilled in a wide range of art techniques and media production skills. They also need creativity, a detail-oriented personality, manual dexterity, good eyesight and color vision, and knowledge of and an interest in general, medical, and biological science.

Medical photographers must have creative talent, an eye for detail, strong interpersonal and communication skills, good eyesight and color vision, the ability to use photo editing and management software, and a willingness to continue to learn throughout their careers.

Self-employed medical illustrators and photographers need good business, marketing, and negotiation skills.

EXPLORING

Here are some interesting ways to explore the world of medical illustration and photography:

✔ Join art and photography clubs in high school and college.

✔ Practice creating your own medical illustrations and photographs.

✔ Talk to medical illustrators and photographers about their careers. Your art teacher or school counselor can help arrange some information interviews.

✔ Read *The Journal of Biocommunication* (www.ami.org/journals -books/journals) and *The Journal of Ophthalmic Photography* (www.opsweb.org/?page=Journal).

✔ Check out the Ophthalmic Photographers' Society Blog!: www.opsweb.org/blogpost/772200/OPS-Blog.

✔ Read the BioCommunication Association's Tips & Techniques website: www.bca.org/resources/tips/tips-techniques.html.

✔ Check out *A Career in Visual Biocommunications in Medicine and Science:* www.bca.org/about/BCA_career_poster.pdf.

EMPLOYERS

Medical illustrators and photographers are employed at hospitals, medical centers, specialty clinics, medical organizations, medical journals, colleges and universities, law firms, private companies, book and magazine publishers, advertising agencies, producers of multimedia and digital content, government agencies, and pharmaceutical, biotech, and medical product companies. Medical photographers may also work for medical examiners' offices and forensic laboratories.

GETTING A JOB

Here are three steps you can take while in college to increase your chances of landing a job:

✔ participate in an illustration- or photography-related internship at a medical-related employer;

✔ begin building your network by joining student organizations and professional associations and networking on LinkedIn and at career fairs; and

✔ develop a portfolio of your work to show to prospective employers or clients.

Additionally, job leads can be obtained directly by contacting potential employers, using the job sites of professional associations (such as www.bca.org/resources/jobs.html and www.opsweb.org/networking), and checking out openings listed on social media sites. Don't forget the resources provided by your college's career service office, which includes information on internships, job openings, and career fairs, as well as advice on resume preparation and interviewing.

ADVANCEMENT

Medical illustrators and photographers who are full-time employees of hospitals, publishing companies, medical schools, and other employers can launch their own freelance businesses. Within a company, they may become art department directors or managers. Some decide to become teachers at the high school or college level.

EARNINGS

The U.S. Department of Labor (USDL) reports that biomedical visualization professionals in the field of health care and social assistance received the following mean annual earnings in May 2015 by specialty:

✔ illustrators, $67,820

✔ photographers, $54,570

✔ multimedia artists and animators, $52,130.

Salaries for photographers employed in all fields ranged from $18,850 to $72,200 or more. Earnings for illustrators, sculptors, and painters in all fields ranged from $19,140 to $99,140 or more.

Salaried medical illustrators had median annual earnings of $62,000 in 2013, according to the Association of Medical Illustrators. Some received salaries of up to $100,000. The Association reports that 46 percent of salaried illustrators supplement their income with freelance work. Self-employed medical illustrators earned median salaries of $82,000. Some illustrators receive substantial royalties from secondary licensing (via stock agencies, publishers, etc.) of existing artwork.

Employers offer a variety of benefits, including the following: medical, dental, and life insurance; paid holidays, vacations, and sick and personal days; 401(k) plans; profit-sharing plans; retirement and pension plans; and educational-assistance programs. Part-time and self-employed workers must provide their own benefits.

EMPLOYMENT OUTLOOK

The U.S. Department of Labor (USDL) predicts that demand for medical illustrators will increase as medical and biological research continues to grow. The Association of Medical Illustrators (AMI) reports that employment opportunities will be good "due to the highly specialized nature of our work and the relatively limited number of medical illustrators graduating each year. The profession remains very viable due to growth in medical research that continually reveals new treatments and technologies that require medical illustrations and animations to explain them."

Demand is also increasing for medical illustrators who are also skilled at computer animation. The AMI reports that a "growing number of medical animators work in research labs analyzing and modeling research data and molecular interactions to guide the data-exploration process as the scientific story is unfolding."

Employment for photographers who work in the health care industry is expected to grow much faster than the average for all careers during the next decade, according to the USDL. Advances in technology, including imaging technology that can capture images at the sub-cellular level, will increase opportunities for medical photographers. Employment may slow if more employers purchase stock photography rather than hiring photographers to take original photos.

FOR MORE INFORMATION

For information on education, careers, and certification, contact
Association of Medical Illustrators
866-393-4AMI
info@ami.org
www.ami.org

Members of the BioCommunications Association include photographers, illustrators, designers, and videographers working in visual communications for the life sciences. Visit its website for information on careers, membership, and certification.
BioCommunications Association
office@bca.org
www.bca.org

For information on certification, contact
Ophthalmic Photographers' Society
800-403-1677
ops@opsweb.org
www.opsweb.org

Interview: John Daugherty

John Daugherty, MS CMI, Clinical Assistant Professor and Director of the Biomedical Visualization Program at the University of Illinois at Chicago

Q. What is biomedical visualization?

A. Biomedical visualization is the process of interpreting or translating the biomedical sciences into visible form. Medical illustrators are innovators in biomedical visualization, applying their creativity, scientific expertise, and interdisciplinary communication skills for those who benefit from the power of medical and scientific understanding like patients, health care providers, researchers, and medical industry.

Biomedical visualization is a multidisciplinary field that draws upon and integrates subject matter from a variety of disciplines (e.g., anatomy, biochemistry, genetics, molecular and cell biology, neuroscience, physiology, and surgery, as well as art, graphic design, animation, and computer science). Professionals in the field are unique individuals with diverse skill sets of artistic problem-solving and scholarly scientific knowledge, standing at the pivotal intersection of biomedical discovery and visualization technologies.

Q. What are a few things that young people may not know about biomedical visualization education and careers?

A. If you are a person who has always had a passion for both art and science, there is a career that is tailor-made for your interests. Your training will include everything from making digital pictures by applying pressure from a stylus moving across a digital tablet to using a scalpel to dissect a human cadaver alongside medical students. New opportunities in the field make use of visual technologies such as animation, interactive media, medical education gaming, holography, virtual reality, and augmented reality.

Q. What personal qualities should students have to be successful in your program and in their post-college careers?

A. Successful medical illustrators must be strong in science and have excellent visualization skills. This would be evidenced by an outstanding GPA, high science grades, and an outstanding art portfolio. Someone who is intellectually curious, creative, organized, and has an interest in lifelong learning is a good fit for a career in biomedical visualization. Storytelling is also important. A good storyteller can use color, clever visual cues, and imagination to transport the viewer into the unseen worlds of science.

Q. What's the employment outlook for your graduates?

A. In the process of today's rapid exchange of information for the purpose of improving health care, one thing is inevitable, and that is the need for competent translators and interpreters of biomedical information. The employment outlook for biomedical visualization graduates has never been better.

Visit www.ahs.uic.edu/bhis/academics/bvis to learn more about UIC's program.

MEDICAL INTERPRETERS AND TRANSLATORS

OVERVIEW

The United States is more of a melting pot than ever. In 2013, a record 61.8 million people (or 20 percent of the U.S. population) spoke a language other than English at home. While some of these people are proficient in English, many are not, which creates communication challenges if they need medical care. As a result, demand has grown for *medical interpreters* (who work with the spoken word) and *medical translators* (who work with the written word) at doctors' offices, hospitals, clinics, imaging facilities, mental health facilities, home health care providers, and in other health care settings. Approximately 9,500 medical and social assistance interpreters and translators are employed in the United States.

THE JOB

Nearly 9 percent of the U.S. population is at risk for an adverse event because of language barriers, according to the Agency for Healthcare Research and Quality. Medical interpreters help physicians, nurses, and other health care professionals to avoid these issues by serving as the language conduit between patients (and sometimes their family members) and health care workers. They most often provide interpreting services for Spanish-language patients, but also interpret for individuals speaking many other languages including Cantonese, Mandarin, Polish, Swahili, and Russian. Medical interpreters are not just proficient in at least two languages, but they are also extremely knowledgeable of health care practices and medical terminology (in both languages), as well as adhere to a code of ethics established by interpreting associations. Many medical interpreters work on site at hospitals, clinics, and physicians' offices, while others work at home or in the offices of interpreting companies, providing interpreting services via telephone or the Internet. Some health care providers, such as hospitals, operate 24/7, which requires interpreters to work at night and on weekends.

Medical translators convert documents and related materials from one language into another. Examples include patient education information sheets, websites, informed consent forms, hospital admission and discharge instructions, prescriptions and medication summaries, and research articles. Some work on site at hospitals and in other health care settings, but many work from home offices. The U.S. Department of Labor reports that "nearly all translation work is done on a computer, and translators receive and submit most assignments electronically. Translations often go through several revisions before becoming final. Translation usually is done with computer-assisted translation (CAT) tools, in which a computer database of previously translated sentences or segments (called a translation memory) may be used to translate new text. CAT tools allow translators to work more efficiently and consistently."

REQUIREMENTS

HIGH SCHOOL

If you are interested in becoming an interpreter or translator, take a wide range of classes that focus on English writing and comprehension, speech, foreign languages, and computer and Internet proficiency. During your high school years, learn about a variety of foreign cultures, join foreign language clubs, and hone your foreign language skills.

POSTSECONDARY TRAINING

A bachelor's degree is often required to work as a translator or interpreter. It's acceptable to major in a field other than a foreign language. If you plan to specialize in health care, it's a good idea to take classes or earn a degree in a medical-related field. Interpreting and translating programs are offered by colleges and universities and in non-university settings such as community centers or the military. Some colleges and universities are adding classes and certificates for students interested in becoming medical interpreters. The International Medical Interpreters Association offers a list of training programs at www.imiaweb.org/education/trainingnotices.asp.

CERTIFICATION AND LICENSING

The National Board of Certification for Medical Interpreters offers the certified medical interpreter credential to medical interpreters. The credential is available in the following languages: Spanish, Mandarin, Cantonese, Russian, Korean, and Vietnamese. The Certification Commission for Healthcare Interpreters also provides certification. Certification is voluntary, but interpreters who are certified typically earn higher pay and enjoy better employment prospects than those who are not certified.

OTHER REQUIREMENTS

To be a successful interpreter, you must have excellent communication, interpersonal, concentration, and listening skills, as well as be detail-oriented and attentive to the nuances of human language and body language (if you're working face-to-face). You should be highly ethical in order to protect the private information of patients and only convey what is being said by medical professionals and patients.

Translators must have good reading and writing skills, the ability to concentrate, and a well-developed vocabulary in multiple languages.

Owners of interpreting and translation firms must have good marketing, business, accounting, and negotiation skills.

Books to Read

Brill, Steven. *America's Bitter Pill: Money, Politics, Backroom Deals, and the Fight to Fix Our Broken Healthcare System.* New York: Random House, 2015.

Burnham, John C. *Health Care in America: A History.* Baltimore, Md.: Johns Hopkins University Press, 2015.

Colbert, Bruce J., and Elizabeth Katrancha. *Career Success in Health Care: Professionalism in Action.* 3rd ed. Farmington Hills, Mich.: Delmar Cengage Learning, 2015.

Kovner, Anthony R., and James R. Knickman (eds.). *Jonas and Kovner's Health Care Delivery in the United States.* 11th ed. New York: Springer Publishing Company, 2015.

Sultz, Harry A., and Kristina M. Young. *Health Care USA: Understanding Its Organization and Delivery.* 8th ed. Burlington, Mass.: Jones & Bartlett Learning, 2014.

EXPLORING

There are many ways to learn more about careers in medical interpreting and translation. First, immerse yourself in a foreign language (ideally, one such as Spanish that is in high demand by the health care industry). Read books and magazines, watch television shows, and listen to broadcasts in your language specialty. Spend time abroad and immerse yourself in different cultures to hone your language and cultural skills. As you gain proficiency, try your hand at interpreting an imaginary conversation between a doctor and a patient. Perhaps friends or family members could play the roles of patient and physician. Translate a document from English to a foreign language. Ask your language teacher to provide feedback.

Check out Discover Interpreting (http://discoverinterpreting.com), a resource from the National Consortium of Interpreter Education Centers that offers information on interpreting careers (including those in health care). Another good resource is Interpreting in Healthcare Settings (www.healthcareinterpreting.org), which is geared toward American Sign Language medical interpreters.

EMPLOYERS

Approximately 9,500 medical and social assistance interpreters and translators are employed in the United States. They work at doctors' offices, hospitals, clinics, imaging facilities, mental health facilities, home health care providers, and in other health care settings. Some work in home offices or for interpreting/translation service firms. Approximately 20 percent of interpreters and translators are self-employed.

Many opportunities are available outside the health care industry. For example, interpreters and translators are employed by government agencies—most commonly at the federal level. Multilingual border patrol agents are needed to communicate with legal and undocumented immigrants. Customs workers need language skills to interact with international travelers. The Department of Homeland Security and intelligence agencies need interpreters and translators who are fluent in languages spoken and written by those who threaten the security of the United States. In addition, there are many opportunities in the diplomatic corps in Washington, DC, and in New York at the United Nations. The court system is in strong need of translators and interpreters. Public and private schools also use the services of interpreters and translators. Corporations are recognizing the benefits of hiring multilingual workers to translate Web sites, provide consulting regarding customs in other countries, and create marketing and sales materials to reach niche market segments.

GETTING A JOB

Successful job-search strategies include networking, attending job fairs, using social media, applying directly to employers, and using the employment sites of professional associations (such as the National Council on Interpreting in Health Care, http://ncihc-jobs.careerwebsite.com). Here are a few additional tips on landing a job and launching an interpreting/translation business:

✔ Check out The Savvy Newcomer blog (https://atasavvynewcomer.org), which provides advice on breaking into and being successful in interpreting and translation.

✔ Study the market in your area to determine which languages are in demand. Spanish-language interpreters/translators are in demand in many areas of the country. Asian-language interpreters and translators are in especially strong demand on the West Coast.

✔ When applying for bilingual medical interpreting and translation jobs, be sure to cite any foreign language skills or experience you have on your resume or cover letter (for example, a book you helped translate from French to English or experience handling customer service complaints from Arabic-speaking customers). The more language experience you have—regardless of industry—the better your chances of landing a job.

✔ Take the long view when breaking into the business. It may take up to two years to establish yourself in the field.

ADVANCEMENT

Skilled and experienced interpreters and translators can advance to manage their departments or even launch businesses that provide interpreting or translation services to hospitals, offices of physicians, and other health care providers.

EARNINGS

Mean annual earnings for interpreters and translators who worked at general medical and surgical hospitals were $47,210 in May 2015, according to the U.S. Department of Labor. Salaries for all interpreters and translators ranged from $23,160 to $78,520 or more.

Employers offer a variety of benefits, including the following: medical, dental, and life insurance; paid holidays, vacations, and sick and personal days; 401(k) plans; profit-sharing plans; retirement and pension plans; and educational-assistance programs. Part-time and self-employed interpreters and translators must provide their own benefits.

EMPLOYMENT OUTLOOK

Opportunities for interpreters and translators who are employed in the health care and social assistance industries are predicted to grow much faster than the average for all occupations during the next decade, according to the U.S. Department of Labor (USDL). In the past, surging immigration to the United States created demand for medical interpreters and telephone interpreting services in hospitals, clinics, and other health care settings. Although the current presidential administration may seek to limit immigration to the U.S., there will still be a strong need for interpreting services for current U.S. residents who do not speak English at all or who are not proficient. The demand for medical interpreters will be especially strong in suburban areas with large immigrant populations.

Although there is growing need for medical interpreters, fewer than 15 states offer Medicare reimbursement for interpreters, which causes many hospitals to have to pay for their services out of their own budgets (which may limit employment opportunities to some degree).

The USDL reports that "demand will likely remain strong for translators of frequently translated languages, such as French, German, Portuguese, Russian, and Spanish. Demand also should be strong for translators of Arabic and other Middle Eastern languages and for the principal Asian languages: Chinese, Japanese, Hindi, and Korean."

FOR MORE INFORMATION

For information on membership and seminars on medical translation, contact
American Translators Association
703-683-6100
ata@atanet.org
www.atanet.org

To learn more about certification, contact
Certification Commission for Healthcare Interpreters
866-969-6665
www.cchicertification.org

To learn more about careers, certification, and membership, contact
International Medical Interpreters Association
info@imiaweb.org
www.imiaweb.org

For information on certification, visit
National Board of Certification for Medical Interpreters
www.certifiedmedicalinterpreters.org

For information on careers, contact
National Council on Interpreting in Health Care
info@NCIHC.org
www.ncihc.org

Interview: Emily Safrin

Emily Safrin, MA, CHI™ is a professional Spanish-English translator-interpreter and the owner of Saffron Translations (www,saffrontranslations.com).

Q. What made you want to become a medical interpreter/translator?

A. Looking back, it's clear to me that I was headed in the direction of becoming a translator and interpreter long before I knew that these professions existed. I have been passionate about language from a very young age. In preschool, I was learning to read upside-down while my classmates were still learning to read right-side up!

I grew up in San Diego, right next to the Mexican border, so when it came time to learn a foreign language in high school I chose Spanish without thinking twice. It quickly became one of my favorite subjects (next to English), especially after I had the chance to spend a summer in Spain at a language academy. In college, I continued taking Spanish classes purely out of personal interest and spent a semester abroad at a Spanish university. I was weeks from graduation when an advisor informed me that I was only two credits short of earning a Spanish major, entirely unbeknownst to me! I realized that when you're really passionate about something, accomplishing your goals comes naturally instead of feeling like work. Nevertheless, I carried on thinking Spanish was just a hobby for me, since I still wasn't aware of any job opportunities requiring language skills other than becoming a Spanish teacher, which I wasn't drawn to.

After college, I started working as the coordinator of an English conversation group for immigrants at a public library. From time to time I was called upon to help Spanish speakers communicate with other library staff, and I found I really enjoyed helping connect people through language. However, I still wasn't aware that there were people who dedicated their careers to doing just that.

After a year of facilitating English conversation groups at the library, I started considering a career in education. I was offered a position as a cultural ambassador and English instructor in Madrid and didn't think twice before moving back across the pond. After spending two years working at a bilingual elementary school, it occurred to me that I wasn't that interested in being a teacher; what I was interested in was languages, especially the delicate and vibrant space between two different languages and cultures.

While I was in Madrid I heard about a master's program in public service translation and interpreting at a nearby university, and for the first time a light bulb went off in my head: it was everything I was passionate about all in one. I worked hard to be admitted and began classes that fall. I haven't looked back since. I feel fortunate not only to have found my passion, but to earn a living from it.

Q. What are one or two things that young people may not know about medical interpreting/translation?

A. When I was young, I didn't even know that the fields of interpreting and translation existed! Here are a couple of things I didn't realize when I began pursuing my career:

1. Not all translators are interpreters and vice versa. In fact, most focus on one profession or the other. Translation and interpreting involve different skillsets, despite that they both require an excellent command of at least two languages and an intimate familiarity with those languages' respective cultures.

2. All translators are writers first and foremost. Medical translators must know how to write like a doctor, medical researcher, drug manufacturer, or whoever else is the author of the texts they work with in order to create an accurate and effective version of the text in the target language.

Q. What are the most important personal and professional skills for medical interpreters? Translators?

A. Some skills are equally important for both translators and interpreters, while each profession has its own more specialized skillset. Both translators and interpreters must possess:

✔ An exceptional command of at least two languages
✔ Intimate familiarity with the cultures tied to their working languages
✔ Outstanding research skills

Furthermore, most translators and interpreters are self-employed, and for that reason interpersonal skills, as well as business and marketing skills, are also key to success. These abilities don't always come naturally-most of us learn them as we go.

Interpreters in particular must have excellent:

✔ Active listening and comprehension skills
✔ Memory retention
✔ Verbal communication skills
✔ Judgment and critical thinking skills

In addition, a good interpreter is:

✔ Quick on her feet
✔ Intuitive
✔ Assertive (when called for-that's where good judgment comes in)

Translators, on the other hand, must have outstanding:
✔ Reading comprehension
✔ Writing skills
✔ Organizational skills
✔ Computer skills

A good translator also:
✔ Pays great attention to detail
✔ Might have specialized knowledge in a particular area, such as health care or even a specialization within health care, such as endocrinology or oncology

Q. What are some of the pros and cons of your job?

A. Interpreting pros

✔ Interpreting is exhilarating and engaging. There's never a dull moment interpreting in the medical field, and you learn something new every day.

✔ Interpreters have the opportunity to witness the inner workings of the health care system and the intimate relationship between medical provider and patient.

✔ Interpreting is fulfilling: interpreters help others access a vital service—sometimes a life-saving one.

Interpreting cons"

✔ Interpreting can be emotionally challenging. It's not uncommon for interpreters to experience vicarious trauma, meaning they sometimes internalize the difficult circumstances and emotions of patients, which can take a toll on their own well-being. While some medical visits are lighthearted or casual, others require the interpreter to break the worst news imaginable to a patient or his or her family, or to synthesize and repeat (in first person) the details of traumatic experiences described by patients.

✔ Interpreting means taking responsibility for making difficult ethical choices; for example, whether to speak up when you witness discrimination or whether to correct a medical professional who makes a mistake. The interpreter must make these decisions while still remaining faithful to the impartiality and confidentiality that are central to the profession's codes of ethics.

✔ Travel time to get to appointments. Staff interpreters (i.e., employees) and telephonic or video interpreters usually work from one place, but those who are self-employed (the majority) often spend significant time getting to and from different jobs. Some appointments are longer than others, but it's not uncommon to interpret for numerous one-hour appointments throughout the day. Not all clients reimburse the interpreter for travel time, gas, or mileage, which means interpreters can end up spending quite a bit of time and money just traveling to appointments.

Translation pros: s

✔ Just like with interpreting, there is no dull day in translation. The excitement for translators comes in the form of research and writing. Translation is gratifying for those who are thirsty for knowledge and who enjoy writing; the translation task involves learning just about everything you can about a text's subject matter, as well as its purpose, audience, and structure.

✔ Like interpreters, translators learn something new every day.

✔ Translation is fulfilling: translators make important information available to patients, researchers, and medical professionals who speak another language.

Translation cons:

✔ Unlike interpreters, translators spend the majority of their time at the computer. Whether you see working at the computer (and usually from home) as a pro or a con depends on your personality, but this is something to keep in mind when considering a career as a translator.

✔ Technical glitches can sometimes be a headache, although most translators are fairly technology-savvy given that their daily work revolves around technology.

A note on self-employment. One last thing to note is that translators and interpreters are usually self-employed—something that has its own advantages and disadvantages.

Self-employment grants you the freedom to:

✔ Create your own schedule
✔ Decide what services to offer
✔ Determine how much to charge for your work

At the same time, self-employment involves:

✔ Added responsibilities, such as finding and covering the cost of your own health insurance, paying taxes that an employer would normally pay on your behalf, and not being able to depend on a consistent paycheck

✔ Accepting that work may come and go in waves: you could be busy for months and suddenly have trouble finding a paid job for weeks or more

For many, the freedom of doing what they love without someone looking over their shoulder and making decisions for them is more than worth it.

Q. What are the best ways to break into the field?

A. There is no one right way to become a translator or interpreter. Some of the best translators and interpreters break into the field after spending a substantial period of time in a different career. This grants them the benefit of bringing specialized knowledge to their translation or interpreting work. (Not surprisingly, some of the most respected medical translators are also doctors!)

Others enter the profession knowing they want to be a translator or interpreter and either earn a degree in translation and interpreting (as was my case), or they take trainings in medical interpreting or translation. There's no shortage of in-person and online classes and certificates that offer a taste of the skills needed without having to make a long-term commitment. Once you decide to pursue a career in translation or interpreting, becoming certified is highly recommended, though not yet a strict requirement for most work and not always a possibility, depending on your language pair.

Another way to break into the professions is to study the field you plan to translate or interpret in (for example, if you want to be a medical interpreter, studying medicine or taking classes on related subject matters like anatomy, chemistry, and biology will be advantageous). Good translators and interpreters must be versed in the subject matter they work within both languages!

MEDICAL SCIENTISTS

OVERVIEW

Medical scientists work to enhance and prolong human life by conducting research on human diseases and conditions. Their research has resulted in advances in the diagnosis, treatment, and prevention of many diseases and conditions. Medical scientists need a Ph.D. in a biological science; some scientists also have medical degrees. Approximately 109,900 medical scientists work in the United States. Employment in the field is expected to be good during the next decade.

THE JOB

The invention of the airplane has made even the remotest reaches of the world accessible. One can fly from the United States to Africa in the better part of a day. However, that new freedom comes with a price. Infectious diseases can also travel the globe via airplane, bringing illnesses such as malaria or yellow fever to populations that have not experienced these diseases in decades. Thankfully we have vaccines for many of these diseases, which has stopped their large-scale spread. We can thank medical scientists for these and other discoveries that help protect our health.

Most medical scientists specialize in a particular discipline. For example, *pharmacologists* study the effects of drugs on biological systems; *cytologic scientists* study cellular materials; *histologic scientists* study tissue structure; and *medical microbiologists* work to identify the microorganisms that cause disease or can be used to fight illness. *Epidemiologists* investigate the causes and spread of disease and try to prevent or control disease out-

---

FAST FACTS

High School Subjects
Biology
Chemistry
Mathematics

Personal Skills
Communication
Complex problem solving
Critical thinking
Scientific
Technical

Minimum Education Level
Doctorate degree (medical scientists, except epidemiologists)
Master's degree (epidemiologists)

Salary Range
$44,000 to $82,000 to $155,000+

Employment Outlook
About as faster as the average

O*NET-SOC
19-1041.00, 19-1042.00

NOC
2121, 3111

breaks. *Research epidemiologists* study diseases in the field and in medical laboratories to find ways to prevent future outbreaks. *Applied epidemiologists* respond to disease outbreaks. They find out what caused the outbreak and suggest ways to contain it. They typically work for state health agencies. *Infectious disease specialists* help physicians and public health workers identify diseases that are difficult to diagnose, are accompanied by a high fever, or do not respond to treatment.

Most medical scientists work in laboratories, preparing samples to study cell structure or studying bacteria or other organisms. They may examine tissues, cells, or microorganisms, often using an electron microscope. Some analyze changes in cells that signal health problems. Medical scientists must understand the behavior of a healthy cell to help diagnose a sick or dying cell. Similarly, they take note of the effects of certain treatments on cells to fine-tune drugs. Medical scientists also try to find ways to prevent health problems. For example, they may study the link between radiation from x-rays and cancer or between alcoholism and liver disease.

Once they finish collecting data, medical scientists use statistical modeling software and other computer-based technologies to analyze their findings. Then they write reports or articles about their findings. Depending on where they work, scientists may also make presentations on their research or write articles for publication in scientific journals.

Emerging Career: Disease Mapper

What do they do?: Disease mappers use satellite imaging technology, inexpensive computer technology, and Internet tools such as Google Earth to track and predict the spread of epidemics (such as malaria) around the world.

Earnings: $40,000 to $150,000

Educational requirements: At least a master's degree in a technical field along with expertise in a particular disease.

Top employers: Government, United Nations, colleges and universities

In hospitals and medical offices, medical scientists conduct tests on blood and tissue samples to diagnosis illnesses. They send their results to *physicians*, who then decide on treatment options. Some medical scientists are also physicians. These individuals interact with patients directly. They administer new or experimental drug treatments to patients, closely monitoring their health during trials. They adjust dosage levels to minimize potential negative side effects or increase levels to maximize the medicine's effectiveness.

Some medical scientists work for pharmaceutical companies. They work to develop new drugs or improve existing ones that are manufactured by their employer. The downside to working in business is these scientists are sometimes limited to the business goals of their company.

A field that has taken off in recent years is biomedical research. *Biomedical scientists* study genetics and DNA to pinpoint their relationship to well-being or illnesses. Biomedical breakthroughs have made it possible to manufacture human substances such as insulin that have improved the lives of millions diagnosed with diabetes. Biomedical scientists hope to apply this same approach to discover the genetic causes of cancers, Alzheimer's disease, and Parkinson's disease, among other diseases.

Medical scientists also do a lot of writing for their job, either mapping out their research approach before they begin their lab work or writing about their end results. They prepare their findings for publication or simply to share with their colleagues and other scientists. Many scientists depend on grant money to conduct their work, so much of their time is spent writing detailed proposals to continue or increase their funding sources. The National Institutes of Health administers many of these grants, and competition for funding is intense. The better that medical scientists can convey the goals of their proposed study, the better their chances of securing a grant.

Medical scientists also do a considerable amount of reading. In order to enhance their own work, they must understand the discoveries and failures that came before them. The field of medical science changes every day, so they must stay on top of the latest breakthroughs.

Most scientists work in laboratories, hunched over a microscope, research article, or computer. Eyestrain and physical stress involved in being stationary for many hours at a time is part of the job. The stereotype of a lone scientist in a dark and windowless lab is not usually accurate. Medical scientists often work with teams of scientists, research subjects, engineers, doctors, and other medical professionals in their work. Because their work can expose them to infectious diseases, medical scientists must follow strict guidelines in the handling of hazardous materials. They often wear a lab coat and may also wear goggles, gloves, and face masks or respirators depending on their work.

Since research funding is often obtained through the awarding of grant money, scientists face the stress of deadlines for applying or, once they receive a grant, reporting results to the grantor agency. Medical scientists typically work standard 9 to 5 hours, but weekend and evening hours may be required when working on certain experiments or projects.

REQUIREMENTS

High School

In high school, take as many health, biology, anatomy and physiology, mathematics, biology, chemistry, physics, English, and speech classes as possible.

Postsecondary Training

Medical scientists need a Ph.D. in a biological science; some scientists also have medical degrees. A growing number of new graduates also complete postdoctoral work in the laboratory of a senior researcher. Epidemiologists need at least a master's degree in public health, although some employers require a doctorate or a medical degree.

To prepare for graduate study, you should earn a bachelor's degree in a biological science. Biology-related degrees are offered by thousands of colleges and universities throughout the United States.

Once students have earned their bachelor's degrees, the U.S. Department of Labor reports that "there are two main paths for prospective medical scientists. They can enroll in a university Ph.D. program in the biological sciences; these programs typically take about six years of study, and students specialize in one particular field, such as genetics, pathology, or bioinformatics. They can also enroll in a joint M.D.-Ph.D. program at a medical college; these programs typically take seven to eight years of study, where students learn both the clinical skills needed to be a physician and the research skills needed to be a scientist." Visit https://students-residents.aamc.org to learn more about M.D.-Ph.D. dual degree training.

The American Society for Pharmacology and Experimental Therapeutics offers a list of graduate-level pharmacology training programs at its website, www.aspet.org/training_programs.

Certification and Licensing

The American Board of Clinical Pharmacology (www.abcp.net) offers voluntary board certification to pharmaceutical scientists. The Certification Board of Infection Control and Epidemiology (www.cbic.org), a subgroup of the Association for Professionals in Infection Control and Epidemiology, offers voluntary certification to epidemiologists. Contact these organizations for more information.

The USDL reports that "medical scientists who administer drugs, gene therapy, or otherwise practice medicine on patients in clinical trials or a private practice need a license to practice as a physician." To become licensed, physicians must pass a licensing examination, graduate from an accredited medical school, and complete one to seven years of graduate medical education.

Other Requirements

Medical scientists should have strong scientific and research skills. They must be extremely focused in order to conduct meticulous, time-consuming research that may or may not result in ground-breaking discoveries. Medical scientists need to be excellent communicators. They frequently convey their findings to colleagues, the press, and the general public in both oral and written format. They also need to have good writing skills in order to craft grant proposals that help them obtain funding for their research. Other important traits include strong organizational skills, the ability to work independently or as part of a team, and an interest in continuing to learn and stay abreast of industry developments throughout their careers.

EXPLORING

There are many ways to learn more about a career as a medical scientist. You can read books and journals about medical scientific research and visit the websites of college programs that offer degrees in pharmacology, genetics, biology, biotechnology, biomedical science, and related fields, and you can ask your teacher or school counselor to arrange an information interview with a medical scientist. Professional associations can also provide information about the field. For example, the American Association of Pharmaceutical Scientists offers videos and interviews with scientists at its website, www.aaps.org/PSI.

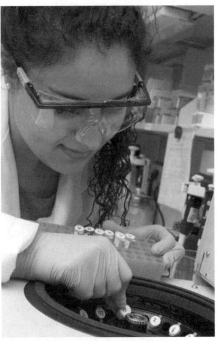

A scientist loads a mini centrifuge. (National Eye Institute)

The American Society for Pharmacology and Experimental Therapeutics provide information on pharmacology and careers at its website, www.aspet.org. The Infectious Diseases Society of America offers *Career Paths in Infectious Diseases Why Choose ID?* at its website, www.idsociety.org. The Association of American Medical Colleges provides information about a career in biomedical research at its website, https://students-residents.aamc.org.

EMPLOYERS

Approximately 109,900 medical scientists are employed in the United States. Medical scientists work for universities, government agencies, medical offices, nonprofit research organizations, and hospitals, and in the private sector for pharmaceutical companies. Thirty-nine percent of medical scientists are employed by scientific research and development services firms; another 21 percent work for colleges and universities; 14 percent are employed by hospitals; and 6 percent work in pharmaceutical and medicine manufacturing. Although opportunities are available throughout the United States, more than half of all medical scientists are employed in five states: California, Massachusetts, New York, Pennsylvania, and Maryland.

GETTING A JOB

Many medical scientists obtain their first jobs as a result of contacts made through postdoctoral positions. Others seek assistance in obtaining job leads from college career services offices, networking events, career fairs, newspaper want ads, and social networking websites. Additionally, professional associations, such as the American Association of Pharmaceutical Scientists and the American Society for Pharmacology and Experimental Therapeutics, provide job listings at their websites. See For More Information for a list of organizations. Those interested in positions with federal agencies—such as the Centers for Disease Control and Prevention, National Science Foundation, and the Food and Drug Administration—should visit www.usajobs.gov.

ADVANCEMENT

Medical scientists advance by receiving higher pay, by working on research projects that are more prestigious or offer larger budgets, by taking on managerial duties, or by becoming college professors and receiving tenure.

EARNINGS

Median annual salaries for medical scientists were $82,240 in May 2015, according to the U.S. Department of Labor (USDL). Salaries ranged from less than $44,510 to $155,180 or more. The USDL reports the following mean annual earnings for medical scientists by employer: federal government, $120,880; pharmaceutical and medicine manufacturing, $114,430; scientific research and development services, $104,310; medical and diagnostic laboratories, $99,150; general medical and surgical hospitals, $86,840; and colleges, universities, and professional schools, $66,910. Salaries for epidemiologists ranged from less than $65,051 to $123,197 or more in 2017, according to Salary.com.

Medical scientists usually receive benefits such as health and life insurance, vacation days, sick leave, and a savings and pension plan. Self-employed scientists must provide their own benefits.

EMPLOYMENT OUTLOOK

Employment for medical scientists and epidemiologists is expected to grow about as fast as the the average for all careers during the next decade, according to the U.S. Department of Labor. The growth of the biotechnology industry has fueled employment opportunities for medical scientists and will continue to do so in the next decade. Other factors that are influencing the strong employment outlook are the increasing number of people age 65 and older, which is creating demand for more drugs and therapies; the expansion in research related to illnesses such as cancer, avian flu, and Zika virus, as well as treatment issues such as antibiotic resistance; and the increasing ease of travel and the growing world population, which will increase the chances of epidemics and pandemics and other global health outbreaks. Medical scientists who have both a Ph.D. and an M.D. will experience the best job prospects.

FOR MORE INFORMATION

For information on education and careers, contact the following organizations
American Association of Pharmaceutical Scientists
703-243-2800
aaps@aaps.org
https://www.aaps.org

American Society for Pharmacology and Experimental Therapeutics
301-634-7060
www.aspet.org

For information on careers, contact
American Society for Microbiology
202-737-3600
service@asmusa.org
www.asm.org

To learn more about the benefits of biotechnology research, visit the BIO website.
Biotechnology Innovation Organization (BIO)
202-962-9200
info@bio.org
www.bio.org

For information on biotechnology careers and industry facts, visit the institute's website.
Biotechnology Institute
202-312-9269
info@biotechinstitute.org
www.biotechinstitute.org

The federation consists of 30 scientific societies with more than 100,000 researcher-members throughout the world. Visit its website for more information.
Federation of American Societies for Experimental Biology
301-634-7000
info@faseb.org
www.faseb.org

For detailed information about biotechnology, visit the center's website.
National Center for Biotechnology Information
info@ncbi.nlm.nih.gov
www.ncbi.nlm.nih.gov

For information on pharmaceutical and biotechnology research, contact
Pharmaceutical Research and Manufacturers of America
202-835-3400
www.phrma.org

For information on epidemiology, contact the following organizations and government agencies
Association for Professionals in Infection Control and Epidemiology
info@apic.org
www.apic.org

Centers for Disease Control and Prevention
800-232-4636
www.cdc.gov/careerpaths/k12teacher-roadmap/epidemiology.html

Council of State and Territorial Epidemiologists
770-458-3811
www.cste.org

Epidemic Intelligence Service
Centers for Disease Control and Prevention
404-498-6110
EIS@cdc.gov
www.cdc.gov/eis

Infectious Diseases Society of America
703-299-0200
www.idsociety.org

For information on career opportunities in Canada, contact
Canadian Medical and Biological Engineering Society
www.cmbes.ca

MENTAL HEALTH COUNSELORS

OVERVIEW

Mental health counselors work with individuals, families, and groups to identify and treat mental and emotional disorders and promote mental health. They help clients address issues such as depression, stress, anxiety, suicidal impulses, low self-esteem, addiction and substance abuse, trauma, and grief. In order to treat the individual, they may collaborate with other mental health specialists and professionals, such as psychiatrists, psychologists, clinical social workers, and school counselors. A minimum of a master's degree in counseling is required to work in the field. There are approximately 128,200 mental health counselors employed in the United States. Employment opportunities for mental health counselors are expected to be very strong during the next decade.

FAST FACTS

High School Subjects
English
Psychology
Sociology

Personal Skills
Active listening
Communication
Helping

Minimum Education Level
Master's degree

Salary Range
$26,000 to $41,000 to $68,000+

Employment Outlook
Much faster than the average

O*NET-SOC
21-1011.00, 21-1014.00

NOC
4153

THE JOB

Many people suffer from anxiety or depression—whether due to stress at the workplace or school, a recent traumatic experience, grief from a death in the family, or low self-esteem resulting from divorce or job loss. Others suffer from drug addiction or alcohol abuse. Those with serious emotional impairments may even have suicidal tendencies. People turn to mental health counselors to help them deal with their various issues and bring them back to mental health.

Mental health counselors encourage patients to express their feelings—sadness, despair, or anger or discuss situations that occurred in their school or workplace, at home, in the military, or in other settings that left them particularly anxious or overwhelmed. Through these counseling sessions, coun-

Shortage of Geriatric Mental Health and Substance Abuse Professionals Predicted

Between 5.6 million and 8 million older Americans—14 percent to 20 percent of the nation's elderly population—have one or more mental health conditions or problems stemming from substance misuse or abuse, according to a report from the Institute of Medicine. Depressive disorders and dementia-related behavioral and psychiatric symptoms are the most common issues faced by the elderly, but rates of accidental and intentional misuse of prescription medications are rising and experts believe that the rate of illicit drug use among older individuals will also grow as the baby boomers age. Unfortunately, the Institute of Medicine reports that "overall, the number of individuals working in or entering fields related to geriatric mental health and substance abuse (G-MH/SA) is disconcertingly small." There are many types of geriatric mental health and substance abuse professionals, including psychologists, psychiatrists, geriatricians, nurses, social workers, and substance abuse counselors.

This shortage of skilled workers is expected to get worse. The number of adults age 65 and older is projected to rise to 72.1 million by 2030—up from 40.3 million in 2010, and the Institute predicts that "millions of baby boomers will likely face difficulties getting diagnoses and treatment for mental health conditions and substance abuse problems unless there is a major effort to significantly boost the number of health professionals and other service providers able to supply this care as the population ages."

Contact the following organizations for information on education and careers in G-MH/SA:

✔ American Association for Geriatric Psychiatry: www.aagponline.org

✔ Geriatric Mental Health Foundation: www.gmhfonline.org

✔ National Coalition on Mental Health and Aging: www.ncmha.org

selors are able to help patients work through their feelings and establish strategies to overcome future episodes. Weekly sessions are typical, though patients, or counselors, may request more frequent sessions as needed.

When working with a new patient, mental health counselors first conduct a patient assessment. They ask the patient questions regarding physical health as well as for any other information that may give them a better picture of his or her mental state. When working with teens or young children, mental health counselors may first meet with the parents or guardians. They maintain detailed records and notes for each patient, which are confidential. During each session, mental health counselors actively listen to the patient, giving full attention to points being made and asking questions or giving prompts only when necessary. Counseling sessions occur one to one, though at times it is necessary to hold group sessions,

Opioid Abuse Epidemic Creates Demand for Addiction Counselors

Drug overdose is the leading cause of accidental death in the U.S., with 55,403 lethal drug overdoses in 2015, according to the American Society of Addiction Medicine. Addiction to opioids (which include illicit drugs such as heroin and prescription pain relievers such as hydrocodone, oxycodone, morphine, and codeine) is fueling this epidemic.

Communities across the United States are struggling to deal with the devastating effects that the abuse of opioids are having on people young and old. Unfortunately, there's a severe shortage of drug treatment counselors to assist people who are addicted to opioids. In 2014, 22.5 million people age 12 or older needed treatment for addiction to illicit drugs or alcohol, but only 2.6 million people received treatment at a specialty facility, according to the 2014 National Survey on Drug Use and Health.

So what's causing the shortage of drug treatment counselors? Addiction rates in the U.S. population are increasing, which is prompting more demand for counselors. Yet, several factors are deterring prospective counselors from entering the field and prompting current professionals to leave the field. This career can be extremely stressful, and some counselors cite the stress of "taking on their clients' pain" as prompting them to leave the profession. Other counselors leave the field because they become frustrated with the level of bureaucracy, paperwork, sometimes long hours, and the lack of government funding for addiction counseling programs. Finally, many counselors cite low pay as a reason why the field is not growing. Fifty percent of substance abuse and behavioral disorder counselors earned between $25,860 and $39,980 in May 2015, according to the U.S. Department of Labor (USDL). Only 10 percent earned $63,030 or more.

The Substance Abuse and Mental Health Association and other professional associations and organizations are developing strategies to encourage more people to pursue careers in addiction counseling.

Demand will continue to be strong for substance abuse and behavioral disorder counselors. In fact, the USDL reports that employment in this field will grow much faster than the average for all careers during the next decade. It says that job opportunities will be particularly strong for those with a bachelor's or master's degree.

Contact the following organizations for more information on a career in addiction counseling:

✔ Addiction Technology Transfer Center Network: Directory of Addiction Study Programs: www.nattc.org/addiction-programs/search.aspx

✔ NAADAC, the Association for Addiction Professionals: www.naadac.org

such as in cases dealing with divorce, in which case entire families may be present. If patients suffer from alcohol or drug dependence, mental health counselors often include family members or close friends in some sessions to identify trigger situations associated with this dependency.

Mental health counselors also collect information through interviews, observation, and testing. They also collaborate with other professionals who are treating or interacting with the patient, such as physicians, nurses, teachers, and social workers. Using this information, they develop and implement a treatment plan for the patient. During the course of the treatment plan and counseling session, mental health counselors often meet with the patient's team of health professionals, as well as with the patient's family members and friends, to keep them abreast of the patient's progress. Some family members may even seek the counselor's advice on how to best deal with the patient's actions and recovery process.

Mental health counselors are excellent listeners. Instead of judging their patients' feelings or actions, counselors help patients by planning, organizing, and leading counseling programs. They teach patients alternative ways to deal with anger or resentment; for example, using behavioral therapy. They may use psychoanalysis to help patients understand their feelings of angst or despair. Mental health counselors also use different methods when working with young children, such as play therapy or art therapy, to learn the children's true emotions or fears.

As the patient improves, mental health counselors begin to shift their sessions toward a plan for maintaining optimum mental health after therapy. This could include follow-up visits or phone calls for a period of time.

Counseling sessions take place in a quiet and private area, with only the patient and mental health counselor present. Mental health counselors take care to maintain a serene environment by providing a counseling area that is softly lit with comfortable couches or face-to-face seating.

Mental health counselors must stay up to date regarding new techniques, studies, or research through continuing-education courses, by attending seminars, or by reading professional literature. Some counselors serve their communities by running workshops to promote mental health issues and programs to prevent substance abuse.

Depending on their specialty, mental health counselors can work in many different environments such as classrooms, health centers, hospitals, day treatment programs, and governmental agencies. Some treat patients in private practice.

Mental health counselors work a standard 40-hour week, though many reserve evening or weekend hours to accommodate patients' work or school schedules. Since emergencies arise at all hours of the day or night, mental health counselors must be on call at all times. Those employed in a group setting may take turns being on call for patient emergencies, either via a pager or phone or through an answering service. Mental health counselors in private practice may take emergency calls through similar measures, as well as taking call turns with other colleagues.

Patient interaction accounts for a large part of a mental health counselor's

Useful Website: GenomicCareers: Find Your Future

GenomicCareers: Find Your Future (www.genome.gov/genomiccareers), which is sponsored by the National Human Genome Research Institute, provides an overview of more than 50 careers in genomics—including bioinformaticians, biomedical engineers, clinical cytogeneticists, environmental geneticists, forensic investigators, genetic counselors, genetic engineers, genetic nurses, nanotechnologists, and reproductive veterinarians. For each career, an overview of job duties, the employment outlook, educational requirements, and earnings are provided. The site also features videos of workers in these fields and a list of additional web resources.

day—either during counseling sessions or during assessments. Many times, mental health counselors assist patients who are severely agitated, depressed, or angry. It's important when working with such patients for mental health counselors to stay calm and professional, no matter the situation.

Oftentimes, patients have more than one health care professional assigned to their care. Mental health counselors may be required to work with nurses, physicians, or social workers to collectively plan the best care and therapy program for the patient. They monitor the patient's prescribed medications and keep in touch with physicians regarding any problems. They many also confer with the patient's family and friends regarding any potential situations or problems at home or in the workplace.

Mental health counselors also supervise other counselors, assistants, or social service staff members. Additional duties depend upon where the mental health counselor is employed—whether at a hospital or agency or self-employed in a private practice. Those in private practice have additional administrative duties such as office maintenance, insurance paperwork, marketing, and billing. A counselor may also hire office assistants to handle these responsibilities.

REQUIREMENTS

HIGH SCHOOL

In high school, take courses in psychology, English, and speech. Take as many science classes as possible, including biology, chemistry, and anatomy and physiology.

POSTSECONDARY TRAINING

You will need a master's degree to become a licensed clinical mental health counselor (LCMHC), which is typically one of the job requirements set by employers. The Council for Accreditation of Counseling and Related Educational Programs accredits counseling programs. Visit its website, www.cacrep.org, for a list of programs. LCMHCs must also complete a minimum of two years of post-master's clinical work under the supervision of a licensed or certified mental health professional.

CERTIFICATION AND LICENSING

Certification and licensing requirements vary greatly based on whether the counselor works for a private or public employer and by state law (although most states have laws requiring counselors to have some form of licensure). Contact the American Mental Health Counselors Association for information about certification and licensing requirements.Some counselors choose to become certified by the National Board for Certified Counselors (NBCC, www.nbcc.org). The NBCC also offers specialty certifications in clinical mental health, addiction, and school counseling.

OTHER REQUIREMENTS

Key traits of mental health counselors include empathy, a strong desire to help others, good listening skills, the ability to communicate well both orally and in writing, strong ethics, the ability to work independently or as part of a team, and physical and mental energy to deal with sometimes stressful and demanding situations (as well as heartbreaking stories).

EXPLORING

To learn more about a career as a mental health counselor, visit the websites of college counseling programs to learn about typical classes and possible career paths, read books and journals (such as the *Journal of Mental Health Counseling,* www.amhca.org/?page=jmhc) about the field, and ask your teacher or school counselor to arrange an information interview with a mental health counselor. Professional associations can also provide information about the field. The American Mental Health Counselors Association provides information on careers at its website, www.amhca.org. You should also try to land a part-time job in the office of a mental health counselor. This will give you a chance to interact with counselors and see if the career is a good fit for your interests and abilities.

EMPLOYERS

There are approximately 128,200 mental health counselors employed in the United States. They work for managed behavioral health care organizations, substance abuse treatment centers, community agencies, hospitals, employee assistance programs, and other organizations and government agencies that provide mental health services. Additionally, some mental health counselors work in private practice or teach counseling at colleges and universities.

GETTING A JOB

Many mental health counselors obtain their first jobs as a result of contacts made through college internships or networking events. Others seek assistance in obtaining job leads from college career services offices, newspaper want ads, and employment websites. Additionally, professional associations, such as the American Counseling Association (ACA), provide job listings at their websites. The ACA also provides helpful articles on writing résumés, acing job interviews, and other career-oriented topics. See For More Information for contact information for the ACA and other organizations.

ADVANCEMENT

Salaried mental health counselors advance by receiving increases in pay and managerial duties. Self-employed counselors advance by developing a strong reputation in their community and attracting more clients. Some counselors become college professors and/or write textbooks about mental health counseling.

EARNINGS

Median annual salaries for mental health counselors were $41,880 in May 2015, according to the U.S. Department of Labor (USDL). Salaries ranged from less than $26,300 to $68,790 or more. The USDL reports the following mean annual earnings for mental health counselors by employer: local government, $55,220; offices of other health practitioners, $50,040; outpatient care centers, $44,310; individual and family services, $43,200; and residential mental retardation, mental health, and substance abuse facilities, $37,680.

Mental health counselors usually receive benefits such as health and life insurance, vacation days, sick leave, and a savings and pension plan. Self-employed workers must provide their own benefits.

FOR MORE INFORMATION

For information on certification and the job search, contact
American Counseling Association
www.counseling.org

To learn more about mental health counseling, contact the following organizations
American Mental Health Counselors Association
www.amhca.org

American Psychotherapy Association
www.americanpsychotherapy.com

For info about mental health issues, contact the following organizations
Mental Health America
www.nmha.org

National Institute of Mental Health
www.nimh.nih.gov

For information on accredited programs, contact
Council for Accreditation of Counseling and Related Educational Programs
www.cacrep.org

For information on certification, contact
National Board for Certified Counselors
www.nbcc.org

To learn more about job opportunities in Canada, contact
Canadian Mental Health Association
613-745-7750
www.cmha.ca

EMPLOYMENT OUTLOOK

Employment for mental health counselors is expected to be strong during the next decade, according to the U.S. Department of Labor. There will be more jobs available (especially in rural areas) than there are people graduating with degrees in counseling. Mental health counselors will enjoy good employment prospects because there is growing demand for mental health services (especially by military veterans and young people) and increasing insurance reimbursements for the services of counselors (which are causing them to be sought after by health care providers as cost-effective alternatives to psychiatrists and psychologists).

Interview: Jennifer Froemel

Jennifer Froemel is the founder/owner of Innovative Counseling Partners, LLC and the President of the Illinois Mental Health Counselors' Association.

Q. What is one thing that young people may not know about the field?

A. No day is ever the same since most clients tend to come in with different issues and one thing can alter how a person is coping, so your days are never dull and boring. The field is definitely open to being able to help others and identify potential issues and fixes to their issues. It does require 6.5 years of education post high school.

Q. What are the most important personal and professional skills for mental health counselors?

A. That you are always in check with your own relationships and yourself. I have found that meditation and mindfulness are key to keeping in touch with what happens with you. I think the other component is that you practice what you preach and can be open and accept criticism.

Q. What do you like most and least about your job?

A. I love getting to meet new people, helping provide them guidance, and seeing them change. Seeing them change and make improved connections is awesome! The thing I like least is having to report abuse and neglect and seeing people drop out of treatment because it is emotionally difficult.

Q. Can you tell us about the Illinois Mental Health Counselors' Association? How important is association membership to career success?

A. Being part of the Illinois Mental Health Counselors Association has been great. We focus on any federal or state changes that may impact our profession, our clients, and our licensure. It is so rewarding to educate our fellow colleagues on issues that are not blatantly out there about our licensure and different laws passed by the federal government. It's important to understand how these pieces of legislation affect our profession. At times, it is also disheartening because you learn that many of the governmental entities do not understand our profession, yet make unilateral decisions that are very uninformed and greatly impact how we can help our clients and community in general.

NURSING AIDES

OVERVIEW

Nursing aides provide care to patients in hospitals, nursing homes, mental health facilities, patients' homes, and other health care settings. They perform routine tasks such as feeding, bathing, dressing, or transporting patients—all under the supervision of nurses or other medical staff. A minimum of a high school diploma is required to work as a nursing aide. More than 1.4 million nursing aides are employed in the United States. Employment is expected to be excellent for nursing aides during the next decade. They are also known as *nursing assistants*, *nurse aides*, *direct care workers*, *certified nursing assistants*, *care assistants*, *hospice assistants*, *patient care assistants*, *restorative aides*, *geriatric aides*, *orderlies*, and *hospital attendants*.

FAST FACTS

High School Subjects
Biology
Health

Personal Skills
Following instructions
Helping

Minimum Education Level
High school diploma

Salary Range
$19,000 to $25,000 to $36,000+

Employment Outlook
Much faster than the average

O*NET-SOC
31-1014.00

NOC
3413

THE JOB

The main duty of nursing aides is patient care. They prepare patients for the day by bathing, grooming, and dressing them. If the patient is unable to stand unassisted, oftentimes nursing aides may need to secure the patient by using specially designed shower seats or bathtub seats before completing the task. Bedridden patients are given a bed bath and changed into fresh hospital gowns. Once patients are dressed, nursing aides help them, depending on their condition, into wheelchairs or wheeled gurneys, or situated into dayrooms or other activity centers. Some patients are transported for therapies, treatments, or appointments.

Nursing aides must be careful when assisting patients out of beds and into wheelchairs. Too quick a movement or not using proper momentum can cause physical harm to the nursing aide as well as the patient. Devices such as the Hoyer lift or other hydraulic mechanisms are helpful in easily and safely transferring obese or physically challenged patients.

Mealtimes are busy for nursing aides. They help distribute meal trays and help patients eat, if necessary. Assistance can range from opening food wrappers and bottle caps, to cutting meat into small pieces, to mixing food and feeding the patient by hand. Nursing aides may test the blood sugar of people with diabetes throughout the day to make sure levels are safe. Nursing aides also pick up food trays after each meal and help patients who need an extra napkin or help washing their hands.

Toilet assistance is another duty of nursing aides. Some patients may call for help in transferring to the bathroom toilet or portable toilet chair, while others prefer to use a bedpan or urinal. Nursing aides clean patients who are incontinent, changing them into fresh clothing.

Nursing aides may take patients' vital signs (such as temperature, pulse, and blood pressure), documenting each reading on the patients' charts or in a database. Some nursing aides are specially trained to assist in exercises as designed by physical and occupational therapists. They may also be asked to participate alongside patients in social activities such as holiday celebrations, birthdays, or other occasions.

Nursing aides keep track of supplies such as gloves, linens, towels, and other patient care items. They change linens and tidy up each patient's room and bathroom area. Nursing aides may also provide fresh ice water and juice or toiletry items, as requested. Other duties of nursing aides include helping patients take daily walks, turning bedridden patients regularly, and moving equipment and supplies in and out of patients' rooms.

If a patient under their care dies, nursing aides clean the patient, gather his or her personal possessions, and prepare the patient for transportation to a funeral home. When a room is vacated, nursing aides clean and disinfect the area before a new patient is brought in.

Nursing aides monitor patients' physical, mental, and emotional status and inform the nursing staff of any changes. In addition to their daily patient care duties, nursing aides may receive other tasks or assignments from their supervising nurse or special requests from patients. Some duties differ according to the nursing aide's work shift. For example, day shift assignments revolve around getting patients ready for their daily activities and eating breakfast and lunch; night shift assignments revolve around eating dinner and preparing patients for bed.

Full-time nursing aides usually work eight-hour shifts, 40 hours a week. Some shifts are scheduled during the evenings, weekends, and holidays.

The work is physically demanding. Nursing aides often stand, stoop, walk, or lift heavy patients. They also risk bodily injury, especially to the back, when lifting and transferring patients from one location to another. It's important for nursing aides to understand and practice the proper procedures for lifting and transferring patients in order to avoid injuries. Nursing aides also are at risk of contracting illnesses (such as HIV or hepatitis) from their patients; they wear protective gloves and masks to reduce this risk.

There are many unpleasant tasks involved in work as a nursing aide, including emptying bedpans, changing soiled linens, and cleaning patients when they are incontinent. At times, nursing aides may work with patients who are depressed, angry, or confused. Some patients may even become violent. Despite these negatives, most nursing aides enjoy their jobs. They find it rewarding to help others. Many times, nursing aides are able to forge caring relationships with their patients, especially those requiring daily, long-term care.

Learn More About It

Carter, Pamela J. *Lippincott's Textbook For Nursing Assistants: A Humanistic Approach to Caregiving.* 4th ed. Philadelphia: Lippincott Williams & Wilkins, 2015.

LearningExpress LLC. *Nursing Assistant/Nurse Aide Exam.* 6th ed. New York: LearningExpress LLC, 2016.

Sorrentino, Sheila A., and Leighann Remmert. *Mosby's Essentials for Nursing Assistants.* 5th ed. Philadelphia: Mosby, 2013.

REQUIREMENTS

HIGH SCHOOL

Recommended classes include health, psychology, biology, anatomy and physiology, computer science, English, and speech. Taking a foreign language such as Spanish will come in handy if you work in an area that has a large population that does not speak English as a first language. Some high schools offer formal training programs for prospective nursing aides.

POSTSECONDARY TRAINING

A minimum of a high school diploma is required to work as a nursing aide. Some nursing aides complete one- to two-year nurse aide programs at community colleges. Others receive their training in formal employer-provided classroom instruction or through on-the-job training. Classes cover topics such as anatomy and physiology, infection control, body mechanics, nutrition, communication skills, personal-care skills, and medical ethics. Students often also complete an internship or clinical experience as part of their studies.

CERTIFICATION AND LICENSING

Nursing aides who work in nursing care facilities must be certified. Aides that satisfactorily complete a state-approved training program of at least 75 hours and pass a competency evaluation can use the designation, certified nurse assistant. Some states have additional requirements. Contact your state's board of professional regulation for information on requirements in your state.

Some nursing aides become certified as national medication aides by completing an exam that is offered by the National Council for State Boards of Nursing.

OTHER REQUIREMENTS

To be a successful nursing aide, you should have empathy and compassion for others. You should work well under pressure, be able to handle multiple—and sometimes repetitive—tasks, be dependable, be good at following instructions, have patience, have excellent communication skills, and be able to work as a member of a team. You should also be in good physical and mental health and be able to pass state-mandated medical tests, as well as background checks administered by potential employers.

EXPLORING

There are many ways to learn more about a career as a nursing assistant. You can read books and magazines (such as *Caring* magazine, www.nahc.org/caringmagazine) about the field, visit the websites of college nurse assistant programs to learn about typical classes and possible career paths, and ask your teacher or school counselor to arrange an information interview with a nursing assistant. Volunteer or land a land a part-time job as a nursing assistant. This will give you a chance to see if the career is a good fit for your interests and abilities.

EMPLOYERS

More than 1.4 million nursing aides are employed in the United States. Nursing care facilities employ 43 percent of nursing aides, and 24 percent work in hospitals. Other employers include home health care agencies, government agencies, outpatient care centers, and residential care facilities.

GETTING A JOB

Many nursing assistants obtain their first jobs via contacts made through college internships or practicums, career fairs, or networking events. Others seek assistance in obtaining job leads from college career services offices, newspaper want ads, and employment and social media websites. Direct application to potential employers is another good job-search strategy. Information on job opportunities at federal agencies is available at www.usajobs.gov.

ADVANCEMENT

There are few advancement opportunities for nursing assistants unless they return to school to continue their education. Career paths for those who complete additional education include licensed practical nurse, registered nurse, and medical assistant.

EARNINGS

Salaries for nursing assistants vary by type of employer, geographic region, and the worker's experience, education, and skill level. Median annual salaries for nursing assistants were $25,710 in May 2015, according to the U.S. Department of Labor (USDL). Salaries ranged from less than $19,390 to $36,890 or more. The USDL reports the following mean annual earnings for nursing assistants by employer:

✔ general medical and surgical hospitals, $29,010;
✔ nursing care facilities, $25,710;
✔ community care facilities for the elderly, $25,130; and
✔ home health care services, $24,720.

Full-time nursing assistants usually receive benefits such as health and life insurance, vacation days, sick leave, and a savings and pension plan. Part-time workers must provide their own benefits.

FOR MORE INFORMATION

For information on home health care careers, visit the association's Web site.
National Association for
Home Care and Hospice
202-547-7424
www.nahc.org

To learn more about careers in nursing homes, contact
National Association of
Health Care Assistants
417-623-6049
www.nahcacareforce.org

For information on careers, contact
National Network of
Career Nursing Assistants
330-825-9342
www.cna-network.org

EMPLOYMENT OUTLOOK

Employment opportunities are expected to be excellent for nursing aides, according to the U.S. Department of Labor. In fact, approximately 262,000 new jobs are expected to be available from 2014 to 2024. Steady increases in the elderly population, whose members typically require more medical care than people in other age demographics, are creating demand for nursing aides. In addition, technological advances are allowing physicians to save more people from diseases and injuries that would have been fatal in the past—creating a need for qualified caregivers for these individuals. Nursing and residential care facilities—especially community care facilities for the elderly—will offer the best employment prospects in coming years.

There is high turnover in the field because it is mentally and physically demanding to work as a nursing aide, there are few advancement opportunities for those who do not receive additional education, and the pay is low. Many people work as nursing aides while attending college programs to prepare for careers in other health care fields such as nursing or physician assisting.

OCCUPATIONAL THERAPISTS

OVERVIEW

Occupational therapists work with patients who are suffering from mentally, physically, developmentally, or emotionally disabling conditions. They help patients improve their ability to perform daily-living and work-related tasks. Using exercises or programs to increase strength, visual acuity, or performance, occupational therapists teach patients how to live independently and have productive lives. A minimum of a master's degree in occupational therapy is required to enter the field. About 114,660 occupational therapists are employed in the United States. Employment opportunities are expected to be strong during the next decade.

THE JOB

People sometimes are physically or mentally limited due to the effects of illness, injury, age, or a physical or psychological condition. These limitations can affect the way they live, work, play, and even learn. People often turn to occupational therapists to help them cope and adjust their activities in a way that makes them more productive, mobile, and independent.

Occupational therapists use games, activities, exercises, and various equipment and tools to improve a patient's basic motor functions and his or her basic reasoning skills. Activities or adaptations may also be designed to compensate for permanent loss of function. Occupational therapists work with patients with a wide range of conditions—from those recuperating from illness or accident, to those with developmental issues—and ages, from infants to senior citizens. While many patients undergo a combination of physical and occupational therapy programs, there is a big difference between the two disciplines. Physical therapy works to restore

Cool Career: Occupational Therapist Assistant

Like their job title implies, *occupational therapy assistants* assist occupational therapists, helping them provide rehabilitative services to patients. Occupational therapy assistants (OTAs) may work with people born with mental or developmental disabilities, or people coping with or recovering from illness or injuries. They help their clients to learn how to perform the skills they need for everyday life, such as eating, dressing, grooming, and working. They may do this by showing their clients how to use adaptive equipment or perform exercises designed to increase their ability to function independently. OTAs help the occupational therapist carry out the client's therapy, document the client's progress, and assist with paperwork and billing issues. They work in a variety of settings, such as hospitals, nursing homes, schools, and clinics. The demand for occupational therapy assistants is expected to grow much faster than average, according to the U.S. Department of Labor, providing a perfect opportunity for students interested in a career that allows them to make a difference in people's lives. Contact the American Occupational Therapy Association (301-652-6611, www.aota.org) for more information.

movement and mobility, while occupational therapy focuses on fine motor skills to restore function.

When working with a new patient, occupational therapists must first assess the patient's needs in all areas—home, work, and recreation. Occupational therapists identify problem areas or activities in their client's home or workplace, and they work to remove the barriers or help the patient make necessary adaptations. For example, when working with a patient who has severe arthritis, occupational therapists may create adaptive equipment for, say, cooking or gardening, to make those particular tasks easier and more productive. Occupational therapists may introduce patients to ergonomic cooking tools, gardening equipment, or other assistive devices to improve mobility and dexterity in these areas.

Once problem areas are identified, occupational therapists assist the patient to develop, maintain, or, in some cases, relearn skills to a more satisfactory level of living and play. Some occupational therapists practice general therapy, meaning they treat people of all ages and conditions. However, most occupational therapists specialize in a particular area, such as pediatrics, gerontology, rehabilitation, or mental/emotional health.

Pediatric occupational therapists work with infants, children, and adolescents with a variety of conditions, including developmental delays; delays in gross, fine, motor, or visual skills; autistic-spectrum delays; and even children with adoption-related concerns. In addition, pediatric occupational therapists work with age-appropriate patients needing help due to illness, disease, or injuries. Early-intervention therapy is important for infants and toddlers who may be at risk for developmental delays as identified by their parents, pediatrician, or teacher.

Tools and equipment, many of which are play based, are often tailored to fit the age, size, and attention span of children. Some sessions may be one on one, while others are held in a group setting. Therapists may have children play with modeling clay, plastic hammers and other tools, or toys to stimulate fine motor skills. They teach children different grasps to help them better hold a pencil or other writing implement. Occupational therapists use therapeutic listening techniques to help children improve their attention spans, behavior, and cognitive processing, which in turn will help them perform better in school. Other therapies help children develop their social skills or teach them skills used for dressing and grooming.

As people age, many find it harder to perform many activities and tasks due to increasing sensory impairment and conditions common with older populations, such as arthritis or Alzheimer's disease. Occupational therapy for gerontology greatly helps the elderly lead more independent and active lives. *Gerontological occupational therapists* may give patients exercises to compensate for difficult movements. Tools such as a bilateral sander—a box with handles on either side—require patients to move the handles backwards and forwards, or side to side, which improves strength and range of motion. Attaching and detaching Velcro blocks can also improve strength and dexterity, both of which are needed for many of the patient's activities of daily living. Cognitive games such as cards, peg boards, or other activities can improve a patient's memory and critical-thinking skills. Other tools and techniques are used to improve patients' cooking, grooming, or dressing skills, as well as other activities that are important to the patients' lives and well-being.

After assessing the patient's home, an occupational therapist may suggest adaptive aides such as safety bars or handles for the bathtub, shower, or toilet area to prevent accidents. They also suggest walking aids or techniques to improve speed and prevent injuries. Some therapists specially trained in driver rehabilitation can teach elderly patients skills to be better and safer drivers.

Rehabilitation is another occupational therapy specialty. Patients recovering from injury or conditions such as a stroke or heart attack often need therapy to help them assimilate back into their everyday lives. For example, stroke patients with short-term memory loss may be taught to make lists or other reminder cues to help in recall. Occupational therapists may use computer games to help patients improve their sequencing, coordination, and problem-solving skills. Exercises done with rubber balls, bands, and other tools can also be implemented to help improve strength and dexterity. Patients suffering from vision loss can be taught techniques to make better use of their remaining vision or can be trained with adaptive equipment such as audio recordings, talking devices, computer technology, or special writing materials. Occupational therapists also help patients use adaptive equipment such as wheelchairs or orthotics. Sometimes, occupational therapists design special tools to better fit a patient's condition,

Top Emerging Niches

Children & Youth

✔ Broader Scope in Schools
✔ Bullying
✔ Childhood Obesity
✔ Driving for Teens
✔ Transitions for Older Youths

Health & Wellness

✔ Chronic Disease Management
✔ Obesity
✔ Prevention

Mental Health

✔ Depression
✔ Recovery and Peer Support Model
✔ Sensory Approaches to Mental Health
✔ Veterans' and Wounded Warriors' Mental Health

Productive Aging

✔ Aging in Place and Home Modifications
✔ Low Vision
✔ Community Mobility and Older Drivers

Rehabilitation, Disability, & Participation

✔ Autism in Adults
✔ Cancer Care and Oncology
✔ Hand Transplants and Bionic Limbs
✔ New Technology for Rehab
✔ Telehealth
✔ Veteran and Wounded Warrior Care

Work & Industry

✔ Aging Workforce
✔ New Technology at Work

Education

✔ Distance Learning
✔ Re-entry to the Profession

Source: American Occupational Therapy Association

needs, or environment including grasping claws to reach items, computer-aided equipment for communication, or other aids to facilitate dressing, eating, grooming, and other daily tasks.

Psychiatric occupational therapists help patients with acute mental health conditions or learning disabilities. Activities, which are geared to improve skills such as time management and socialization, give patients the confidence to live independently or take part in social activities. Occupational therapists also work with patients suffering from alcoholism, drug addiction, depression, eating disorders, or stress-related conditions. They can help patients improve their skills to do everyday tasks such as shopping, cooking, cleaning, using public transportation, or even holding a job.

Occupational therapists also have administrative duties. After each session, they track and chart a patient's progress. They often consult with physicians, nurses, social workers, and other health care professionals regarding a patient's condition or treatment plan. Some occupational therapists supervise occupational therapy assistants, medical assistants, or volunteers.

Approximately 25 percent of occupational therapists employed in the United States work part-time, with some working for more than one employer at various times. Full-time therapists work about 40 hours a week, with some evening and weekend hours scheduled. Occupational therapists can expect to work indoors in large, spacious, well-lit workrooms. Some work is done outdoors, especially when conducting activities such as gardening, games, exercises, or perhaps practice visits to various stores. At times, occupational therapists make follow-up visits to patients' homes, schools, or workplaces to determine their rate of progress.

This career can be demanding and tiring; occupational therapists spend much of their day on their feet or walking from activity to activity. They also run the risk of injury—especially to their back—when supporting, lifting, or shifting patients, or when moving heavy equipment.

REQUIREMENTS

HIGH SCHOOL

Take courses in anatomy and physiology, biology, chemistry, health, physics, psychology, art, computer science, and the social sciences.

POSTSECONDARY TRAINING

There are no baccalaureate-level occupational therapy programs. Aspiring occupational therapists typically earn undergraduate degrees in anatomy, anthropology, biology, kinesiology, liberal arts, psychology, or sociology.

You will need a minimum of a master's degree in occupational therapy to work in the field. Combined bachelor's/master's degree programs are available for those who have not earned a bachelor's degree before entry into an occupational therapy educational program. Visit the American Occupational Therapy Association's website, www.aota.org/Education-Careers/Find-School.aspx, for a list of approximately 200 occupational therapy programs that are accredited by the Association.

Typical classes include Introduction to Occupational Sciences and Occupational Therapy, Kinesiology for the Occupational Therapist, Theoretical Foundations of Occupational Therapy, Technologies in Occupational Therapy, Occupations of Infants and Children, Applied Neuroscience for Occupational Therapy, Research and Occupational Therapy, Occupations of Adolescents and Young Adults, Pathophysiology: Impact of Conditions on Occupation, Occupations of Adults and Older Adults, and Professional Trends and Issues in Occupational Therapy. In addition to classes, students participate in at least 24 hours of fieldwork, where they work with patients under the supervision of experienced occupational therapists.

CERTIFICATION AND LICENSING

National certification is available from the National Board for Certification in Occupational Therapy. Certification is required as one criterion of becoming licensed. To become certified, you must graduate from an accredited occupational therapy program, complete the clinical practice period, and pass a written test. Those who meet these requirements are awarded the designation, occupational therapist, registered. In addition, the American Occupational Therapy Association offers several specialty certifications, including board certification in gerontology, mental health, pediatrics, and physical rehabilitation, as well as specialty certification in driving and community mobility; environmental modification; feeding, eating, and swallowing; and low vision.

All states and the District of Columbia require occupational therapists to be licensed or meet other forms of professional regulation. To become licensed, you must graduate from an accredited occupational therapy program, and then take and pass the NBCOT certification exam. In some states, you must meet additional requirements, such as passing an exam that measures your knowledge of state statutes and regulations.

OTHER REQUIREMENTS

The ability to communicate well is important for occupational therapists, who teach, instruct, and motivate their patients when working with them one on one. In addition, they frequently write reports detailing their treatment plans for patients and document their progress. A successful occupational therapist will remain emotionally calm and stable when dealing with sometimes stressed, angry, or uncooperative patients. Other important traits for occupational therapists include patience, imagination, creativity, and good problem-solving skills.

EXPLORING

Does the career of occupational therapist sound interesting? If so, there are many ways to learn more. You can read books and journals (such as *OT Practice,* www.aota.org/Publications-News/otp.aspx) about the field, visit the websites of college occupational therapy programs to learn about typical classes and possible career paths, and ask your teacher or school counselor to arrange an information interview with an occupational therapist. Professional associations can also provide information about the field. The American Occupational Therapy Association provides a lot of helpful information on education and careers at its website, www.aota.org/Education-Careers/Considering-OT-Career.aspx. You should also try to land a part-time job in the office of an occupational therapist. This will give you a chance to interact with therapists and assistants and see if the career is a good fit for your interests and abilities.

EMPLOYERS

Approximately 114,660 occupational therapists are employed in the United States. Occupational therapists are employed by hospitals; nursing homes; intermediate-care facilities; public and private schools; mental-health centers; rehabilitation hospitals; home health agencies; group homes; individual and family services; community care facilities for the elderly; offices of physicians and other health care practitioners; government agencies; and outpatient clinics. A small number of occupational therapists work in private practice.

GETTING A JOB

Aspiring occupational therapists should be sure to use the resources of their college's career center to improve their resume and interviewing skills and learn about recruiter visits and career fairs. Other job-search strategies include participating in internships, checking out newspaper want ads, and searching for jobs on LinkedIn and other social networking sites. Additionally, the American Occupational Therapy Association provides job listings at its website, http://aota.otjoblink.org/jobseekers.

ADVANCEMENT

Occupational therapists advance by receiving increases in salary and managerial duties. Others become sought-after specialists in gerontology, mental health, pediatrics, physical rehabilitation, or other areas. Occupational therapists also work as professors at colleges and universities.

EARNINGS

Salaries for occupational therapists vary by type of employer, geographic region, and the worker's experience, education, and skill level. Median annual salaries for occupational therapists were $80,150 in May 2015, according to the U.S. Department of Labor (USDL). Salaries ranged from less than $53,250 to $116,030 or more. The USDL reports the following mean annual earnings for occupational therapists by employer: home health care services, $91,860; nursing care facilities, $88,670; offices of other health care practitioners, $83,790; general medical and surgical hospitals, $81,110; and elementary and secondary schools, $71,470.

Employers offer a variety of benefits, including the following: medical, dental, and life insurance; paid holidays, vacations, and sick and personal days; 401(k) plans; profit-sharing plans; retirement and pension plans; and educational-assistance programs. Self-employed therapists must provide their own benefits.

EMPLOYMENT OUTLOOK

An increase in the number of people who have disabilities or who have limited function, growth in the number of individuals age 65 and over (who often have a higher incidence of illness and disability), and advances in medical technology and therapy techniques will create strong opportunities for occupational therapy professionals during the next decade, according to the U.S. Department of Labor (USDL). The USDL predicts that job opportunities "should be good for licensed occupational therapists in all settings, particularly acute hospital, rehabilitation, and orthopedic settings, because the elderly receive most of their treatment in these settings." The American Occupational Therapy Association reports that opportunities should be good in early-intervention programs and in schools for children with disabilities served by the federal Individuals with Disabilities Education Act. Occupational therapists who have specialized knowledge in an area such as gerontology and autism spectrum disorder will have the best job prospects.

Interview: Melissa Winkle

Melissa Winkle, OTR/L, FAOTA, the owner of Dogwood Therapy Services, Inc. (www.dogwoodtherapy.com) in Albuquerque, New Mexico

Q. How long have you worked in the field? What made you want to enter this career?

A.   I graduated from the University of New Mexico in 2001. I became an occupational therapist after volunteering in a variety of therapeutic disciplines for four years. I watched the interactions of patients and clients with each discipline and loved the functionality of the scope of practice found in occupational therapy. When people work with occupational therapists, they are able to return to doing something that they have not been able to do for a period of time. Other clients learn how to do something that they have never been able to do before. Occupational therapists work with people of all ages and stages of life, who have encountered a disability due to birth, injury, illness, or aging. The goal is for them to become as independent as possible, or to regain their dignity and self-sufficiency. I was attracted to occupational therapy because it is the study of people and their roles, patterns, and habits. It encompasses extensive knowledge about the body and how it all works together so that people can establish or return to roles, patterns, and habits.

Q. What is one thing that young people may not know about a career in occupational therapy?

A.   Occupational therapists are actually health care providers. The term "occupation" refers to what people do with their time—at different ages and stages of life, we all have different things that occupy our time. As children, our occupation is to play, grow, and learn. An occupational therapist may work with a child who has a disability in a hospital or clinical setting, at school, at home, or in the community. Their goals may be to learn how to use their fingers to manipulate buttons, zippers, and snaps; to learn play skills like climbing, to learn social skills, or to maintain standing balance to reach items on a table top; or to transition to new environments without having a behavioral outcome as a result of sensory processing issues. An occupational therapist (OT) might also work with a teen or an adult who suffered a spinal cord injury as the result of an accident. In this case therapies may take place in similar settings, and the client may even need skills to get back into the work setting. This person may need stretching, strengthening, and memory and other thinking skills. They may also need assistive technology such as splints or wheelchairs, or even voice-activated computers so they may resume normal activities or occupations. OTs may serve in the role of life coaching, as people begin making interesting life changes such as vocations, family status, returning from serving in the military, etc. Later in life, individuals may find themselves with diagnoses that are more common with aging. A person may have a stroke and lose the use of one side of his or her body and some thinking skills. In this case, an occupational therapist offers strategies for strength, balance, dressing, cooking, visual issues (loss of peripheral vision, etc), problem-solving strategies, etc.

FOR MORE INFORMATION

Visit the association's Web site to learn more about accredited occupational therapy programs, career information, and news related to the field.
American Occupational Therapy Association
301-652-6611
www.aota.org

To learn more about certification, contact
National Board for Certification in Occupational Therapy
301-990-7979
info@nbcot.org
www.nbcot.org

For information on career opportunities in Canada, contact
Canadian Association of Occupational Therapists
800-434-2268
www.caot.ca

Q. **What are the most important personal and professional qualities for occupational therapists?**

A. An occupational therapist must be able to work as an individual and as part of an interdisciplinary team alongside physicians, nurses, social workers, other therapy professionals, teachers, corrections officers, etc. It is critical that OTs be able to take perspective of others' situations, socioeconomic status, spiritual beliefs, and lifestyle. Disability happens to people from all walks of life and with little or no warning. OTs should be chameleons, and be able to blend into a person's home and family life, into a prison situation, into a daycare, or into a crowd on a bus. This is where people live and occupy their time. The best OTs are creative and flexible, and they spend a lot of time watching and listening.

Q.   What are some of the pros and cons of your job?

A.   For me, the best part of occupational therapy is seeing people make progress, working in a variety of environments. I have worked in schools, homes, community centers, places of employment, clinics, hospitals, skilled nursing facilities, corrections facilities, and the greater community. I have worked with clients to drive, and to schedule transportation. I have taken clients on buses, taxis, trains, planes, and automobiles. I get to become part of people's lives; sometimes for a brief period, and others for much longer. Sometimes clients attend sessions with a friend or a family member—so our network can be rather large. I have been very fortunate to open a private practice and have a special interest in individuals with developmental disabilities and integrated services. Individuals are typically referred to us for our modalities of nature therapy, animal-assisted therapy, and assistance dogs as assistive-technology options. It is great to be working in the community, and later that afternoon, be working on research to prove the efficacy of our preferred modalities and methodologies.

Another exciting part of occupational therapy is that you are never done learning. There are always advances in health care, and there is always a lot to learn.

The most difficult part of occupational therapy is that services may be severely limited or there may be a waiting list for people to get funding for services. For example, it is not realistic for an individual who has received a traumatic brain injury and physical injuries to be able to return to daily routines after just 12 visits. In addition, the amount of documentation, which is different for each funding source, can feel overwhelming. There are evaluations, reports, intervention plans, support plans, progress reports, daily contact notes, and client working files to keep. Another downfall to occupational therapy is that people do not know what the profession really does.

Q.   What advice would you give to young people who are interested in becoming occupational therapists?

A.   Anyone interested in occupational therapy should volunteer in at least three different settings. Each will be totally different from the next. Each facility is as unique as the individuals who seek services. As I reflect on my career, I would advise young people to learn all you can in volunteer settings, in college, and on the job. But remember that there is no such thing as a textbook client.

Q.   What is the employment outlook for occupational therapists? How is the field changing?

A.   Occupational therapy is up and coming. While the field began its emergence in the 1700s, mainly in the psychiatric/psychosocial arena, the field has evolved into a strong holistic profession. OTs now have working knowledge and skills to facilitate self-help skills and independence in the triad of mind, body, and spirit in any environment that is meaningful to the individuals we serve.

ORTHOTIC AND PROSTHETIC PROFESSIONALS

OVERVIEW

The U.S. Department of Labor defines orthoses as "externally applied devices used to modify the structural and functional characteristics of the neuromuscular and skeletal system," and prosthetics as "the evaluation, fabrication, and custom fitting of artificial limbs, known as prostheses." Orthoses are used to provide external support to patients with sports injuries, back strain, foot conditions (caused by diabetes, high or flat arches, repetitive stress, etc.), spina bifida, stroke, traumatic brain injury, multiple sclerosis, cerebral palsy, and scoliosis. Prostheses are created for patients who have experienced amputation due to trauma, infection, abnormalities in nerves or blood vessels, or cancer, or those who have been born with missing limbs or a limb deficiency. *Prosthetists* and *orthotists* work with prostheses and orthoses that help improve the lives of individuals in need of such assistive devices. They work as members of a patient's

rehabilitation team, along with physicians, nurses, physical and/or occupational therapists, dietitians, and social workers. The prosthetist/orthotist may be involved with evaluating the individual in need of an orthosis or prosthesis, and the original design, construction, and fitting of the device for that individual. *Prosthetic and orthotic technicians* and assistants help prosthetists and orthotists in their work. Many are responsible for the actual construction of the orthosis or prosthesis. Other career paths include *therapeutic shoe fitters, mastectomy fitters, orthotic fitters,* and *pedorthists.* Approximately 7,100 orthotists and prosthetists and 16,100 medical appliance technicians (including those who specialize in creating orthoses and prostheses) are employed in the United States.

Did You Know?

✔ People with diabetes have a 15 to 40 percent higher risk of losing a foot or leg than those without diabetes.

✔ More than 3,000 patient-care facilities in the United States offer prosthetic and orthotic services.

✔ Each year, orthotic and prosthetic businesses provide patient services that are worth $3.5 million to $4 billion.

✔ The states of California, Ohio, New York, Michigan, and North Carolina employ the highest number of orthotists and prosthetists.

Sources: American Diabetes Association, American Orthotic and Prosthetic Association, U.S. Department of Labor

THE JOB

Orthotists and prosthetists work directly with patients who need orthoses and prostheses. They meet with, examine, and evaluate patients to determine what type of orthosis or prosthesis is necessary. Then they take measurements or impressions of the area of the patient's body that will be fitted with a brace or artificial limb. Orthotists and prosthetists may recommend standard orthoses and prostheses, or they use computer-aided design software to create specialized products. Orthotic assistants and technicians construct orthopedic braces for people with disabilities. Prosthetic assistants and technicians design, fit, and construct artificial limbs for people who have lost limbs due to disease or injury. They fabricate these devices using thermoplastics, titanium, silicone, urethane, foams, carbon fiber, plaster, and leather. Technicians and assistants use power tools such as drill presses, band saws, and heat guns, as well as technology such as computer-aided design software, 3-D printers, robotics, and myoelectrics. These allied health professionals work under the supervision of certified orthotists and prosthetists.

After the devices are constructed, orthotists and prosthetists fit them onto patients and instruct them regarding their use and care. They may adjust, repair, or replace prosthetic and orthotic devices, or technicians and assistants may handle these duties.

Prosthetic and orthotic professionals often have the opportunity to work in varied environments, spending time with individuals in need of assistive devices, as well working in labs to create new orthoses and prostheses. Some specialize in working with patients in specific age groups (e.g., the elderly or youth) or in a specific interest area (such as sports medicine).

REQUIREMENTS

HIGH SCHOOL

In high school, take classes in human anatomy and physiology, biology and chemistry, physics, mathematics, shop, English, speech, psychology, and computer science (especially computer-aided design).

POSTSECONDARY TRAINING

A minimum of a master's degree in orthotics and prosthetics and a residency in one or both areas is required to become an orthotist and prosthetist. Orthotic and prosthetic education programs are accredited by the National Commission on Orthotic and Prosthetic Education (NCOPE) and the Commission on Accreditation of Allied Health Education Programs (CAAHEP). Common undergraduate majors include engineering, bioengineering, kinesiology, biology, and athletic training.

Typical classes in an orthotic/prosthetic training program include Introduction to Orthotics and Prosthetics; Plastics, Materials and Processes; Upper Limb Orthotics; Lower Extremity Orthotics; Upper Extremity Orthotics; Spinal Orthotics; Lower Extremity Prosthetics; Upper Extremity Prosthetics; Upper Limb Prosthetics Lab; Musculoskeletal Pathologies for Orthotics and Prosthetics; Kinesiology-Biomechanical Basis of Orthotic and Prosthetic Management; Clinical Gait Analysis; Clinical Affiliation; Applied Patient Practicum in Orthotics and Prosthetics; Research Methods for Orthotics and Prosthetics; Applied Patient Practicum in Orthotics and Prosthetics; Advanced Techniques and Procedures in Orthotics and Prosthetics; Administration of Orthotics and Prosthetic Facilities; and Capstone Project in Orthotics and Prosthetics.

Technicians require an associate degree or two years of work experience under the supervision of a certified practitioner or technician. Only a few training programs are accredited by NCOPE and CAAHEP.

Visit www.opcareers.org/education for a listed of accredited orthotic and prosthetic practitioner and technician programs.

To become an orthotic and prosthetic assistant, you'll need a minimum of a high school diploma (but, ideally, some college), with coursework in human anatomy, medical terminology, physics, and mathematics.

CERTIFICATION AND LICENSING

The American Board for Certification in Orthotics, Prosthetics & Pedorthics offers voluntary certification for the following orthotic and prosthetic (O&P) professions: orthotist, prosthetist, O&P technician,

O&P assistant, pedorthist, orthotic fitter, mastectomy fitter, and therapeutic shoe fitter.

The Board of Certification/Accreditation provides certification in six professional areas: orthotists, prosthetists, pedorthists, orthotic fitters, mastectomy fitters, and durable medical equipment specialists.

Most certifications require a combination of educational achievement, experience, and the passage of an examination.

Orthotists and prosthetists must be licensed in some states. Certification is typically a requirement of receiving licensure, but prerequisites vary by state.

Learn More About It

Coppard, Brenda M., and Helene Lohman. *Introduction to Orthotics: A Clinical Reasoning and Problem-Solving Approach.* 4th ed. Philadelphia: Mosby, 2014.

Crawford, Cassandra S. *Phantom Limb: Amputation, Embodiment, and Prosthetic Technology.* New York: NYU Press, 2014.

Jacobs, MaryLynn A., and Noelle M. Austin. *Orthotic Intervention for the Hand and Upper Extremity: Splinting Principles and Process.* 2nd ed. Philadelphia: Lippincott Williams & Wilkins, 2013.

Lusardi, Michelle M., Millee Jorge, and Caroline C. Nielsen. *Orthotics & Prosthetics in Rehabilitation.* 3rd ed. Philadelphia: W. B. Saunders, 2012.

Palastanga, Nigel, and Roger W. Soames. *Anatomy and Human Movement: Structure and Function.* 6th ed. Waltham, Mass.: Churchill Livingstone, 2012.

OTHER REQUIREMENTS

Orthotists and prosthetists must have a strong interest in helping others and excellent interpersonal and communication skills. They frequently interact with people who have experienced trauma or serious illness, and they must be caring and compassionate. Orthotists and prosthetists also need an aptitude for math and science, creativity, dedication, excellent hand skills, problem-solving abilities, and a willingness to continue to learn throughout their careers.

Technicians and assistants must have dexterity and good eye-hand coordination, the ability to follow instructions and do precise work, a detail-oriented personality, and strong communication and interpersonal skills. They must enjoy working with their hands and be able to use power tools and digital scanners, 3-D printers, myoelectrics, and microprocessors.

EXPLORING

A good way to break into orthotics and prosthetics (O&P) is to participate in an information interview with or job shadow an O&P professional. Ask your health teacher or school counselor to help arrange such an opportunity. By job shadowing, you might learn that you're more interested in behind-the-scenes, hands-on fabrication and maintenance of orthotic and prosthetic devices rather than working directly with patients as an orthotist or prosthetist—or vice versa. Additionally, check out the following resources to learn more about orthotics and prosthetics:

✔ Orthotics & Prosthetics: Make a Career of Making a Difference: www.opcareers.org

✔ *Journal of Prosthetics and Orthotics:* www.oandp.org/jpo

✔ Profiles of the Profession: www.opcareers.org/professionals/profiles.

EMPLOYERS

Approximately 7,100 orthotists and prosthetists and 16,100 medical appliance technicians (including those who specialize in creating orthoses and prostheses) are employed in the United States. Orthotic and prosthetic (O&P) professionals work at O&P patient care facilities, offices of physicians, fabrication laboratories (technicians), hospitals, rehabilitation facilities, specialty clinics, patients' homes, long-term care facilities, Veterans Affairs facilities, and cancer care centers.

GETTING A JOB

Some orthotists and prosthetists enter the field after first working as physical therapists, occupational therapists, or in related careers. Others work their way up by starting out as assistants, technicians, fitters, or pedorthists. Through a combination of experience and additional education, they become eligible for higher-level positions.

Many people land their first positions in orthotics or prosthetics by working as interns or volunteers during college. Other job-search strategies include using the resources of one's college career services office, networking online and at in-person events, joining and becoming involved in professional associations, applying to employers to directly, and utilizing job sites offered by associations (such as the American Orthotic and Prosthetic Association, http://jobs.aopanet.org).

ADVANCEMENT

Orthotic and prosthetic assistants and technicians who earn a master's degree in orthotics and prosthetics and complete a residency can become orthotists and prosthetists. A skilled and experienced orthotist or prosthetist may choose to launch his or her own business. Others become college professors.

EARNINGS

Salaries for orthotists and prosthetists ranged from less than $35,160 to $107,550 or more in May 2015, according to the U.S. Department of Labor (USDL). The USDL reports the following mean annual earnings for orthotists and prosthetists by employer: medical equipment and supplies manufacturing, $75,590; offices of physicians, $73,520; federal government, $68,700; health and personal care stores, $68,050; offices of other health practitioners, $67,870; and general medical and surgical hospitals, $56,320.

In 2017, orthotic and prosthetic technicians earned median salaries of $39,670, according to PayScale.com. Salaries ranged from $24,107 to $77,955 or more.

Orthotic and prosthetic professionals who are certified typically earn higher pay and have better job prospects than those who are not certified. The American Orthotic and Prosthetic Association reports that certified O&P technicians earned average salaries of $45,000 in 2013, as compared to $36,000 for non-certified technicians.

Employers offer a variety of benefits, including the following: medical, dental, and life insurance; paid holidays, vacations, and sick and personal days; 401(k) plans; profit-sharing plans; retirement and pension plans; and educational-assistance programs. Part-time and self-employed workers must provide their own benefits.

EMPLOYMENT OUTLOOK

Employment for orthotists and prosthetists is expected to grow by 23 percent during the next decade, according to the *Occupational Outlook Handbook,* or much faster than the average for all careers. Job opportunities for medical appliance technicians (including those who work in orthotics and prosthet-

FOR MORE INFORMATION

For information on education, careers, and certification, contact
American Academy of Orthotists and Prosthetists
www.oandp.org

To learn more about certification, contact
American Board for Certification in Orthotics, Prosthetics & Pedorthics
www.abcop.org

For job listings, visit
American Orthotic and Prosthetic Association
www.aopanet.org

For information on certification, contact
Board of Certification/Accreditation
www.bocusa.org

For information on accredited educational programs, contact
National Commission on Orthotic and Prosthetic Education
info@ncope.org
www.ncope.org

To learn more about education, careers, and certification in Canada, contact
Orthotics Prosthetics Canada
www.opcanada.ca

ics) are expected to increase faster than the average. Several factors are fueling demand. The number of people with diabetes and cardiovascular disease, which are two leading causes of limb loss, is rising. Additionally, more people who need orthotics or prosthetics have obtained access to health insurance, which has created demand for O&P workers. Finally, 24 percent of O&P professionals are age 55 and older and likely to retire over the next decade—which will spur demand for qualified O&P workers.

Interview: Leigh Davis

Leigh Davis, MSPO, CPO, FAAOP is the Vice President of the American Academy of Orthotists & Prosthetists.

Q.   What made you want to enter this career?

A.   My younger brother has arthrogryposis, a musculoskeletal disorder that causes multiple joint contractures. Arthrogryposis is notoriously difficult to brace and tends to recur. Growing up, my brother spent many hours with his orthotist and tried many different brace designs. Helping put them on in the morning was one of my childhood chores.

When I was in college, I pursued a degree in mechanical engineering, and I knew that I wanted to have a career that helped people. I started looking for a profession that would be a blend of engineering and medicine. I spent two summers in a rehab engineering lab doing research about wheelchair cushions. Some of the other students in the lab were working on their master's degrees in orthotics and prosthetics. Meeting them, the pieces came together. Orthotics and prosthetics was the perfect choice for me. This is a profession where every day you are engineering devices for individual patient needs and seeing firsthand how you are impacting their lives. Every patient has their own unique challenges and warrants their own unique solution. Seeing someone come in in a wheelchair and walk out on a prosthesis never gets old.

Q.   What is one thing that young people may not know about the field?

A.   Orthotists and prosthetists perform all aspects of patient care, including the design and fabrication of the devices. We evaluate patients, help select the design and components that fit their presentation and goals, fit the devices, and follow up regularly. There is a fair amount of hands-on work in the construction and adjustment of the devices. Most of our devices are still made by hand using hand casting and modification in plaster, followed by thermoforming or laminating. While many facilities utilize technicians for the bulk of the fabrication, clinicians need to be able to understand the fabrication process and perform their own adjustments and finishing. There aren't too many health care jobs where you regularly get to use power tools!

Q.   What are the key skills for orthotists and prosthetists?

A.   An aptitude for mechanics is important in this profession. Few patients are "by the book," and thus most require an understanding of how the body moves and the forces involved to individually design devices. Personal skills are essential as the patient/practitioner relationship is crucial for success.

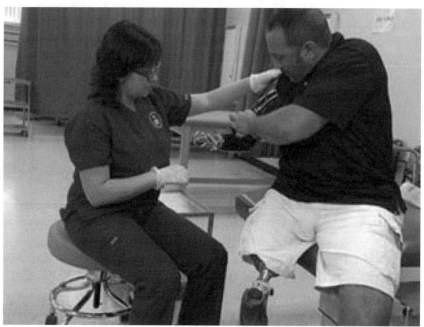

A prosthetist makes adjustments to the prosthetic lower and upper arm of a patient.
(American Academy of Orthotists & Prosthetists)

Q. What is the employment outlook for orthotists and prosthetists? How is the field changing?

A. The orthotic/prosthetic patient population continues to grow as the incidence of diabetes and vascular disease, as well as life expectancy, rises. There is great opportunity right now to enter the profession. Trained clinicians are always in demand.

This used to be a profession that emphasized the physical. Women who entered the profession years ago tell stories of being asked in job interviews if they would feel comfortable lifting heavy casts or large bags of plaster. While hand skills are still important at all levels, we don't see physical strength as an entry requirement anymore.

Q. What's the best way to land a job in the field?

A. O&P is a very small profession. The best way to get in is to start making connections. Job shadow at a local office, communicate with a practitioner, volunteer with an organization for people with disabilities. A good resource: www.opcareers.org.

Q. Can you tell us about the American Academy of Orthotists & Prosthetists? How important is association membership to career success?

A. As a small profession, networking is key to advancement. Academy membership connects practitioners around the country and opens doors for opportunity. Also, as with all health care professions, evidence and standards of care change quickly. The Academy provides the highest level of education focused on keeping practitioners up-to-date so they can provide their patients with the best possible care.

PHARMACISTS

OVERVIEW

Pharmacists are health care professionals who provide pharmaceutical care. They take medicinal requests written by a medical provider, evaluate the appropriateness of the requests, and dispense medicine to the patient. They also spend a considerable amount of time counseling patients regarding the proper use of medicine or medical supplies, and advising them of any possible adverse side effects. A doctor of pharmacy (Pharm.D.) degree is required to practice as a pharmacist. Approximately 295,620 pharmacists are employed in the United States. Job opportunities for pharmacists who work in the health care and social assistance sectors are expected to be good during the next decade.

FAST FACTS

High School Subjects
Biology
Chemistry
Mathematics

Personal Skills
Critical thinking
Judgment and decision making
Scientific

Minimum Education Level
Doctorate

Salary Range
$86,000 to $121,000 to $154,000+

Employment Outlook
Faster than the average

O*NET-SOC
29-1051.00

NOC
3131

THE JOB

Pharmacists do more than just count pills. At retail pharmacies, they evaluate the type of medicine prescribed by your doctor, make sure the dosage is correct, check for any incompatibility with existing prescriptions, and warn people about any adverse effects. Sometimes they may contact the doctor, especially with new prescriptions, to verify the type of medicine and dosage, to suggest a generic equivalent, or to get more information from the provider. Pharmacists may compound—combine or change from a solid form to a liquid form—ingredients or medicines to create the desired prescription. This practice is rarely done today, since many medicines are now delivered in their final form by the manufacturer. However, pharmacists may add flavorings, such as fruit or bubblegum, to some juvenile medicines to make them more palatable. Most pharmacists work in community settings, such as a retail drugstore, or in a health care facility, such as a hospital or clinic.

Pharmacists are often a source of valuable health care information. They provide advice on prescription drugs and over-the-counter medications. Many people rely on their expertise regarding a variety of health care prod-

Learning About Great Employers

Here are a few publications that provide lists of the best health care companies:

✔ *Modern Healthcare* publishes a list of "The 100 Best Places to Work in Healthcare" at www.bestplacestoworkhc.com.

✔ *Becker's Hospital Review* publishes an annual list of "100 Great Hospitals in America" at www.beckershospitalreview.com/lists/100-great-hospitals-in-america-2016.html.

✔ *Fortune* publishes a variety of industry best lists (such as the "100 Best Workplaces for Millennials," "World's Most Admired Companies," and "100 Best Companies to Work For") at http://fortune.com/rankings.

✔ *Forbes* publishes an annual list of best employers (which features many companies in the health care industry) at www.forbes.com/best-employers.

✔ DiversityInc publishes "The DiversityInc Top 5 Hospitals and Health Systems," "The DiversityInc Top 50 Companies for Diversity," and other lists at www.diversityinc.com/top-5-hospitals-and-health-systems.

✔ Newspapers and magazines in many large cities publish lists of the best places to work. For example, the *Chicago Tribune's* 2016 list (www.chicagotribune.com/business/careers/topworkplaces) included large health care employers such as the Rush-Copley Medical Center, Thresholds, Medline Industries, and Advocate Health Care. The *Boston Globe, Los Angeles Business Journal, Crain's New York Business, Seattle Business, The Denver Post,* and *The Atlanta Journal-Constitution* also publish lists.

ucts—from the most effective eye drops to help irritated eyes to the most potent topical allergy creams. Pharmacists also provide information on other products such as medical equipment or home health care supplies. Since they recognize the importance of total well-being, many pharmacists also provide general health advice about diet, nutrition, exercise, as well as ways to alleviate stress. Some of their duties are administrative. They maintain computerized records for customers/patients in order to avoid possible drug interactions, as well as complete insurance documents to submit for reimbursement. Pharmacists keep track of all medicine, vaccines, and other supplies, and they place orders when necessary. Some pharmacists are trained to administer vaccinations. Depending on the size of the pharmacy, they may supervise the work of pharmacy technicians, assistants, and interns. In large pharmacy departments, they manage the work of other pharmacists.

Pharmacists who are employed at hospitals or clinics often team up with other health care professionals to monitor patients' drug therapies.

They may interpret medical lab results in order to design and implement the proper treatment plan, such as a nuclear medicine course or intravenous nutrition support. Often changes must be made in the type of medicine given or the dosage before obtaining the desired results. There are many pharmaceutical specialties, including the following:

Nuclear pharmacists, along with other members of a nuclear medicine team, use radioactive drugs for diagnosis and therapy of different diseases. Their duties include procuring, compounding, testing, administering, and monitoring the use of radioactive drugs such as isotopes that are used for cardiac stress tests or radioactive iodine that is used to treat certain cancers.

Nutrition support pharmacists help critically ill patients receive nutrition either by gastric tubes, by nasogastric-feeding tubes, or through intravenous feedings. They design or modify nutrition plans for patients and help them maintain optimal nutrition.

Oncology pharmacists work with *oncologists* (cancer doctors) to help design, implement, and monitor pharmacotherapeutic plans, and they make changes as needed.

Pharmacotherapists are responsible for the safe, proper, and economical use of various drugs for patient care. While they work as part of a medical professional team, they are often the primary source of drug information.

Working in consultation with other health care professionals, *psychiatric pharmacists* design and implement treatment plans for patients who have psychiatric illnesses. They make patient assessments, monitor their response to a type of drug, and identify drug-related reactions.

Managing health care information electronically and using information technology and computers is becoming an important part of pharmacy care. According to the American Society of Health-System Pharmacists, *pharmacist informaticists* "use and integrate data, information, knowledge, technology, and automation in the medication-use process for the purposes of improving health outcomes." They design and promote systems and approaches such as electronic medical records, e-prescribing, computerized prescriber order entry, bar code dispensing and administration systems, and automated dispensing cabinets.

Consulting pharmacists provide distributive, administrative, and clinical services to people in nursing facilities, prisons, psychiatric facilities, and adult day-care facilities, as well as those in their own homes. *Senior care pharmacists* are specialized consulting pharmacists who work at nursing facilities, hospices, and other long-term care facilities. They provide and oversee the implementation of drug therapy regimens for the elderly.

In addition to working at hospitals, clinics, and privately owned and chain pharmacies, pharmacists work in other settings. One example is a pharmaceutical manufacturing company. In this capacity, pharmacists conduct research to develop new drugs and test them before they are offered to the public. For example, pharmacists employed at Pfizer Inc. may be in charge of a research and development trial for a new drug to control hypertension. Working with a study group, they adjust dosages and keep track of changes in blood pressure, or any negative side effects. Once the drug passes all testing—which can take many years—pharmacists may help create and launch a marketing campaign for the new drug.

Some pharmacists choose to work for insurance companies. They develop patient cost analysis studies, or they may help develop a new drug benefits package. Another career path is in the field of education. Pharmacists teach at colleges and universities or conduct in-service seminars and certification classes for pharmacists. Some pharmacists pursue legal training to become patent attorneys or pharmaceutical law consultants. There are also opportunities in marketing and sales.

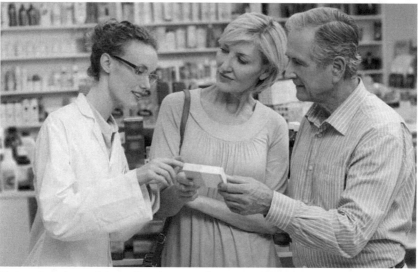

Pharmacists who work in retail settings must have strong communication and interpersonal skills. (Adobe Stock)

Full-time pharmacists work about 40 hours a week, with some evening, weekend, and holiday hours required. Some pharmacies are open 24 hours a day; pharmacists employed at such facilities should expect to work some overnight shifts. Twenty percent of pharmacists work part-time.

Pharmacists wear professional attire, often including a lab coat. Comfortable shoes are a must, since they spend the majority of their workday standing or walking to different areas of the pharmacy. Pharmacists wear gloves, masks, and other protective equipment when working with sterile products or potentially hazardous chemicals.

Attention to detail is a must for this job. Pharmacists are careful when mixing or dispensing medicine, in order to avoid costly, and potentially harmful, mistakes. Customers rely on pharmacists for advice regarding when and how to take medications, as well as potential side effects. Many times, pharmacists speak with physicians or nurses regarding a patient's prescription, either to verify a new prescription or to consult regarding generic forms of the medication. It is important for pharmacists to stay abreast of any new pharmaceutical developments as well as any changes in Medicare, Medicaid, or health insurance coverage for prescription drugs.

Some pharmacists provide consultations to different health facilities, such as nursing homes or rehabilitation centers. In such cases, a reliable means of transportation is needed in order to travel from one facility to another.

REQUIREMENTS

HIGH SCHOOL

You should take a college-preparatory track in high school that includes classes in mathematics (especially calculus and statistics) and science (especially anatomy, biology, chemistry, and physics). Additionally, you should take English and speech classes because developing good communication skills is key to success in the field. If you plan to work as a retail pharmacist or own your own drugstore, you should take business and accounting courses. Finally, taking one or more foreign languages (especially Spanish) will help you effectively interact with people who do not speak English as a first language.

POSTSECONDARY TRAINING

A doctor of pharmacy (Pharm.D.) degree is required to practice as a pharmacist. The six-year doctor of pharmacy, the degree most commonly offered by pharmacy programs, trains pharmacists to help patients monitor chronic illnesses, to administer immunizations, and to host public education activities. The American Association of Colleges of Pharmacy offers a director of pharmacy training programs at its website, www.aacp.org/RESOURCES/STUDENT/Pages/SchoolLocator.aspx.

Pharmacists who own their own businesses might augment their training in pharmaceutical science by earning a master's degree in business administration. Others earn degrees in public administration or public health.

CERTIFICATION AND LICENSING

The Board of Pharmacy Specialties, which was created by the American Pharmacists Association, offers voluntary certification in the following areas: ambulatory care, critical care, geriatric, nuclear, nutrition support, oncology, pediatric, pharmacotherapy, and psychiatric. The Commission for Certification in Geriatric Pharmacy also provides certification. Contact these organizations for more information about certification requirements.

All states and the District of Columbia, as well as Guam, Puerto Rico, and the U.S. Virgin Islands, require pharmacists to be licensed. Licensing requirements include earning a Pharm.D. degree from a college of pharmacy that has been approved by the Accreditation Council for Pharmacy Education and passing a series of examinations. The North American Pharmacist Licensure Exam (NAPLEX) is required by all states, U.S. territories, and the District of Columbia. The Multistate Pharmacy Jurisprudence Exam (MPJE) is required by 44 states and the District of Columbia. States and territories that do not require the MPJE have their own pharmacy law exams. The NAPLEX and MPJE are offered by the National Association of Boards of Pharmacy.

OTHER REQUIREMENTS

To be a successful pharmacist, you should have excellent communication and interpersonal skills, be very attentive to detail, have a desire to help others live healthier lives, be conscientious, have scientific aptitude, and be willing to continue to learn throughout your career.

EXPLORING

Does a career as a pharmacist sound interesting? If so, there are many ways to explore the field. You can read books and periodicals about the field, visit the websites of college pharmacy programs to learn about typical classes and possible career paths, and ask your teacher or school counselor to arrange an information interview with a pharmacist. Professional associations also provide information about the field. Here are a few examples of available resources:

✔ *Mapping Your Career in Managed Care Pharmacy*: http://amcp.org

✔ Pharmacy is Right For Me: http://pharmacyforme.org

✔ *Is Pharmacy for You?*: www.aacp.org/resources/student/pharmacyforyou

Additionally, you should try to land a part-time job at a retail pharmacy. This will give you a chance to watch pharmacists at work and determine if this career is a good match for your abilities and interests.

EMPLOYERS

Approximately 295,620 pharmacists are employed in the United States. Fifty-five percent work at retail pharmacies, and 23 percent are employed in hospitals. Other employers include mail-order and Internet pharmacies, pharmaceutical wholesalers, pharmaceutical manufacturers, insurance companies, offices of physicians, government agencies (including the Food & Drug Administration, Departments of Defense and Veterans Affairs, Indian Health Service, and Public Health Service), and colleges and universities.

GETTING A JOB

Many pharmacists obtain their first jobs as a result of contacts made through college internships, residency programs, or fellowships. Others obtain job leads via college career services offices, newspaper want ads, and employment websites (such as RX Career Center, www.rxcareer-center.com). Additionally, professional associations, such as the American Pharmacists Association and the American Society of Health-System Pharmacists, provide job listings at their websites. See For More Information for a list of organizations.

Those interested in positions with the federal government should visit the U.S. Office of Personnel Management's website, www.usajobs.gov.

ADVANCEMENT

Advancement options for pharmacists vary by employment setting. Pharmacists in retail pharmacies may be promoted to the positions of pharmacy supervisor or store manager. Others become district, regional, or corporate managers. Hospital pharmacists can become supervisors or administrators. Some pharmacists go into business for themselves and open their own pharmacies. Others become professors at colleges and universities.

EARNINGS

Salaries for pharmacists vary by type of employer, geographic region, and the worker's experience level and skills. Median annual salaries for pharmacists were $121,500 in May 2015, according to the U.S. Department of Labor (USDL). Salaries ranged from less than $86,790 to $154,040 or more. The USDL reports the following mean annual earnings for pharmacists by employer:

✔ offices of physicians, $132,870;

✔ outpatient care centers, $126,980;

✔ health and personal care stores, $119,620;

✔ general medical and surgical hospitals, $119,460;

✔ department stores, $117,850; and

✔ grocery stores, $115,830.

Employers offer a variety of benefits, including the following: medical, dental, and life insurance; paid holidays, vacations, and sick days; personal days; 401(k) plans; profit-sharing plans; retirement and pension plans; and educational assistance programs.

EMPLOYMENT OUTLOOK

Employment for pharmacists who work in the health care and social assistance sectors is expected to grow faster than the average for all careers during the next decade, according to the U.S. Department of Labor (USDL). It predicts that there will be rapid employment growth at medical care establishments (such as doctors' offices, outpatient care centers, and nursing care facilities) and mail-order pharmacies. Some growth will also occur at hospitals, drug stores, mass retailers, and grocery stores because pharmacists in these settings still dispense the majority of prescriptions. Pharmacists in these settings are also beginning to administer vaccinations and offer other patient care services.

Factors that are fueling demand include the growing elderly population (whose members traditionally need more prescriptions than other demographic groups), continuing scientific advances (which are creating more pharmaceutical treatment options), and the growing number of people who are becoming eligible for prescription drug coverage as a result of health care reform.

The duties of pharmacists have changed in recent years. Pharmacists are spending less time dispensing drugs and more time "advising patients on drug therapies, evaluating the safety of drug therapy, administering vaccines, and counseling patients on services ranging from self-care to disease management," according to the American Pharmacists Association.

The USDL says that "students who choose to complete a residency program gain additional experience that may improve their job prospects. Certification from the Board of Pharmacy Specialties or as a certified diabetes educator also may be viewed favorably by employers."

FOR MORE INFORMATION

Visit the academy's website to read *Mapping Your Career in Managed Care Pharmacy.*
**Academy of Managed
Care Pharmacy**
www.amcp.org

To learn more about pharmacy education, contact
**Accreditation Council
for Pharmacy Education**
info@acpe-accredit.org
www.acpe-accredit.org

For information on postsecondary training, contact
**American Association
of Colleges of Pharmacy**
703-739-2330
mail@aacp.org
www.aacp.org

For information on education, careers, and licensing, contact
American Pharmacists Association
202-628-4410
www.pharmacist.com

To learn more about careers and certification, contact
**American Society
of Consultant Pharmacists**
800-355-2727
http://ascp.com

For information on careers, contact
**American Society
of Health-System Pharmacists**
custserv@ashp.org
www.ashp.org

For more information about pharmacy specialties, contact
Board of Pharmacy Specialties
202-429-7591
www.bpsweb.org

For information on state boards of pharmacy, contact
**National Association
of Boards of Pharmacy**
help@nabp.pharmacy
www.nabp.net

To learn more about pharmacy education and careers, contact
**National Association
of Chain Drug Stores**
contactus@nacds.org
www.nacds.org

To learn more about careers at community pharmacies, contact
**National Community
Pharmacists Association**
703-683-8200
www.ncpanet.org

For information on career opportunities in Canada, contact
Canadian Pharmacists Association
www.pharmacists.ca

PHYSICAL THERAPISTS

OVERVIEW

Physical therapists, also known as *physiotherapists*, provide health care services to individuals suffering from functional problems caused by arthritis, burns, amputations, stroke, back and neck injuries, traumatic brain injuries, sprains/strains and fractures, headaches, carpal tunnel syndrome, incontinence, multiple sclerosis, cerebral palsy, spina bifida, limitations caused by old age, and work- and sports-related injuries. They evaluate, design, and implement individualized programs to help reduce pain, improve mobility, and increase the quality of life for patients of all ages. Physical therapists use many different techniques for their work including exercise equipment, massage, and electrotherapy. A minimum of a doctorate in physical therapy is required to work in the field. Approximately 209,690 physical therapists are employed in the United States. Employment for physical therapists is expected to grow much faster than the average for all careers during the next decade.

FAST FACTS

High School Subjects
Biology
Chemistry
Health

Personal Skills
Communication
Helping

Minimum Education Level
Doctorate

Salary Range
$57,000 to $84,000 to $119,000+

Employment Outlook
Much faster than the average

O*NET-SOC
29-1123.00

NOC
3142

THE JOB

Many individuals suffer from functional limitations due to injury, disease, surgery, advanced age, or other medical conditions. Their limitations may include difficulty in walking, problems shifting weight, a limited range of motion in their arms or legs, a weak grip, or even decreased endurance. Physical therapists provide therapy services to help patients eliminate or reduce these problems. They also develop and implement therapy programs to help people retain their mobility and flexibility and generally have a healthy lifestyle.

When working with a new patient, physical therapists must first evaluate the individual. They conduct a physical assessment to determine the patient's physical condition and limitations, as well as a short interview to learn more about the patient's lifestyle, work habits, degree of pain, degree of mobility, and therapy goals. Oftentimes, physical therapists consult with other health care professionals such as doctors, nurses, speech-language pathologists, audiologists, dentists, and social workers, as well as members of the patient's family, to complete the assessment. Once a diagnosis of the patient's movement dysfunction is made, physical therapists design a therapy plan to suit the patient's capabilities and schedule. Therapy plans, depending on the extent of the patient's disability or injury, can include a series of exercises, muscle manipulation and massage, traction, hot or cold therapy, ultrasound, and electrotherapy. Physical therapists use many different tools and techniques to achieve positive results such as hand weights, exercise balls and bands, risers, and cardiovascular equipment (treadmills, stationary bicycles, etc.).

Many physical therapists specialize in a specific clinical area and may develop and implement therapy plans that are customized to meet different needs and goals. Patients suffering from cardiopulmonary disease or those who have undergone recent cardiac or pulmonary surgery often have decreased endurance or lung function. For example, physical therapists use manual therapy to help remove excess secretions from the lungs, or they use chest mobilization exercises to increase lung capacity.

Physical therapists often work with elderly patients who have arthritis, osteoporosis, balance disorders, joint replacements, or Alzheimer's disease. Techniques used with geriatric patients include water aerobics, stretching exercises, and light weight lifting to improve their mobility. Physical therapists also teach geriatric patients better ways to conduct daily activities, such as the proper way to safely climb and descend stairs or how to use a walker or other aid.

Pediatric physical therapy is another specialty. When working with infants, children, and young adolescents, physical therapists create a plan to address not only areas of concern, but also the capabilities and attention spans of their young patients. Infants needing physical therapy may be those born with a congenital disorder such as spina bifida. Physical therapists may suggest leg braces or specific exercises and massages to keep limbs flexible and avoid contracting. Children with developmental delays also benefit from physical therapy. For example, balls and other squeezable toys may be incorporated into an exercise plan to increase mobility and strength.

Orthopedic physical therapy, the most common and identifiable specialty, treats patients suffering from injuries sustained at home, on the athletic field, or at the workplace as well as those needing rehabilitation after orthopedic surgery. Most orthopedic therapy is conducted on an outpatient basis. For a patient recovering from a sports injury to a muscle in his or her arm, for example, physical therapists may use techniques such as therapeutic exercises, hot or cold packs, and even electrotherapy to expedite neuromuscular stimulation and retraining. They may use arm pulleys or resist-a-bands to increase strength. Continuous passive motion machines can be used to increase a patient's rotator cuff flexibility and strength.

Physical therapists are responsible for charting their patients' scheduled therapy sessions and progress. They consult with other health care professionals to keep them abreast of the patient's progress or to discuss or update them regarding changes in therapy plans. Depending on their employer, physical therapists may also complete and submit billing sheets for services rendered, maintain equipment, and order supplies and equipment.

The work of physical therapists is physically demanding. They spend a considerable amount of time each day standing, stooping, walking, bending, reaching, lifting, and operating equipment or using various tools.

A normal workweek for a full-time physical therapist is 40 hours, with time off on weekends or holidays. However, many physical therapists have some weekend and evening hours in order to accommodate patient loads. Approximately 20 percent of physical therapists work part-time. Some travel may be necessary, especially for those providing home health therapy.

Physical therapists may be required to wear a uniform, which often consists of hospital scrubs, pants, and smock, and comfortable, non-skid shoes.

Books to Read

Goodman, Catherine C., and Kenda S. Fuller. *Pathology: Implications for the Physical Therapist.* 4th ed. Philadelphia: W.B. Saunders, 2014.

Jewell, Dianne V. *Guide to Evidence-Based Physical Therapist Practice.* 3rd ed. Burlington, Mass.: Jones & Bartlett Learning, 2014.

Pagliarulo, Michael A. *Introduction to Physical Therapy.* 5th ed. Philadelphia: Mosby, 2015.

REQUIREMENTS

HIGH SCHOOL

In high school, take science courses (especially anatomy, biology, chemistry, and physics), as well as classes in mathematics, statistics, physical education, social science, psychology, computer science, English, and speech. If you plan to work in an area with a large number of people who do not speak English as a first language, you should take a foreign language—especially Spanish.

POSTSECONDARY TRAINING

A minimum of a doctor of physical therapy degree from an accredited physical therapy program is required to work in the field. The Commission on Accreditation of Physical Therapy Education (www.capteonline.org/home.aspx), which accredits entry-level academic programs in physical therapy, has accredited more than 230 education programs. Typical courses in a doctorate program include Intro to Physical Therapy, Gross Human Anatomy, Physiology, Clinical Applications, Functional Histology, Neuroanatomy, Joint Function and

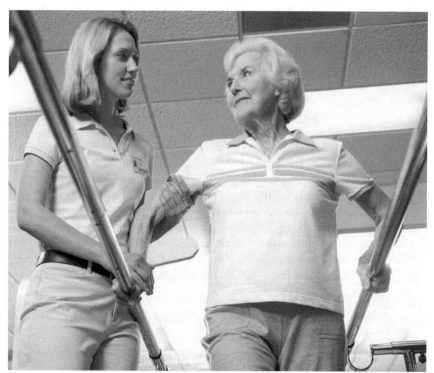

A physical therapist helps a patient re-learn how to walk. The U.S. Department of Labor predicts that more than 71,800 new jobs will be available for physical therapists through 2024. (Thinkstock)

Movement, Applied Pathophysiology, Psychosocial Theory and Practice, Applied Pathophysiology, Biophysics, Case Management in Physical Therapy Practice, Musculoskeletal Dysfunction, Clinical Fieldwork, Cardiopulmonary Dysfunction, and Neuromuscular Dysfunction.

Aspiring physical therapy students can use the Physical Therapist Centralized Application Service (www.ptcas.org), which allows one to apply to multiple accredited physical therapy programs at one time.

Some licensed physical therapists choose to pursue a fellowship or residency program to improve their knowledge and skills.

CERTIFICATION AND LICENSING

Certification, while voluntary, is highly recommended. It is an excellent way to stand out from other job applicants and demonstrate your abilities to prospective employers. The American Board of Physical Therapy Specialities offers certification in the following specialties: cardiovascular and pulmonary, clinical electrophysiology, geriatrics, neurology, oncology, orthopaedics, pediatrics, sports, and women's health. Contact the board for more information.

All states require physical therapists to be licensed. Licensing requirements vary by state but typically include graduation from an accredited physical therapy education program; passing the National Physical Therapy Examination, which is administered by the Federation of State Boards of

Physical Therapy (www.fsbpt.org); and fulfilling state requirements (which may involve passing additional examinations).

OTHER REQUIREMENTS

Physical therapists must be in optimum physical condition in order to lift patients and assist them in turning, standing, or walking. A positive disposition is also helpful when working with patients who are suffering from chronic pain or who have limited mobility. Physical therapists must often motivate their patients during therapy sessions, and this is best done with a smile and encouraging words. Other important traits include compassion, an interest in helping others, and good time-management skills.

EXPLORING

There are many ways to learn more about a career as a physical therapist. You can read books and journals about the field (such as *Physical Therapy* and *Perspectives* (for PTs and PTAs in the first five years of their careers), which are published by the American Physical Therapy Association, APTA), visit the websites of college physical therapy programs to learn about typical classes and possible career paths, and ask your teacher or school counselor to arrange an information interview with a physical therapist. Professional associations can also provide information about the field. The APTA, the leading physical therapy association in the United States, provides a wealth of information on education and careers at its website, www.apta.org. You should also try to land a part-time job in a setting where physical therapists are employed. This will give you a chance to interact with physical therapists and see if the career is a good fit for your interests and abilities.

EMPLOYERS

Approximately 209,690 physical therapists are employed in the United States. About 60 percent of physical therapists work in hospitals or in offices of health practitioners. Employment opportunities also exist at nursing homes, home health services providers, outpatient care centers, adult day-care programs, industrial settings, schools, and government agencies (such as the Departments of Defense and Veterans Affairs and the Indian Health Service). Other physical therapists work as professors and researchers at colleges and universities. Some have their own businesses. In fact, the American Physical Therapy Association reports that nearly 22 percent of physical therapists are owners of, or partners in, a physical therapy practice.

GETTING A JOB

Many physical therapists obtain their first jobs as a result of contacts made through college internships, clinical experiences, or networking events. Others seek assistance in obtaining job leads from college career services offices, newspaper want ads, and employment websites. Additionally, the American Physical Therapy Association provides job listings at its website, www.apta.org/apta/hotjobs. Those interested in positions with the federal government should visit the U.S. Office of Personnel Management's website, www.usajobs.gov.

ADVANCEMENT

At large therapy providers, physical therapists may advance to managerial and supervisory positions. Others start their own businesses and offer their services on a contract basis to hospitals, nursing facilities, and other therapy providers.

EARNINGS

Salaries for physical therapists vary by type of employer, geographic region, and the worker's experience level and skills. Median annual salaries for physical therapists were $84,020 in May 2015, according to the U.S. Department of Labor (USDL). Salaries ranged from less than $57,060 to $119,790 or more. The USDL reports the following mean annual earnings for physical therapists by employer: home health care services, $96,560; nursing care facilities, $91,480; general medical and surgical hospitals, $85,190; offices of physicians, $83,810; and offices of other health practitioners, $83,800.

Physical therapists usually receive benefits such as health and life insurance, vacation days, sick leave, and a savings and pension plan. Self-employed workers must provide their own benefits.

EMPLOYMENT OUTLOOK

Employment for physical therapists is expected to grow by 34 percent during the next decade, according to the U.S. Department of Labor—or much faster than the average for all careers. Factors that are fueling growth include an increasing elderly population, which has a strong need for physical therapy services; changes in insurance reimbursement, which will allow more people to have access to physical therapy services; the implementation of the Individuals with Disabilities Education Act, which ensures that disabled students will

---

FOR MORE INFORMATION

For information on education and careers, contact
American Physical Therapy Association
800-999-2782
www.apta.org

To learn more about accredited programs, contact
Commission on Accreditation in Physical Therapy Education
accreditation@apta.org
www.capteonline.org

For information on career opportunities in Canada, contact
Canadian Physiotherapy Association
613-564-5454
information@physiotherapy.ca
https://physiotherapy.ca

have better access to physical therapy and other rehabilitative services in schools; and advances in medicine and technology that are allowing people with severe trauma, serious illness, and birth defects to survive, which will create the need for more physical therapists to treat these patients.

Physical therapists who specialize in treating the elderly will have especially strong job prospects. Typical employers for these workers include acute care hospitals, skilled nursing facilities, and orthopedic settings. Opportunities will also be good in rural areas, where there is a shortage of trained physical therapists.

Interview: Steven W. Forbush

Steven W. Forbush, PT, Ph.D., an Assistant Professor of Physical Therapy at the University of Central Arkansas in Conway, Arkansas

Q. What made you want to enter this career?

A. I was in a pre-medical program in my undergraduate school, majoring in biology and minoring in chemistry and psychology. I was planning on going into some form of medical-based field and was thinking of dentistry. I then realized I didn't want to spend my life with my hands in other person's mouths. I had already decided I didn't want to be a doctor as I did not want to prescribe medicine, or have life and death decisions weighing on me at critical times. Some of my classmates (ones I respected) had decided on going on with physical therapy programs, and I decided to look into this field in the summer between my junior and senior years. I met a gentleman in my hometown who was in private practice (men were not common in the profession at that time and private practice was also an unusual setting) in physical therapy and was doing well. I already had all of the prerequisite courses to apply and decided this was where I wanted to be. After 25 years in the profession, I went back to school to gain a Ph.D. in physical therapy so I could continue to advance the profession through the educational realms.

Q. What do you like most and least about your career?

A. I am really excited about my field and my career, even after over 30 years of working in this area. I enjoy knowing that I am making an immediate, and sometimes a life-long, difference in my patient's lives. I also am now able to improve the skills and knowledge of students at my Doctor of Physical Therapy Program and established therapists through other continuing education offerings so that they may influence the lives of countless other patients and clients. I am truly excited to go to work each and every day and daily learn more to become a better therapist and person through my patient and peer interactions. I also enjoy being active in the American Physical Therapy Association and its components as this is the only organization representing the profession of physical therapy and its interests on a state or federal level.

I don't enjoy watching all the medical professions protect turf in every legislative session rather than working together to improve all aspects of health care. I also don't enjoy fighting for continuing payment for the services we provide as a profession through the constant cost-cutting that is occurring on the state and federal levels.

Q. What is the one thing that young people may not know about a career in physical therapy?

A. I am not sure the public really understands the field of physical therapy and all that it offers. I have people come up to me all the time and, after I tell them I am a physical therapist, suggest they need a massage, have other misconceptions they relate to me, or suggest that they would like to see me but feel they need to see a physician first to find out what is wrong with them. Young persons (and old persons in the general public) do not understand that our profession should be the profession to visit for any neurological, musculoskeletal, or other functional or movement problem they may have. Very few of the problems anyone experiences in their lifetime are from a serious pathology...and if these pathologies are present, the physical therapist is trained to recognize that the problem needs to be addressed by another medical specialty and refer them accordingly.

Q. Can you please tell us about your program?

A. The University of Central Arkansas, where I am now a professor, offers a Doctor of Physical Therapy Program, which is the program that is the expected program for a graduating physical therapist anywhere in the United States. It is a full three-year program encompassing 126 graduate credit hours of education, including 43 hours of clinical practicum, in order to graduate. To get into a typical physical therapy program (including our's) one needs to have 48 credit hours of specific undergraduate pre-requisite courses to prepare them for the program. Most programs around the U.S. are very similar to ours, and all programs must be accredited through the same national body, the Commission on Accreditation in Physical Therapy Education.

Q. What type of students pursue study—and find success—in your program?

A. The typical person finding their way to physical therapy as a profession is relatively academically gifted (average entrance GPA in our program is a 3.73, with a science GPA of 3.53), usually like the field of biology, have an altruistic interest and wish to help others, are relatively social and can interact and communicate well with persons of all ages, and usually have had some connection to the field of physical therapy in their life history. If a person is willing to accept change and adapt to a constantly changing environment and is service oriented in the typical business model, they will be even more successful. I like the student who is willing to smile, politely challenge what is told to them, be willing to admit they are wrong, and be humble in the process.

Q. What advice would you offer physical therapy majors as they graduate and look for jobs?

A. I am very active in advising new graduates on jobs and areas of interest as they graduate. Almost every student has an area where they have found the most reward as they have worked through their varied practicum experiences, and I always suggest they start and stay in the area where they have the most passion. I suggest they find a workplace with ethical and work standards that most closely resembles their own; a setting where they will have the proper mentorship to continue to grow; a setting in the area of the country where they are eager to live and work; and a setting where they will be challenged on a regular basis. Jobs are available in almost any set-

Interesting Career: Ocularist

When people lose one or both of their eyes as a result of illness or injury (such as those occurring to soldiers involved in combat), it is necessary to replace them with an ocular prostheses. An *ocularist*, according to the American Society of Ocularists (ASO), is a "carefully trained technician skilled in the arts of fitting, shaping, and painting ocular prostheses." They also show patients "how to handle and care for the prosthesis and provide long-term care through periodic examinations."

It is a very demanding task to create a custom ocular prosthesis. Ocularists must replicate the color and shape of the patient's natural eye or eyes to ensure the closest match to the new prosthetic eye(s). They must have artistic ability, fine hand skills, and compassion for those who have been through traumatic circumstances.

Individuals who are interested in becoming ocularists receive their training through an apprenticeship with an approved ocularist. The ASO offers a five-year apprenticeship program for aspiring ocularists. Visit the ASO's website, www.ocularist.org, for more info.

ting, in almost any town with a population over 25,000, and in almost any region in the country so job scarcity is rarely an issue.

Q.   What is the employment outlook for physical therapy? Have certain areas of this field been especially promising (or on the decline) in recent years?

A.   Physical therapy is consistently rated as one of the fastest-growing professions with one of the highest demands in the medical arena. In the past 30 years there has only been one short period of time when supply of physical therapists has exceeded the demand of the society (just after the passage of the BBA in 1997, which greatly limited the payments for any rehabilitative professionals) and this self-corrected within less than five years. The population of the U.S. has been aging according to all statistics and this demographic typically needs more rehabilitative care than other areas of the population. The population is also participating in more youth-based organized competitive sport (leading to more acute and chronic injury), getting heavier (leading to more joint and muscle problems), and living a more sedentary lifestyle in middle age (also a predictor for more pain complaints), and all of these predict a greater need for a group of professionals specializing in neuromusculoskeletal differential diagnosis and persons specialized in the correction of movement disorders. Also, the state and federal governments have emphasized care of children in all the medical payment systems leading to a rapid growth in the field of pediatric physical therapy.

PHYSICAL THERAPY ASSISTANTS AND AIDES

OVERVIEW

Physical therapy assistants and aides help physical therapists provide health care services to individuals suffering from functional problems caused by arthritis, burns, amputations, strokes, back and neck injuries, traumatic brain injuries, sprains/strains and fractures, headaches, carpal tunnel syndrome, incontinence, multiple sclerosis, cerebral palsy, spina bifida, limitations caused by old age, and work- and sports-related injuries. Physical therapy assistants are responsible for services including exercises, massages, electrical stimulation, and therapeutic baths. Physical therapy aides can assist physical therapists and assistants with simple therapy procedures but tend to have a more clerical role in the therapy team. Physical therapy assistants train for the field by earning an associate's degree in physical therapy assisting; physical therapy aides learn their skills on the job. Approximately 81,230 physical therapist assistants are employed in the United States. Physical therapist aides hold 50,540 positions. Assistants and aides should expect very good job prospects during the next decade.

FAST FACTS

High School Subjects
Biology
Health

Personal Skills
Communication
Following instructions
Helping

Minimum Education Level
Associate's degree (assistants)
High school diploma (aides)

Salary Range
$32,000 to $55,000 to $76,000+ (assistants)
$18,000 to $25,000 to $38,000+ (aides)

Employment Outlook
Much faster than the average

O*NET-SOC
31-2021.00, 31-2022.00

NOC
3237, 3414

THE JOB

People with various illnesses, diseases, or injuries often seek the help of physical therapists to help them regain strength and mobility, as well as find relief from pain. While physical therapists evaluate patients' needs and design and implement therapy programs, they turn to physical therapy

Cool Career: Massage Therapist

Although not new, the field of massage therapy has steadily gained in popularity in recent years. Using soft-tissue manipulation techniques, massage therapists provide medical benefits to their clients, treating disorders of the human body or helping them recover from injuries. Or massage therapists may simply promote relaxation or provide an energizing experience for their clients, depending upon the goal of the client. Students enrolling in an accredited massage therapy program will likely take a survey of general massage therapy classes, then choose electives depending on which areas of massage therapy they wish to specialize in—reflexology, shiatsu, Swedish massage, and deep tissue massage are just a few of the options. Massage techniques are also geared towards different populations, such as sports massage for athletes, or massage specifically for infants, pregnant women, or the geriatric population. Because many therapists are self-employed, they need to know about the business and legal aspects of the career. Some massage therapy programs offer classes to address those aspects of the profession. According to the U.S. Department of Labor, the need for massage therapists is likely to grow much faster than average—providing a perfect opportunity for students who want a "hands-on" career, would like to help others, and desire the opportunity for self-employment.

Contact the following organizations for more information: American Massage Therapy Association (877-905-0577, info@amtamassage.org, www.amtamassage.org) and Associated Bodywork and Massage Professionals (800-458-2267, expectmore@abmp.com, www.abmp.com or www.massagetherapy.com).

assistants and aides to oversee some basic therapy procedures and much of the administrative work.

Physical therapy assistants work with patients and perform procedures as selected and supervised by physical therapists. Their patients include those with physical disabilities resulting from disease or injury or a disabling condition due to chronic illness such as arthritis, heart disease, or cerebral palsy.

When assessing a new patient, physical therapy assistants help physical therapists conduct tests and measurements to better gauge the patient's limitations. Some tests may have the patient reach or bend to determine his or her range of motion, or perhaps work with pulleys and weights to assess his or her muscle strength. Physical therapy assistants also perform gait and functional analyses to identify any weaknesses. They help patients improve their speed and adapt for many different walking surfaces and for different activities. Physical therapy assistants use gait strategies to retrain patients, especially those affected by a stroke, or teach them to use walking devices.

Physical therapy assistants help patients through a series of exercises to improve muscle strength and function. They also use therapeutic massages, both deep-tissue and surface techniques, to maintain muscle function. Physical therapy assistants administer treatments using hot or cold packs, ultraviolet and infrared lamps, or electrical stimulation equipment to improve muscle function. Traction devices and incline surfaces are also used to relieve neck or back pain. Hydrotherapy is a treatment used by physical therapy assistants to treat conditions such as osteoarthritis, osteoporosis, Parkinson's disease, or strokes. The buoyancy of the water and warmth from the pool or tub helps combat muscle stiffness and spasms or pain. Sometimes physical therapy assistants also enter the pool, especially when helping patients with water exercises.

Physical therapy assistants also help patients with cardiovascular exercises, especially those who are recuperating from a heart attack or heart surgery. They monitor patients as they go through an interval training series using recumbent bicycles, treadmills, or elliptical machines.

Physical therapy assistants also provide education and instruction. They train patients and their family members regarding the proper way to do exercises while at home. They also help patients become familiar with the use of new prosthetic or orthotic devices. Physical therapy assistants often work with other members of the patient's medical team, noting any changes or improvements in the patient's therapy progress.

Depending upon the facility and the type of physical therapy offered, physical therapy assistants may work with a variety of patients and conditions. Some physical therapy assistants work with children, those with special needs, or, in the case of a sports rehabilitation facility, they may specialize in sports-related injuries and conditions.

Physical therapy aides also help with some basic procedures, done under the direct supervision of physical therapists and assistants. They often help during hydrotherapy sessions by assisting patients into whirlpools or tubs, or even entering the pool as patients do their exercises. Aides also apply hot and cold packs to soothe tightened muscles and use paraffin baths to relieve patients' pain from arthritis, bursitis, or other chronic joint inflammation. Some aides are trained to give massages and other such treatments. They prepare patients for their treatments, including helping them undress (if necessary), removing supportive devices such as braces and slings, and getting them properly situated on machinery.

A large part of their job involves clerical duties. Aides often maintain the front office, including answering the phone, greeting and processing patients as they enter the facility, and filling out insurance forms or other paperwork. They keep track of supplies and equipment and reorder these materials when necessary.

Aides also clean and maintain treatment areas, including hydrotherapy pools and spas, and request necessary repairs. They often transport patients from one area of the facility or hospital to another, sometimes moving patients in wheelchairs or other equipment.

Full-time assistants and aides typically work 40 hours a week. Shifts vary depending on the facility and its patient load—some evening and weekend hours should be expected in order to accommodate patients' schedules and needs.

Many physical therapy assistants and aides wear scrubs, smocks, or other clothing that allows easy movement. Assistants and aides wear bathing suits when helping patients engaged in water therapy exercises. Comfortable, skid-resistant shoes are a must, since a great part of their day is spent standing or walking with patients.

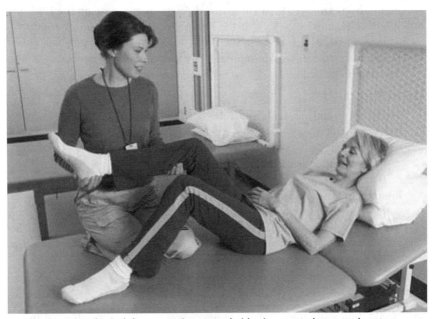

Employment for physical therapy assistants and aides is expected to grow by 40 percent during the next decade, according to the U.S. Department of Labor.
(Hemera Technologies/Thinkstock)

REQUIREMENTS

HIGH SCHOOL

In high school, take anatomy and physiology, biology, health, physics, chemistry, social sciences, computer science, physical education, English, and speech classes.

POSTSECONDARY TRAINING

Physical therapy assistants train for the field by earning an associate's degree in physical therapy assisting, which is required by most states as one of the criteria for licensing. The Commission on Accreditation in Physical Therapy Education (www.capteonline.org), which accredits postsecondary physical therapy assistant programs, has accredited 340 educational programs. Students complete both classroom and clinical instruction. Typical classes include Introduction to Physical Therapy, Medical Terminology, First Aid and CPR, Applied Kinesiology, Human Anatomy and Physiology, Principles of Biological Science, and Patient Management. Physical therapy aides do not need a college degree. They learn their skills through on-the-job experience and training.

CERTIFICATION AND LICENSING

Most states require physical therapy assistants to hold a license, certification, or registration to work. Requirements for most states include graduating from an accredited educational program and passing the National Physical Therapy Exam. Visit the Federation of State Boards of Physical Therapy website, www.fsbpt.org, for more information about licensure/certification requirements. Physical therapy aides do not need to be certified or licensed.

OTHER REQUIREMENTS

Physical therapy assistants and aides need to be in good physical condition to work with patients of all ages and sizes as they undergo procedures and exercises. Oftentimes, they must kneel, stoop, walk, or otherwise physically assist patients during sessions.

It is important for physical therapy assistants and aides to have good interpersonal skills, especially when working with patients who may be suffering from injury or pain. They should be patient and have compassion for their patients. Other important traits include the ability to follow instructions, good organizational skills, a detail-oriented personality, and an interest in helping others.

EXPLORING

Do the following things to learn more about a career as a physical therapist assistant or aide:

✔ Read books (Dreeben-Irimia's *Introduction to Physical Therapist Practice For Physical Therapist Assistants*) and journals about the field (such as *Physical Therapy* and *Perspectives* (for PTs and PTAs in the first five years of their careers), which are published by the American Physical Therapy Association, APTA). The APTA, the leading physical therapy association in the United States, provides a wealth of information on education and careers at its website, www.apta.org.

✔ Visit the websites of college physical therapy assisting programs to learn about typical classes and possible career paths

✔ Ask your teacher or school counselor to arrange an information interview with a physical therapist assistant or aide.

✔ Land a part-time job in a setting where physical therapists, assistants, and aides are employed.

EMPLOYERS

Approximately 81,230 physical therapist assistants are employed in the United States. Physical therapist aides hold about 50,540 positions. They work in hospitals, clinics, offices of physicians and other health care professionals, inpatient and outpatient rehabilitation facilities, skilled nursing homes, fitness centers, sports facilities, corporate or industrial health centers, pediatric centers, elementary and secondary schools, colleges and universities, hospice facilities, and private homes.

GETTING A JOB

Many assistants and aides obtain their first jobs as a result of contacts made through career fairs, college internships, or networking events. Others seek assistance in obtaining job leads from college career services offices, newspaper want ads, and employment websites. Additionally, the American Physical Therapy Association provides job listings and career planning resources at its website, www.apta.org/apta/hotjobs. Information on job opportunities at federal agencies is available at www.usajobs.gov.

FOR MORE INFORMATION

For detailed information on education and careers, contact
American Physical Therapy Association
800-999-2782
www.apta.org

For information on accredited programs, contact
Commission on Accreditation in Physical Therapy Education
accreditation@apta.org
www.capteonline.org

To learn more about career opportunities in Canada, contact
Canadian Physiotherapy Association
613-564-5454
information@physiotherapy.ca
https://physiotherapy.ca

ADVANCEMENT

With further college education, physical therapist assistants can become physical therapists. Aides can become assistants and eventually physical therapists. Other means of advancement include salary increases, taking on managerial duties, or becoming a college professor at a physical therapy education program.

EARNINGS

Median annual salaries for physical therapist (PA) assistants were $55,170 in May 2015, according to the U.S. Department of Labor. Salaries ranged from less than $32,640 to $76,940 or more. PA assistants who worked in skilled nursing facilities earned mean annual salaries of $63,200. The median annual salary for physical therapy aides was $25,120. Ten percent earned less than $18,720, and 10 percent earned more than $38,040. PA aides who worked in psychiatric and substance abuse hospitals had the highest mean annual salary ($64,910).

Health Care Career Resources on the Web

Here are a few useful websites to help you explore health care careers:

✔ **Careers in Aging: Consider the Possibilities:**
www.aghe.org/resources/careers-in-aging

✔ **ExploreHealthCareers.org:** http://explorehealthcareers.org

✔ **Health Professions:** www.ama-assn.org/education

✔ **HRSA Health Professions:** http://bhpr.hrsa.gov

✔ **National Health Service Corps** (scholarships/loans): https://nhsc.hrsa.gov

Employers offer a variety of benefits, including the following: medical, dental, and life insurance; paid holidays, vacations, and sick and personal days; 401(k) plans; profit-sharing plans; retirement and pension plans; and educational-assistance programs. Part-time workers must provide their own benefits.

EMPLOYMENT OUTLOOK

Employment for physical therapist assistants and aides is expected to grow much faster than the average during the next decade, according to the U.S. Department of Labor (USDL). Employment is expected to grow by 40 percent—far faster than the average of 7 percent for all careers. The growing population (especially elderly people who need rehabilitation services); breakthroughs in medical technology and treatments that are allowing more babies to survive serious birth defects and people to survive illnesses and injuries; and the aging of the large Baby Boomer population, which will require an increasing amount of cardiac and physical rehabilitation, will create very good employment prospects. The USDL reports that employment opportunities should be particularly strong in home health, skilled nursing homes, and outpatient orthopedic settings—practice areas in which a large number of elderly patients are treated.

PHYSICIAN ASSISTANTS

OVERVIEW

*Physician assistants (PAs) pro-
vide medical care that ranges
from basic primary health care
to specialty and surgical procedures.* They work under the
supervision of physicians.
Physician assistants work in
almost all medical and surgical
specialties and in every medical setting. Thirty-two percent
of PAs specialize in primary
care medicine, according to
the American Academy of
Physician Assistants (AAPA).
Other popular practice areas
include surgical subspecialties
(27 percent), emergency
medicine (11 percent), and
internal medicine subspecialties (10 percent). A minimum
of a master's degree in physician assisting is required to
work in the field. According to
the AAPA, there are more than 93,000 practicing physician assistants
(PAs) in the United States. Employment for PAs is expected to be excellent during the next decade.

THE JOB

The emergency room is filled to capacity, with many more patients waiting
to be triaged. A boy with a possible broken arm, an elderly woman with a
bad case of the flu, and a young woman having an asthma attack are just a
few of the cases that the emergency room staff is facing. With the help of
a physician assistant, patients with less-critical cases are seen, diagnosed,
treated, and, hopefully, sent home. Physician assistants play an important
role in these situations. They help speed the flow of patients through the
emergency department. But PAs don't just work in emergency rooms.

Wherever there are patients in need of health services, there are physician assistants to provide key support to physicians.

PAs are trained to provide diagnostic, therapeutic, and preventive health care services, working under the supervision of physicians. When taking a new case, they consider the patient's medical history—what medicines the patient is currently taking, his or her family medical history, and all presenting symptoms and complaints. They give the patient a complete examination and, depending on the patient's symptoms, order blood work and other laboratory tests or diagnostic procedures such as x-rays, MRIs, or CT scans. With such information, PAs are able to make a diagnosis and begin to treat the patient's condition. PAs prescribe the proper medication or refer the patient to a physician for further evaluation. PAs can prescribe medications in all 50 states, the District of Columbia, Guam, and the Commonwealth of the Northern Mariana Islands. In the majority of employment settings, prescriptions and laboratory test requests written by the PA must be evaluated and approved by the attending physician. PAs working in the inner city or in a rural setting may not be constantly supervised by a physician. They sometimes may be the sole care provider in the clinic. Such settings may have physicians present only some days of the week or for only a few hours a day. In these cases, the PA is responsible for seeing patients and conferring with medical physicians as needed or as dictated by state law.

Learn More About It

Ballweg, Ruth, Edward M. Sullivan, et al. *Physician Assistant: A Guide to Clinical Practice.* 5th ed. Philadelphia: W.B. Saunders, 2013.

Rodican, Andrew J. *The Ultimate Guide to Getting into Physician Assistant School.* 4th ed. New York: McGraw-Hill Education, 2017.

Wittner, Seth. *True Tales from a Physician Assistant.* Seattle: CreateSpace, 2015.

PAs also practice preventive health care services by counseling patients about health care issues. They advise patients on potential side affects or adverse reactions from certain medications. When diagnosing a patient with hypertension, for example, a PA may give nutritional advice such as limiting salt intake, changing dietary habits, and participating in cardiovascular exercise, as well as continuing to take prescribed medications.

PAs can also perform certain procedures, depending on their area of specialty. When working in an orthopedic practice setting, for example, PAs can apply a splint to a badly sprained finger or cast a fractured elbow. In a pediatric setting, PAs can suture a child's facial laceration. PAs working in a dermatological office can perform procedures ranging from wart excisions to medical and cosmetic Botox injections, as well as lipodissolve treatments.

Many PAs choose to practice in a surgical setting. When conducting pre-operative care, PAs take patient histories, record vital signs, and handle other tasks that prepare the patient for the surgical procedure. During major surgery, PAs may work as the first or second assistant to the surgeon. Their duties, depending on the type of surgery, could include placing indwelling catheters and tubes such as Foley catheters, intravenous lines, or arterial lines. They may also be called on to assist in the closure of the surgical incision. PAs may be responsible for post-operative care of their patient. Duties include the insertion or removal of lines and catheters and chest tubes or changing dressings and bandages. PAs also answer questions from patients and their families regarding the patient's status after the surgery.

Nursing homes, assisted-living communities, and long-term rehabilitation centers are other settings in which PAs practice. In these settings, PAs conduct weekly or monthly assessments of geriatric patients (many of whom have chronic conditions); monitor prescription medicines, nutrition, or any needed inpatient therapy; and order outpatient services or tests. They start treatment on any new illnesses or injuries common with their patients' age group, such as pneumonia, pressure sores, heart problems, or even dementia. If working with patients in rehab, PAs monitor the types of exercise programs used or track the progress of therapy sessions. Some PAs, especially those working in rural areas, make house calls. Whether making a monthly patient assessment at a nursing home, a house visit, or daily rounds at a hospital, PAs must report back to their attending physician and give their findings and recommendations.

PAs also have administrative duties. Charting—writing or electronically recording information regarding the patient's conditions, findings, and any recommended treatment—is part of the job, no matter the physician assistant's specialty. Some PAs order the office or clinic's medical supplies or equipment such as stethoscopes, syringes, vaccines, drugs, and culture kits. They meet with drug representatives or medical supply salespeople to discuss new drugs and equipment. Some PAs, especially those working in a large clinical practice, train and supervise medical technicians and assistants.

Full-time physician assistants work about 40 hours a week, including evenings, weekends, and overnight shifts.

REQUIREMENTS

HIGH SCHOOL

Recommended high school classes include those in anatomy and physiology, biology, chemistry, mathematics, English, speech, computer science, health, psychology, nutrition, the social sciences, and statistics.

POSTSECONDARY TRAINING

A minimum of a master's degree in physician assisting is required to work in the field. The American Academy of Physician Assistants reports that the average PA program takes 26.5 months to complete. Typical courses in the first year of study include Anatomy and Physiology, Biochemistry, Clinical Laboratory, Clinical Medicine, Medical Ethics, Microbiology, Pathology, and Pharmacology. Second-year classes include Emergency Medicine, Family Medicine, Geriatric Medicine, Internal Medicine, Obstetrics/Gynecology, Orthopedics, Pediatrics, Psychiatry, Radiology, and Surgery. Students also complete clinical rotations in these various practice areas.

Nearly 220 physician assistant training programs in the United States are accredited by the Accreditation Review Commission on Education for the Physician Assistant (www.arc-pa.org/accreditation/accredited-programs). Associate, baccalaureate, and master's degree programs in physician assisting are available.

The Physician Assistant Education Association offers the Central Application Service for Physician Assistants, a Web-based application service that allows students to apply to more than one program by using the same application. Visit https://caspa.liaisoncas.com/applicant-ux for more information.

Physician assistants can also attend postgraduate educational programs in internal medicine, surgery, pediatrics, neonatology, rural primary care, emergency medicine, and occupational medicine.

CERTIFICATION AND LICENSING

All states and jurisdictions require physician assistants to pass the Physician Assistant National Certifying Examination, which is administered by the National Commission on Certification of Physician Assistants. Applicants must have graduated from an accredited physician assistant training program. Those who become certified can use the title, physician assistant-certified.

OTHER REQUIREMENTS

Hospital and clinical settings often include many different health care workers. PAs must be team players and be able to work with a variety of workers and personalities. They should have excellent communication skills to interact well with patients and coworkers. Since medical technology is ever changing, PAs must be willing to continue to learn throughout their careers. They often attend seminars, conventions, or continuing-education classes as a requirement for licensure. Other important traits for physician assistants include emotional stability, the ability to make decisions under pressure, a desire to serve others, and compassion for people who are in pain or other discomfort.

EXPLORING

There are many ways to learn more about a career as a physician assistant. You can read books and magazines about the field, visit the websites of college physician assisting programs to learn about typical classes and possible career paths, and ask your teacher or school counselor to arrange an information interview with a physician assistant. Professional associations can

Did You Know?

From 2014 to 2024, 11 of the top 20 jobs adding the most positions that require an associate's degree or postsecondary vocational award are in the health care industry. They are:

✔ Nursing Aides: +262,000 jobs
✔ Medical Assistants: +138,900 jobs
✔ Licensed Practical Nurses: +117,300 jobs
✔ Dental Assistants: +58,600 jobs
✔ Emergency Medical Technicians: +58,500 jobs
✔ Dental Hygienists: +37,400 jobs
✔ Massage Therapists: +36,500 jobs
✔ Physical Therapist Assistants: +31,900 jobs
✔ Medical Records and Health Information Technicians: +29,000 jobs
✔ Medical and Clinical Laboratory Technicians: +29,000 jobs
✔ Phlebotomists: +28,100 jobs

Source: U.S. Department of Labor

also provide information about the field. The American Academy of Physician Assistants (AAPA) provides information on education and careers at its website, www.aapa.org/career. Many professional associations also have a presence on social media. For example, the AAPA has Twitter, LinkedIn, Instagram, YouTube, and Facebook pages at which you can learn more about the career of physician assistants and association events.

Try to land a part-time job in a medical office. This will give you a chance to interact with physician assistants and see if the career is a good fit for your interests and abilities.

EMPLOYERS

There are more than 93,000 practicing physician assistants in the United States, according to the American Academy of Physician Assistants (AAPA). The AAPA reports that nearly 26 percent of physician assistants work at hospitals. Other major employers include single-specialty physician group practices, 26.1 percent; multi-specialty physician groups, 10.3 percent; and solo physician practices, 9.4 percent.

GETTING A JOB

Many physician assistants obtain their first jobs as a result of contacts made through college internships or clinical rotations, career fairs, or networking events. Others seek assistance in obtaining job leads from newspaper want ads, college career services offices, and employment websites. Additionally, the American Academy of Physician Assistants (AAPA) provides job listings at its website, www.aapa.org/career. Student and professional members of the AAPA can participate in Huddle, the organization's members-only online community for sharing ideas and networking. Those interested in positions with the federal government should visit the U.S. Office of Personnel Management's website, www.usajobs.gov.

ADVANCEMENT

Physician assistants advance by receiving pay raises and managerial responsibilities. Some pursue postgraduate education and become specialists in internal medicine, emergency medicine, and other areas. Other physician assistants continue their education to become physicians or college professors.

EARNINGS

Salaries for physician assistants vary by type of employer, geographic region, and the worker's experience, education, and skill level. Salaries for physician assistants ranged from less than $62,760 to $139,540 or more in May 2015, according to the U.S. Department of Labor.

Full-time clinically practicing PAs had mean annual incomes of $93,800 in 2014, according to the American Academy of Physician Assistants (AAPA). In 2008, PAs earned the following median annual salaries by practice area: cardiovascular and cardiothoracic surgery ($117,000), interventional radiology ($105,500), emergency medicine ($102,960), and pediatric surgery ($102,500).

Physician assistants usually receive benefits such as health and life insurance, vacation days, sick leave, and a savings and pension plan. Part-time workers must provide their own benefits. The AAPA reports that, in 2014, more than 50 percent of all PAs "received monetary bonuses and more than 75 percent of PAs received some other form of additional compensation, such as research stipends, profit sharing, student loan repayment, paid relocation, tuition reimbursement, or signing bonuses."

FOR MORE INFORMATION

For more information on educational programs and careers, contact
American Academy of Physician Assistants
aapa@aapa.org
www.aapa.org

To learn more about certification, contact
National Commission on Certification of Physician Assistants
678-417-8100
www.nccpa.net

For information on accredited educational programs, contact
Physician Assistant Education Association
info@paeaonline.org
www.paeaonline.org

To learn more about career opportunities in Canada, contact
Canadian Association of Physician Assistants
https://capa-acam.ca

EMPLOYMENT OUTLOOK

Employment for physician assistants is expected to grow much faster than the average for all careers during the next decade, according to the U.S. Department of Labor. Physician assistants are in strong demand as a result of the growing U.S. population and the health care industry's attempts to contain costs (physician assistants are a cost-effective alternative to physicians). Opportunities will be best in rural and inner-city health care facilities. In addition to jobs in traditional office-based settings, an increasing number of opportunities will be available in hospitals, public clinics, academic medical centers, and prisons.

Interview: Lara Mack

Lara Mack is an emergency medicine physician assistant in Chicago, Illinois. She has worked in the field for six years.

Q. What made you want to enter this career?

A. I was always interested in biology, and in college I was a biology major with a public health policy focus. I didn't think I wanted to practice clinically, until I spent a week in the hospital with my little sister when she had spinal fusion surgery for scoliosis. I realized I was fascinated with everything that was happening around me. Her 12-year-old roommate had had a stroke. I read about everything I encountered and realized I wanted to learn more. I spoke to a family friend, an orthopedic surgeon, who told me about the career.

Q. What is one thing that young people may not know about the field?

A. I'm not sure if this stands true today, but young people may not even know the field exists. This is not a career path I knew was a possibility until I had graduated from college. Working as a physician assistant is great because you can do what the docs do with much less schooling. Of course, the ultimate paycheck is also less.

Q. What are the most important personal and professional skills for emergency medicine PAs?

A. Some of the most important skills are being smart, organized, and able to prioritize. You also need to have compassion—that's more of a character trait than a skill. This is basically the customer service industry, but for patients. You have to balance many tasks at once, do the most urgent thing first, while keeping all of your patients happy and healthy. It is definitely a career for someone who can handle a fast-paced work environment.

Q. What are some of the pros and cons of your job?

A. Pros: You get to be a part of an interdisciplinary team working to care for patients. You work very closely with doctors, nurses, techs, and pharmacists to treat a patient. Many jobs require only three or four days a week of work. The work is fast-paced and shifts go by quickly. Often, patients' stories are entertaining.

Cons: We are open 24 hours a day. There are some undesirable shift times including weekends and holidays. Being very busy can lead to burnout.

Interview: Kara D. Larson

Kara D. Larson, MSPAS, PA-C, a physician assistant and a member of the American Academy of Physician Assistants' Judicial Affairs Commission

Q. What made you want to enter this career?

A. I wanted to practice medicine since my seventh-grade life science course. That was the easy decision; the hard decision was what medical career was right for me. Going into college, I labored over the decision between a nursing or pre-med major. After much time comparing both fields, I realized I was more interested in the medical decision-making of taking care of a patient and chose pre-med.

When I graduated from college, I again was faced with a tough decision: medical school or physician assistant (PA) school. Both programs are fundamentally the same, learning multiple disease processes and their treatments while assimilating the vast number of patient skills. I chose to become a PA instead of a M.D., not because I couldn't handle the rigors of medical school, but because of the difference in lifestyle I would have as a physician assistant.

Becoming a PA takes 2.5 years after college whereas becoming an M.D. takes four years after college for medical school and then three to seven years of residency before you are prepared to enter the medical field. This shorter time frame for PA school, with a corresponding lower amount of student loans for repayment, made the profession very attractive to me. I had the ability to start working with a practice as well as start my family sooner without being overwhelmed with large loan repayments.

Another attractive aspect of the PA profession is the flexibility to work in various medical specialties. A physician must decide in medical school what specialty he will devote his entire life to, whereas a PA has the ability to work in different specialties throughout his career. Also, the PA shares the pressure of being the "final decision-maker." A PA works within the medical team, making decisions together with the physician and always has the ability to consult with his supervising physician for final decisions.

Q. What is one thing that young people may not know about a career as a physician assistant?

A. Young people may have encountered PAs in the primary care fields (family practice, pediatrics, women's health) as their health care providers. Therefore, they may not be aware that PAs practice in such diverse specialties as emergency medicine, internal medicine, neurology, dermatology, multiple surgical specialties, and many others. Numerous fields are open to PAs, leading to a wonderful career in which they will never be bored!

Q. If you could do anything differently in preparing for your career in college/high school, what would it be?

A. I would shadow PAs in various specialties for a better understanding of the flexibility of PAs throughout the medical field. I didn't understand this flexibility (a great plus for the profession) until I was on clinical rotations during PA school.

Q. Can you please describe a day in your life on the job?

A. I work in a family medicine/urgent care office with two physicians and two other PAs. We work 12-hour shifts, with two days on and two days off. I begin my day by looking over lab and x-ray reports from my last shift, determining if a patient needs to return to discuss lab results and have more testing or if the nurse on duty should notify the patient of normal results.

At 8 A.M. patients are triaged and placed in exam rooms. Our office does not take appointments, so I never know the next problem I will encounter, and I spend the next 12 hours treating complaints ranging from sore throat to chest pain to prescription refills, charting as I go and seeing patients of all ages and stages. I spend the day ordering and interpreting labs and x-rays and writing numerous prescriptions for antibiotics, diabetes and high blood pressure medicine, and pain medicine, as well as sometimes just reassuring a patient that his or her symptoms will subside with just a little bit of time and patience.

As a part of the practice we see many urgent-care cases, so I get lots of opportunities to suture lacerations, cast broken bones, and drain abscesses. I work alongside my supervising physician but have autonomy in my work. The physician is there for help when I need it for a difficult patient scenario, but I am not required to have his approval for my plan or to have

> "Compassion is the number-one quality for all physician assistants. It is the source of all other qualities exhibited by the best physician assistants."

him sign my chart or prescriptions. I may go through the entire day without needing consultation or may have several complicated patients requiring his assistance. In these cases, we always work as a team, making the best decision together. Though I have a large amount of autonomy during the day, I must always remember one of the most important pieces of information I learned in PA school: "Know what you don't know and when you need help." At the end of a normal day I've seen and treated 20-30 patients. I'm tired, but I always finish with the overwhelming satisfaction of having made a difference.

Q. What are the most important personal and professional qualities for people in your career?

A. Compassion is the number-one quality for all PAs. It is the source of all other qualities exhibited by the best PAs. It is the guide during the difficult days of school when you feel like giving up the overwhelming task of learning the mountain of medical information. It is the quality that spurs you into studying and reading so you can provide the best information to your patients, and it is the quality that endears your patients to you.

Q. What are some of the pros and cons of your job?

A. Pros:

✔ Having the responsibility to guide patients and help them make life-changing decisions (a pro because of the amazing privilege).

✔ Building a relationship with patient and their families.

✔ Working in a growing profession—it's only headed up!

✔ Having the availability to work in multiple specialties. Physicians must decide in medical school which specialty they will work in for the rest of their lives; however, PAs are free to navigate the medical field and work in any specialty (family practice, neurology, surgery, etc.), with only on-the-job training required.

Cons:

✔ Having the amazing responsibility to guide patients and help them make life-changing decisions (a con because of the stress involved in decision-making).

✔ Long hours and very busy days. There is a shortage of medical providers, which leads to pressure to see a large number of patients per day, leading to less comprehensive care.

✔ Jobs in certain specialties are limited by the number of physicians who are entering the field, since PAs must work in a team with physicians.

Q.   What advice would you give to young people who are interested in becoming physician assistants?

A.   Study hard, and work harder! Due to the small number of PA schools compared to medical schools, as well as the exponential growth of the profession, admission is very competitive.

Shadow multiple PAs in various specialties and settings (i.e., hospital and outpatient) to understand how PAs function. The PA role is variable based on specialty. The family-practice PA is relatively autonomous, whereas the surgical PA may work closer to his supervising PA in the surgical setting.

> "Study hard, and work harder! Due to the small number of PA schools compared to medical schools, as well as the exponential growth of the profession, admission is very competitive."

If possible, work as a medical assistant or patient care technician in a hospital. This is not the most glamorous job (it involves bed changes and patient baths), but it will give you a glimpse into the health care setting as well as teach you basic skills. You will be ahead of your classmates if you already know how to take vital signs (blood pressure, pulse, respirations), start IVs, and perform blood-draws. This experience will help you develop one of the most important skills in medicine—patient assessment. Patient assessment is the ability to determine the overall condition of a patient with simple observation of external signs (i.e., the subtlety of determining breathing difficulty and ill-appearing features of patients). This skill cannot be taught; it is developed with experience.

PHYSICIANS

OVERVIEW

Physicians, also known as *doctors,* assess, diagnose, and treat patients of all ages and with many different conditions. Their methods of treatment may include prescribing medications and diagnostic tests, offering counseling on nutrition and exercise, and conducting surgery and other medical procedures. Many physicians specialize by focusing on a particular system, a part of the body, or patients in a particular age group. A medical degree is necessary to enter the field. Approximately 642,720 physicians are employed in the United States. Employment opportunities for physicians should be good during the next decade.

THE JOB

Physicians play an important role in our society. We rely on their knowledge of medical technology and treatment methods to help us when we are sick, or in order to stay healthy. There are two types of physicians: the

designation, M.D., for Doctor of Medicine, and D.O., for Doctor of Osteopathic Medicine. M.D.s, also known as *allopathic physicians,* use surgery and drugs to treat patients, while D.O.s, also known as *osteopathic physicians,* practice holistic patient care in addition to prescribing medicine and surgery. They pay special attention to the body's musculoskeletal system when examining patients and stress preventive medicine.

Physicians diagnosis illnesses, prescribe medications, and/or administer treatments. Sometimes they perform diagnostic tests to help confirm a diagnosis or refer patients to a *medical specialist* (such as an *oncologist* if they suspect that a patient has cancer) or laboratory for additional testing. Physicians may see patients suffering from injuries or pain, and they perform procedures ranging from suturing lacerations, to setting broken bones, to prescribing medications to help alleviate pain and discomfort. Physicians also counsel patients on health and may suggest dietary or lifestyle changes to improve their patients' conditions.

Cancer Doctors in Short Supply

The growing elderly population (which is often more susceptible to certain types of cancer), a rising number of cancer survivors, and a large number of predicted retirements by oncologists is expected to create a shortage of these medical specialists by 2025, according to a study by the *Journal of Oncology Practice*. In fact, the journal predicts a shortage of 2,258 oncologists by 2025.

In addition to encouraging more physicians to pursue careers in oncology, medical associations suggest the following steps to alleviate the predicted shortage: encouraging existing oncologists to continue to practice past the typical retirement age, improving the efficiency of oncologists via technology, and increasing the use of other health care professionals (such as general practitioners, physician assistants, and nurse practitioners) in oncology-related settings.

Some physicians are *primary care doctors,* providing a wide range of general services. They often have a group of long-term patients that they see on a regular basis. Primary care doctors see patients for a variety of reasons including wellness care, routine physicals and immunizations, and the treatment of minor injuries, infections, or diseases. If the patient has more specific health needs, primary care physicians will then refer him or her to a specialist. Some examples of primary care doctors are those practicing *family and general medicine, internal medicine,* and *pediatrics. Family and general medicine practitioners* are typically the first physician practitioners an individual sees when ill or injured. They diagnose and treat a wide variety of illnesses or injuries—from broken bones, to the flu, to respiratory infections. *General internists* treat problems that affect the internal organ systems, such as the liver, stomach, kidneys, and digestive tract. *General pediatricians* provide health care services to infants, children, teens, and young adults.

Physician specialists are trained to focus on a particular system or part of the body. Some specialties, especially those involving surgery or other procedures, require additional training during residency or fellowship.

Specialists work with primary care doctors in treating patients for a particular medical condition, or for complete care throughout life. Examples of medical specialties include *neurology, obstetrics and gynecology, anesthesiology,* and *orthopedic surgery.*

The following paragraphs detail some of the largest medical specialties:

Anesthesiologists are specially trained in anesthesia and peri-operative medicine. They treat patients before, during, and after surgery or any other medical procedure that requires anesthesia. Before a surgery begins, anesthesiologists assess the patient and consult with the surgical team to create an anesthesiology plan customized for the patient's needs. They take into account airway management and provisions for pain management. During surgery, they administer anesthesia and monitor the patient's vital life functions—heart rate, blood pressure, body temperature, and breathing. After surgery, they make sure the patient is stabilized and monitor him or her for any adverse reactions to the anesthesia.

Dermatologists treat conditions and diseases of the skin, scalp, hair, and nails. They treat patients suffering from conditions ranging from acne to cancerous lesions.

Emergency medicine physicians, also known as *emergency room physicians,* are specially trained to care for patients with illnesses or injuries that require immediate medical attention. Emergency medicine covers the field of general medicine, but it also involves practically all fields of medicine, surgery, and surgical sub-specialties. Emergency medicine physicians diagnose, treat, and stabilize patients with conditions ranging from lacerations to heart attacks. They may also treat patients suffering from injuries caused by sports or trauma (such as a car accident or a gunshot wound). Some emergency physicians also train staff members regarding cardiopulmonary resuscitation, advanced cardiac life support, and advanced trauma life support. Some participate in mock disaster drills with other health care professionals in order to be ready when a real emergency occurs.

In the 1990s, a movement to introduce medical professionals who focused solely on the care of hospital inpatients began. These physicians are known as *hospitalists.* Since that time, there has been much debate about whether their existence is a good thing. But one thing is certain: their numbers are growing, from approximately 800 in 1990 to more than 35,000 today, partly due to the increasing number of people admitted to hospitals nationwide and partly due to the movement to reform health care. Ninety-eight percent of large hospitals (200+ beds) employ hospitalists, according to the Society of Hospital Medicine (SHM) which provides a wealth of information about the field at www.hospitalmedicine.org). Hospitalists are doctors who work only in hospitals. They take over for primary care physicians or internists who have to juggle their inpatient and outpatient workloads. In addition to patient care, hospitalists handle administrative tasks such as ordering tests and medications and ensuring that their orders are carried out correctly, filling out paperwork that details patient care, and overseeing patient discharge. Approximately 82.1 percent of practicing hospitalists are trained in general internal medicine, 17.2 percent in family practice, and 0.7 percent in geriatric medicine, according to the SHM.

Obstetricians and gynecologists (OB/GYNs) are responsible for the general health of women. They also provide care related to pregnancy and the reproductive system. OB/GYNs give patients annual physicals and important tests such as Pap smears or breast exams. They try to catch early occurrences of cancer in the breast, cervix, or reproductive system. OB/GYNs also specialize in prenatal care, delivery, and postnatal care.

Psychiatrists are trained in the study and treatment of mental disorders. Their patient assessment includes a mental status examination and compilation of case history. Diagnostic tests may be prescribed, including neuroimaging and other neurophysiological techniques. Psychiatrists can prescribe treatments such as medication, psychotherapy, or transcranial magnetic stimulation. Depending on the severity of the patient's condition, treatment can be conducted during hospitalization or on an outpatient basis.

Radiologists are specially trained to take and interpret medical images. Through the use of x-rays, radioactive substances, sound waves, or the body's natural magnetism, radiologists can determine the presence and severity of injuries and diseases. Some radiologists sub-specialize in a particular area of the body or system, such as head and neck radiology or breast imaging. Others sub-specialize in interventional radiology, which allows them to treat patients with minimally invasive interventional techniques. Angioplasty, angiography, stent placement, and biopsy procedures are some examples of interventional radiology techniques.

Surgeons specialize in the treatment of injury or disease through surgical procedures. Physicians perform general surgery or may specialize in surgery on a specific area of the body or system. For example, *orthopedic surgeons* perform procedures related to the musculoskeletal system, *neurosurgeons* specialize in surgical procedures on the brain and nervous system, and *cardiothoracic surgeons* specialize in conducting surgeries on the chest, heart, and lungs. Other surgical specialists include *otolaryngologists* (treatment and surgery for conditions or injuries to the ear, nose, and throat) and *plastic or reconstructive surgeons.*

Physicians, regardless of their specialty, have additional duties including charting patients' progress and treatments; consulting with other physicians, health care workers, and patients and their families; and participating in staff meetings. Depending on the size and scope of their medical practice, some physicians may be responsible for other office management duties including billing, staff education, and administrative tasks. Some physicians, especially those employed by university or teaching hospitals, may supervise, train, and mentor medical students, interns, and residents. Some physicians also teach at medical schools or conduct scientific research and publish their findings in medical journals or other scholarly publications. Physicians sometimes provide expert testimony in legal proceedings.

Physicians work in hospitals, private offices, or clinics. Certain specialties, such as family medicine, pediatrics, or obstetrics/gynecology, lend themselves to private practice, while others—such as radiology, emergency medicine, and urology—are practiced in physician groups, hospitals, or other health care settings.

Physicians work in clean and sterile conditions. Their uniform consists of either hospital scrubs and gown, or other professional attire. They are often aided by a staff of other health care professionals such as nurses, physician assistants, nurse aides, therapists, technicians, and medical secretaries. Their days are often stressful; physicians can expect to work with multiple patients with varying degrees of illness.

Many physicians work long and irregular hours. More than 40 percent of all doctors working in the United States log 50 or more hours a week, including evening, weekend, and holiday hours. Depending on their specialty, physicians are "on call" day and night and deal with many patient complaints or emergencies outside the office.

REQUIREMENTS

HIGH SCHOOL

You will need to study for many years before you can become a physician. In high school, take a college-preparatory track that includes as many science classes as possible (especially chemistry, biology, and anatomy and physiology), as well as courses in mathematics, computer science, psychology, English, speech, foreign languages (especially Latin), and social studies.

POSTSECONDARY TRAINING

A medical degree is necessary to enter the field. Preparation for this career is very demanding. Medical students must complete eight years of training after high school, plus three to eight years of internship and residency. Applying to and succeeding in medical school can be challenging. Aspiring medical students must also take and pass the very demanding Medical College Admission Test (https://students-residents.aamc.org/applying-medical-school/taking-mcat-exam), a national examination that is administered by the Association of American Medical Colleges (AAMC). To assist students in this process, the AAMC has developed the following publications and websites:

✔ *The Road to Becoming a Doctor:*
www.aamc.org/download/68806/data/road-doctor.pdf

✔ *Navigate Your Journey from Pre-Med Through Residency:* https://students-residents.aamc.org

✔ Aspiring Docs Diaries: http://aspiringdocsdiaries.org

Approximately 65 percent of medical school applicants major in biology or another physical science at the undergraduate or graduate levels. Others major in pre-med.

More medical schools are reaching out to students with nonscience backgrounds, including those in the humanities. By accepting students from nonscience backgrounds, medical schools are trying to create more well-rounded students "who can be molded into caring and analytical doctors," according to an article about the trend in *Newsweek*.

Nearly 150 medical schools in the United States are accredited by the Liaison Committee on Medical Education, which accredits M.D. medical education programs. The American Osteopathic Association accredits colleges that award a D.O. degree. It has accredited 33 schools at 48 teaching locations.

A Statistical Snapshot of Medical School Applicants and Enrollees

✔ 88,304 people were enrolled in medical school in 2016-17—an increase of about 7 percent in 2012-13.

✔ Forty-eight percent of students were female in 2016-17.

✔ In 2015, the total number of applicants to medical school increased by 6.2 percent to 52,550, double the percentage increase from the previous year. First-time applicants—an important indicator of interest in medicine—grew by 4.8 percent to 38,460.

Source: Association of American Medical Colleges

According to the AAMC, a typical medical school curriculum is as follows: Year 1—biochemistry, cell biology, medical genetics, gross anatomy, structure and function of the organ systems, neuroscience, and immunology; Year 2—infectious diseases, pharmacology, pathology, clinical diagnoses and therapeutics, and health law; Years 3 and 4—generalist core (family and community medicine, obstetrics and gynecology, surgery, etc.), neurology, psychiatry, subspecialty segment (anesthesia, dermatology, orthopedics, urology, radiology, ophthalmology, otolaryngology), continuity-of-care segment (sub internships, emergency room and intensive-care experiences), and electives.

As they approach their fourth year of school, medical students choose a specialty area in which they want to practice and begin applying to graduate medical education programs, which are known as residencies. Students obtain residencies through the National Resident Matching Program (www.nrmp.org). Residencies can last anywhere from three to seven years depending on the specialty.

Students who plan to conduct biomedical research often attend joint M.D./Ph.D. programs. In these programs, which typically last seven or eight years, students learn the research skills that will help them as scientists and the clinical skills that will allow them to practice medicine. Visit

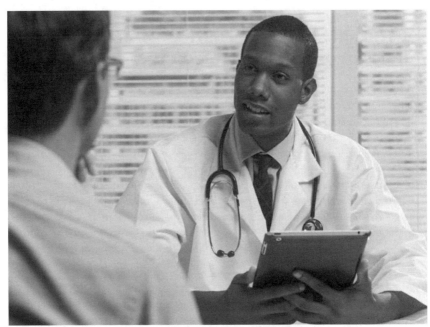

A pediatrician talks with a patient about proper nutrition. (DPC)

https://students-residents.aamc.org to learn more about M.D./Ph.D. dual degree training.

Medical school tuition is high. The AAMC reports that the average annual cost of tuition, fees, and health insurance at state medical schools in 2016-17 was $34,592 for state residents and $58,668 for non-residents. At private schools, tuition and fees averaged $55,534 for residents and $56,862 for non-resident students. Housing and living expenses were not included in these figures. A number of private and government financial aid programs are available to help students pay for medical school. Visit the websites of the associations in the For More Information section for details.

Certification and Licensing

Physicians can earn voluntary board certification in a variety of medical specialties. They must participate in medical residencies and pass an examination by a member board of the American Osteopathic Association or the American Board of Medical Specialties.

Once they complete their medical training, physicians must take an examination in order to be licensed to practice medicine. Licensing is required in all 50 states and U.S. territories. The board of medical examiners in each state administers the examinations.

Other Requirements

Physicians must be able to think quickly and clearly and must stay calm—especially when dealing with patient emergencies. Good bedside manners

A Closer Look: Alternative and Complementary Medicine

A growing number of Western medical doctors, therapists, counselors, and other health care professionals are incorporating alternative and complementary medicine into their practices, often prescribing or recommending alternative or complementary therapies or dietary supplements in conjunction with traditional Western medical treatments. Disciplines such as acupuncture, massage therapy, and herbal medicine are now grouped under the umbrella term of complementary and alternative medicine (CAM), which is sometimes also referred to as integrative medicine. CAM is usually grouped into four main categories: natural products, energy medicine, manipulative practices, and mind-body medicine. More than 33 percent of adults reported having used a complementary health approach in 2012 (the most recent year for which data is available), according to the National Center for Health Statistics.

While the CAM movement is only now gaining in popularity with the U.S. medical community, holistic medicine has been practiced for almost a thousand years throughout the world. Why are Western doctors jumping on board considering they were among the biggest skeptics only a decade or so ago? While they still believe that the effectiveness of CAM practices must be confirmed via scientific study and research, they also now understand the benefits of combining proven CAM therapies with traditional Western medical approaches. For example, if a patient suffers from chronic back pain, a doctor might prescribe pain medicine as well as suggest breathing exercises, acupuncture, or massage therapy. Others may hold off on prescribing prescription medicine to treat diarrhea or headaches, first suggesting dietary changes or vitamin or herbal supplements. Doctors also believe in using CAM as a preventive measure. They may recommend exercise and nutritional changes to help patients prevent heart disease or high blood pressure.

A better understanding and continued use of CAM is expected, especially since the National Center for Complementary and Integrative Health is continuing to fund grants for CAM research.

Contact the following organizations for more information on careers in CAM:

- ✔ **Academy of Integrative Health & Medicine:** www.aihm.org
- ✔ **American Association of Integrative Medicine:** www.aaimedicine.com
- ✔ **American Association of Naturopathic Physicians:** www.naturopathic.org
- ✔ **American Herbalists Guild:** www.americanherbalistsguild.com
- ✔ **American Holistic Health Association:** http://ahha.org
- ✔ **National Association for Holistic Aromatherapy:** www.naha.org
- ✔ **National Ayurvedic Medical Association:** www.ayurvedanama.org

are a must—meaning physicians should have empathy toward their patients' conditions, be good listeners, and be able to have a kind and sincere disposition when counseling patients and their families.

EXPLORING

One good way to learn more about a career as a physician is to read books about the field. Here is one suggestion: *White Coat Wisdom,* by Stephen J. Busalacchi (Apollo's Voice, 2011). You can also visit the websites of medical schools to learn about typical classes and medical specialties, and you can ask your teacher or school counselor to arrange an information interview with a physician or talk to your doctor about his or her career. Professional associations are good sources of information for aspiring physicians. For example, the Association of American Medical Colleges (AAMC) offers AspiringDocs.org (www.aspiringdocs.org), which aims to increase diversity in medicine. It also offers an annual career fair for students who are interested in learning more about careers in medicine. Visit the AAMC website for more information. Additionally, the American Medical Association provides a wealth of information at its website, www.ama-assn.org. You should also try to land a part-time job in a doctor's office. This will give you a chance to interact with physicians and see if the career is a good fit for your interests and abilities.

EMPLOYERS

Approximately 642,720 physicians are employed in the United States. About 47 percent of physicians and surgeons work in medical offices. Thirty percent are employed by hospitals. Other physicians are employed by government agencies, schools, correctional facilities, and outpatient care centers. Approximately 9 percent are self-employed.

According to the American Medical Association, the following medical areas employed the most physicians: internal medicine, 20.1 percent; family medicine/general practice, 12.4 percent; pediatrics, 9.6 percent; obstetrics and gynecology, 5.6 percent; anesthesiology, 5.5 percent; psychiatry, 5.2 percent; general surgery, 5.0 percent; and emergency medicine, 4.1 percent.

GETTING A JOB

Many physicians obtain their first jobs as a result of contacts made during their residencies. Others seek assistance in obtaining job leads from medical school career services offices, newspaper want ads, and employment websites. Some professional associations, such as the American Academy of Family Physicians, provide job listings at their websites. See For More Information for a list of organizations. Job listings can also be found at the *Journal of the American Medical Association*'s website, www.jamacareercenter.com. Some new graduates start their own solo private practices, enter into a partnership with other physicians, or enter into a group practice. Those interested in positions with federal agencies—such as the Veterans Health Administration and Indian Health Service—should visit www.usajobs.gov.

ADVANCEMENT

Physicians advance by assuming managerial duties, by becoming experts in their medical specialty, or by opening their own practices. Some physicians become medical administrators or college professors.

EARNINGS

Salaries for physicians vary by type of employer, geographic region, and the employee's experience level, specialty, and skills. The U.S. Department of Labor (USDL) reports the following mean annual earnings for physicians by specialty in May 2015:

- ✔ anesthesiology, $258,100;
- ✔ family and general practice, $192,120;
- ✔ internal medicine, $196,520;
- ✔ obstetrics/gynecology, $222,400;
- ✔ pediatrics, $183,180;
- ✔ psychiatry, $193,680; and
- ✔ surgery, $247,520.

Mean annual salaries for physicians and surgeons, not otherwise classified were $197,700. Some physicians earned less than $57,820.

While work in these careers is lucrative, earnings are offset by high medical malpractice insurance and the higher-than-average number of hours worked.

Employers offer a variety of benefits, including the following: medical, dental, and life insurance; paid holidays, vacations, and sick and personal days; 401(k) plans; profit-sharing plans; retirement and pension plans; and educational assistance programs. Physicians who own their own practices or who are in a partnership with other doctors must provide their own benefits.

EMPLOYMENT OUTLOOK

Employment opportunities for physicians should be good during the next decade. The rapidly growing U.S. population, the predicted doubling of the number of people over age 65 between 2000 and 2030, rising expectations about the quality and ready availability of health care services, an aging physician workforce, the increasing availability of health insurance as a result of health insurance reform, a trend toward reduced hours for physicians, and an expected wave of retirements of doctors in the next decade have created a potential physician shortage in coming years, according to the Association of American Medical Colleges, which predicts that there will be a shortage of 61,700-94,700 doctors by 2025. Here's an overview of the expected shortfall:

FOR MORE INFORMATION

For information on accredited post-M.D. and -D.O. medical training programs in the United States, visit the council's website.
**Accreditation Council
for Graduate Medical Education**
312-755-5000
www.acgme.org

For information on family medicine, contact
**American Academy
of Family Physicians**
800-274-2237
aafp@aafp.org
www.aafp.org

To read the *Osteopathic Medical College Information Book,* and for information on careers and financial aid, visit the AACOM website.
**American Association of Colleges
of Osteopathic Medicine (AACOM)**
301-968-4100
www.aacom.org

To learn more about board certification, contact
American Board of Medical Specialties
312-436-2600
www.abms.org

For comprehensive information on medical education and careers, contact
American Medical Association
800-621-8335
www.ama-assn.org

To learn more about osteopathic medicine, contact
American Osteopathic Association
800-621-1773
www.osteopathic.org

For information on accredited medical schools in the U.S. and Canada, contact
**Association of
American Medical Colleges**
202-828-0400
www.aamc.org

Bureau of Health Workforce
U.S. Department of Health and Human Services
http://bhpr.hrsa.gov

To learn more about the career of hospitalist, contact
Society of Hospital Medicine
800-843-3360
www.hospitalmedicine.org

For information on career opportunities in Canada, contact
Canadian Medical Association
www.cma.ca

✔ Primary Care Physicians Shortage: 12,500 to 31,100
✔ Non-Primary Care Physicians Shortage: 28,200 to 63,700
  —Medical Specialists Shortage: 5,100 to 12,300
  —Surgical Specialists Shortage: 23,100 to 31,600
  —Other Specialists Shortage: 2,400 to 20,200.

Physicians who are willing to work in rural and low-income areas will have the best job prospects. Opportunities will also be good for physicians who specialize in caring for the elderly because this segment of the population is growing rapidly and its members require more medical care than people in other demographics. As a result, demand for geriatricians, cardiologists, and oncologists will be strong.

RADIOLOGIC TECHNICIANS AND TECHNOLOGISTS

OVERVIEW

Radiologic technicians operate and maintain x-ray machinery and equipment, while *radiologic technologists* perform more complicated diagnostic imaging procedures such as magnetic resonance imaging scans and computed tomography scans. They are sometimes referred to as *radiographers*. Educational requirements vary by specialty, but radiologic technicians and technologists typically require education ranging from a certificate to a bachelor's degree to enter the field. There are more than 325,000 radiologic technicians and technologists and related workers in the United States. Employment opportunities in the field are expected to be good during the next decade.

FAST FACTS

High School Subjects
Biology
Mathematics

Personal Skills
Helping
Technical

Minimum Education Level
Two-year training program at
a hospital or college

Salary Range
$38,000 to $56,000 to $100,000+

Employment Outlook
Faster than the average

O*NET-SOC
29-1124.00, 29-2032.00,
29-2033.00, 29-2034.00,
29-2099.06

NOC
3215, 3216

THE JOB

Radiologic technicians and technologists operate and maintain diagnostic imaging equipment and provide radiologists with detailed images used in the diagnosis and treatment of patients. Before starting a procedure, technicians and technologists first prepare the examining room. They make sure equipment is in working condition and ready for use and that all sterile and non-sterile supplies, including contrast materials, catheters, film, and chemicals, needed for the procedure are available. Equipment and supplies are determined by the types of images ordered by the physician.

When the patient arrives, technicians and technologists take a brief medical history, explain the procedure, and answer any questions the patient may have. Then they position the patient in order to achieve the best angle for exposure. They angle or adjust the height of instruments to concentrate on a particular area of the body. They use measuring sticks or tapes to gauge the thickness of the area to be imaged. Patients are draped with lead aprons or shields as a protective measure against radiation exposure. Technicians and technologists place x-ray film under the area, then expose and develop the film using film processors or use computer-generated methods to capture the image.

Technicians and technologists produce x-rays of proper density, detail, or contrast as presented in the physician's orders. They repeat exposures as needed, rejecting any work that does not meet established requirements or standards.

Radiologic technologists complete advanced training in order to operate and maintain equipment that produces more specialized images. They often specialize in one or more imaging modalities. The following paragraphs detail these specialties.

Bone densitometry technologists use special x-ray equipment to measure bone mineral density. Usual sites for this procedure include the wrist, spine, heel, or hip. Physicians use this information to determine if patients have or are at risk for osteoporosis, to track general bone loss, or for other reasons.

Cardiovascular-interventional technologists use biplane fluoroscopy (i.e., real time x-rays) and other techniques to guide small instruments, such as catheters, vena cava filters, or stents during interventional or therapeutic procedures. Examples of some procedures are angioplasty, embolizations, and biopsies, all minimally invasive treatments done to cure or alleviate symptoms of vascular disease, stroke, or cancer.

Computed tomography (CT) technologists use x-ray equipment that rotates around the patient during the imaging procedure to obtain cross sections, or slices, of a particular part of the body. Using a computer, these slices are stacked together, creating a three-dimensional image. Since the complete image allows a view of an organ's interior, physicians may order a CT to rule out possible brain hemorrhages or appendicitis, among other diseases and conditions.

Diagnostic medical sonographers use ultrasound equipment to obtain images of organs, tissues, and blood vessels in the body, or in the case of pregnancy, to assess the health and development of a fetus. This technology is increasingly being used to detect heart attacks and heart and vascular disease. Specialties in the field include abdominal, breast, echocardiography, neurosonography, obstetrics/gynecology, ophthalmology, pediatric echocardiography, and peripheral vascular doppler.

Magnetic resonance imaging technologists operate machinery that uses strong magnetic fields or radio frequency waves to image body tissues. These signals are measured by a computer and processed into a detailed three-dimensional image of a particular part of the patient's body. MRIs are often ordered to identify the extent of injury to the ligaments or locate tumors in the brain.

Mammographers operate special low-dose x-ray equipment that produces images of the breast. They complete comprehensive education and training, as mandated by federal law, namely the Mammography Quality Standards Act.

Job Growth in the Health Care Industry by Employment Sector, 2014-24

Home Health Care Services: +48 percent

Outpatient Care Centers: +41 percent

Offices of Other Health Practitioners: +38 percent

Offices of Physicians: +19 percent

Offices of Dentists: +17 percent

Source: U.S. Department of Labor

Nuclear medicine is used to diagnose, manage, treat, and prevent diseases. *Nuclear medicine technologists* use small amounts of radioactive materials, or radiopharmaceuticals, to obtain information about organs, tissues, or bones, and their degree of health. According to the American Society of Radiologic Technologists, common nuclear medicine applications include "diagnosis and treatment of hyperthyroidism (Graves' Disease), cardiac stress tests to analyze heart function, bone scans for orthopedic injuries, lung scans for blood clots, and liver and gall bladder procedures to diagnose abnormal functions or blockages." Nuclear medicine technologists prepare radiopharmaceutical solutions for patients to drink; once ingested, these images allow special cameras to create an image of a particular organ, bone, or tissue area. These solutions may also be administered by injection or other methods.

Some technologists, after additional training and much experience, work as part of the radiation oncology team. They help radiation oncologists, medical physicists, and nurses diagnose and treat many different types of cancers. *Medical dosimetrists* calculate and measure the dose of radiation delivered to the site of a tumor, using treatment plans developed by an oncologist. They use three-dimensional computer models to determine how and where to deliver the radiation. Before treatment begins, the dosimetrist runs computer simulations to ensure that his or her treatment plan will work as envisioned. Then the dosimetrist instructs the *radiation therapist* to deliver the radiation. Other duties for dosimetrists include documenting treatment plans, calibrating radiation oncology equipment, conducting research, and teaching medical dosimetry students at colleges and universities. Radiation therapists, using treatment plans developed by a radiation oncologist and medical dosimetrist, dispense targeted radiation doses to the patient's body. Repeated exposure to radiation doses often shrinks and destroys malignant sites or cancerous cells. Treatment duration varies for cancer patients, but it typically lasts three to five days a week for four to seven weeks.

Depending on the size of the office or practice, radiologic technicians and technologists may have additional duties including calling for equipment maintenance when needed, ordering additional supplies, scheduling work shifts, and handling other administrative duties.

Full-time radiologic technologists and technicians work about 40 hours a week. Some technologists and technicians work during the evenings, on weekends, and some may be on call to accommodate patients' needs. This job can be physically demanding, as technologists and technicians are on their feet most of the day. While most procedures are done in examining rooms, some are conducted at the patient's bedside using portable imaging equipment. Some travel is also required when working with home health patients. In these cases, portable diagnostic equipment is usually transported in vans or other large vehicles to the patient's home.

Radiologic technicians and technologists face an enhanced risk of exposure to radiation. Technologists and technicians wear protective lead aprons, gloves, and other shielding devices to minimize this hazard. Their work stations are located behind protective glass windows or doors to help alleviate exposure. Technicians and technologists wear badges that measure radiation levels in the radiation area, as well as keep detailed records on their cumulative lifetime exposure to radiation.

REQUIREMENTS

HIGH SCHOOL

In high school, take physics, algebra, anatomy and physiology, science, chemistry, and biology courses. Classes in English and speech will help you develop your communication skills, and computer science courses will help you become adept at using computers and software programs.

POSTSECONDARY TRAINING

Radiologic technologists must complete a minimum of two years of training at a hospital or a community college. An associate's degree is the most common educational award for technicians and technologists, although some earn bachelor's degrees.

Radiography, magnetic resonance, medical dosimetry, and radiation therapy educational programs are accredited by the Joint Review

Committee on Education in Radiologic Technology (www.jrcert.org/cert/Search.jsp). The Joint Review Committee on Education in Diagnostic Medical Sonography (www.jrcdms.org) and the Commission on Accreditation of Allied Health Education Programs (www.caahep.org/Find-An-Accredited-Program) accredit programs in diagnostic medical sonography. The Joint Review Committee on Education Programs in Nuclear Medicine Technology (http://jrcnmt.org) accredits nuclear medicine technology educational programs.

CERTIFICATION AND LICENSING

The American Registry of Radiologic Technologists (ARRT, www.arrt.org) offers certification to those who have graduated from an ARRT-approved program and pass an examination. The American Registry for Diagnostic Medical Sonography (www.ardms.org), the ARRT, and Cardiovascular Credentialing International (www.cci-online.org) offer certification to diagnostic medical sonographers. Certification for nuclear medicine technologists is offered by the ARRT and the Nuclear Medicine Technology Certification Board (www.nmtcb.org). The Medical Dosimetrist Certification Board (www.mdcb.org) awards certification to dosimetrists. Certification, while voluntary, is highly recommended. It is an excellent way to stand out from other job applicants and demonstrate your abilities to prospective employers.

Most states require radiologic technicians and technologists to be licensed. Licensing requirements vary by state and specialty. Contact your state's department of regulation for information on requirements in your state.

OTHER REQUIREMENTS

To be a successful radiologic technician or technologist, you should have excellent hand-eye coordination in order to effectively operate equipment and create quality images; physical stamina, since you will be on your feet for long periods of time and be required to turn and lift patients; and good communication skills because you will have to carefully explain procedures to patients and interact closely with doctors and other medical professionals to understand imaging procedures and treatment goals. You should also have compassion and empathy because you will often work with sick and sometimes scared or angry patients who need encouragement as they face health challenges. Other important traits for technicians and technologists include strong observation skills, an analytical mind, proficiency with computers and technology, and a willingness to continue to learn throughout your career.

EXPLORING

There are many ways to learn more about a career as a radiologic technician or technologist. You can read books and journals (such as *Radiologic Technology* and *Radiation Therapist,* www.asrt.org/main/news-research)

Health Care Information Technology Security Professionals in Demand

Rapid advances in the use of technology (e.g., electronic medical records, wearables, data analytics, health-monitoring devices, etc.) are making the delivery of health care easier and allowing medical facilities to collect more data about patient health. But the collection of this data, and the wide variety of technologies used to do so, are creating data security nightmares for health care executives. These fears were recently reinforced when the computer systems of Hollywood Presbyterian Medical Center in Los Angeles were locked up by ransomware. The hospital ended up paying $17,000 in bitcoins to the "data-knappers" to regain access to its data.

Despite the ongoing need to keep information technology (IT) systems updated and working and with the aforementioned concerns about security, *Network World* reports that there's a "skills gap when it comes to finding IT and security professionals that are well versed and have the right background and experience."

Additionally, *CIO* magazine has identified the following health care IT careers as fast growing:

1. Clinical Applications Analysts
Duties: "Work as a liaison of sorts between patient care and clinical technologies…they help to design, implement, maintain, and train to support clinical and/or business systems."
Average Annual Salary: $71,000

2. Clinical Informatics Specialists
Duties: Collect and analyze medical data and help medical professionals use it to improve clinical results
Average Annual Salary: $89,000

3. HL7 Interface Analysts and Developers
Duties: HL7 is a nonprofit organization that provides a common standard that allows health care systems/technology from different health care organizations to communicate. Analysts troubleshoot and identify issues and trends related to HL7. Developers use programming languages such as Cloverleaf and Rhapsody to create the messages themselves.
Average Annual Salary: $91,000

4. Clinical Application Trainers
Duties: These professionals teach doctors, nurses, and other health care professionals how to use software applications and other technologies.
Average Annual Salary: $73,000

about the field and visit the websites of college radiology educational programs to learn about typical classes and possible career paths. Ask your teacher or school counselor to arrange an information interview with a radiologic technician or technologist. Professional associations can also provide information about the field. The American Society of Radiologic Technologists offers information on education and careers at its website, www.asrt.org/main/careers/careers-in-radiologic-technology. Many other associations are listed in the For More Information section of this article. You should also try to land a part-time job in a medical office that employs radiologic technicians and technologists. This will give you a chance to interact with workers in the field and see if the career is a good fit for your interests and abilities.

EMPLOYERS

There are more than 325,000 radiologic technicians and technologists and related workers in the United States. Hospitals employ 58 percent of radiologic technologists. Other employers include clinics, medical and diagnostic laboratories, offices of physicians, outpatient care centers, cancer care facilities, and other health care facilities.

GETTING A JOB

Many radiologic technicians and technologists obtain their first jobs as a result of contacts made through college internships, career fairs, or networking events. Others seek assistance in obtaining job leads from college career services offices, newspaper want ads, and employment websites. Additionally, professional associations, such as the American Society of Radiologic Technologists, the American Institute of Ultrasound in Medicine, the Society for Nuclear Medicine and Molecular Imaging, and the American Society of Echocardiography, provide job listings at their websites. Many associations and potential employers have a presence om LinkedIn, Facebook, YouTube, and other social media sites. Visit www.usajobs.gov to learn more about job opportunities at federal agencies.

ADVANCEMENT

General radiologic technicians and technologists with experience and additional educational training can become specialists in bone densitometry, mammography, magnetic resonance imaging, and other areas. The typical managerial track for technicians and technologists is promotion to supervisor, chief radiologic technologist, and department administrator or director. Radiology department directors may require the completion of classes or a master's degree in business or health administration. Other possibilities include working as a sales representative or college educator.

EARNINGS

Median annual salaries for radiologic technologists and technicians were $65,756, according to the American Society of Radiologic Technologists (ASRT) Wage and Salary Survey 2016. The ASRT reports the following average salaries for other specialties: medical dosimetrists, $106,777; radiation therapists, $82,798; nuclear medicine technologists, $75,819; magnetic resonance imaging technologists, $71,063; and radiographers, $56,071.

Salaries for radiologic technicians and technologists ranged from less than $38,110 to $81,660 or more in May 2015, according to the U.S. Department of Labor (USDL). The USDL reports the following mean annual earnings for radiologic technologists and technicians by employer: federal government, $61,100; outpatient care centers, $60,510; general medical and surgical hospitals, $59,820; medical and diagnostic laboratories, $57,830; and offices of physicians, $54,290.

In May 2015, salaries for nuclear medicine technologists ranged from less than $52,950 to $100,080 or more, according to the USDL. They had median annual earnings of $73,360.

Radiation therapy technologists earned salaries that ranged from less than $63,774 to $95,483 or more in 2017, according to Salary.com. They had median earnings of $78,060.

Employers offer a variety of benefits, including medical, dental, and life insurance; paid holidays, vacations, and sick and personal days; 401(k) plans; profit-sharing plans; retirement and pension plans; and educational-assistance programs. Part-time workers must provide their own benefits.

EMPLOYMENT OUTLOOK

The U.S. Department of Labor predicts that employment in the field will grow faster than the average for all careers during the next decade. Demand will increase as the U.S. population grows and ages, creating a need for more diagnostic procedures. In addition, radiation technology has become safer in recent years, and more procedures are being done—especially to detect diseases earlier and to reduce health care insurance costs. Technicians and technologists who are skilled in more than one imaging modality—such as magnetic resonance imaging (MRI) and computed tomography (CT)—will have the best job prospects. In fact, MRI and CT technologists and technicians will be in especially strong demand in coming years due to the accuracy of these imaging technologies.

The ASRT reports that the job market is currently very competitive for new graduates, but job opportunities are available. Workers who are willing to relocate to areas of the United States that are experiencing shortages of workers, or work nontraditional shifts (such as nights and weekends), will have stronger employment prospects. "Right now we are in a period of decreased demand, but these periods are generally followed by a demand surge," says Sal Martino, chief executive officer and executive director of the ASRT.

FOR MORE INFORMATION

Contact the following organizations for more information on education, careers, and certification.

**Alliance of
Cardiovascular Professionals**
www.acp-online.org

**American Association
of Medical Dosimetrists**
www.medicaldosimetry.org

**American Institute of
Ultrasound in Medicine**
800-638-5352
www.aium.org

**American Society
for Radiation Oncology**
www.astro.org

**American Society of
Echocardiography**
919-861-5574
www.asecho.org

**American Society
of Radiologic Technologists**
800-444-2778
customerinfo@asrt.org
www.asrt.org

**Association of Vascular and
Interventional Radiographers**
www.avir.org

**International Society
for Clinical Densitometry**
www.iscd.org

**International Society for
Magnetic Resonance in Medicine**
www.ismrm.org

**Society for Cardiovascular
Magnetic Resonance**
www.scmr.org

**Society for Nuclear Medicine
and Molecular Imaging**
www.snm.org

Society for Vascular Ultrasound
www.svunet.org

**Society of Diagnostic
Medical Sonography**
www.sdms.org

For information on educational training and careers in Canada, contact
**Canadian Association of Medical
Radiation Technologists**
www.camrt.ca

Interview: Sal Martino

Sal Martino, Ed.D., R.T.(R), FASRT, CAE, Chief Executive Officer and Executive Director of the American Society of Radiologic Technologists (ASRT)

Q. What is one thing that young people may not know about a career in medical imaging and radiation therapy?

A. Radiologic technologists should possess excellent patient care skills. It's not uncommon for prospective students to become enamored with the technology related to medical imaging and radiation therapy and forget that radiologic technologists work hard every day to improve patient outcomes. Although the profession is extremely high-tech and exciting, it's the human side of the radiologic science profession that's most significant. A technologist who has a great deal of technical expertise won't provide the best overall examination for a patient if he or she fails to include the human touch.

Q. What is the employment outlook for medical imaging and radiation therapy professionals? How is the field changing, and what are the most promising career paths in the field?

A. The job market for medical imaging and radiation therapy professionals is fairly tight right now. About 15 years ago there was a major shortage of radiologic technologists, but it evaporated in just five or six years. We believe that the downturn in the economy in 2008 was a major factor. Hospitals and outpatient clinics slowed hiring and started doing more with less. We don't know if another shortage of radiologic technologists will occur in the near future. It's important to note that ASRT has conducted a great deal of research on radiologic technology hiring trends and history shows the demand for radiologic technologists fluctuates. Right now we are in a period of decreased demand, but these periods are generally followed by a demand surge.

Q. What advice would you offer radiologic technology students as they graduate and look for jobs?

A. The radiologic technology job market has been tight for a number of years. We've seen some loosening in job vacancy rates in the past couple of years, but it's still a very competitive job market for new graduates. That being said, there are some jobs out there if a graduate is willing to relocate or work during off hours. The most important step graduates can take is to get a foot in the door at a health care institution. The job may not be the desired shift or location, but it may lead to increased opportunities as radiologic technologists retire and the field expands in the future. In addition, this is a wonderful time for graduates to build their skills and prepare themselves for the future. Advancements in computed tomography, magnetic resonance, imaging informatics, and many other practice areas offer exciting professional opportunities in the future for those technologists who take the initiative to learn about different specialty areas.

Q. Can you tell us about the American Society of Radiologic Technologists? How important is membership in the ASRT for career success?

A. The American Society of Radiologic Technologists represents health care professionals who perform medical imaging examinations or deliver radiation therapy treatments. The ASRT's role is to ensure that its 153,000 members keep up with the technological advances, regulatory changes, and economic forces that are transforming their profession. ASRT's educational resources, career development tools, practice standards, and advocacy efforts help radiologic technologists improve the quality of patient care. It's the leading provider of continuing education in the radiologic sciences and the principal source for research data on the profession.

The ASRT provides its members with a variety of opportunities to strengthen their skills and advance their careers. Whether keeping up-to-date with the latest professional news or staying ahead with continuing education, ASRT members have access to the information they need to succeed. There's no better investment a radiologic technologist can make than becoming an ASRT member.

REGISTERED NURSES

OVERVIEW

Registered nurses work to promote health, prevent disease, and help patients who are sick or injured. They also serve as health educators for patients, families, and communities. Registered nurses train for the field by earning a bachelor's degree, an associate degree, or a diploma in nursing from an approved nursing program. Registered nurses who decide to become advanced practice nurses (clinical nurse specialists, nurse anesthetists, nurse-midwives, and nurse practitioners) must earn master's degrees and industry certifications. Registered nurses (RNs) make up the largest occupational group in the health care industry, comprising more than 2.7 million jobs. Employment opportunities for RNs are expected to be good during the next decade.

THE JOB

Most RNs provide direct patient care. They observe, assess, and record patient symptoms, reactions, and progress. Nurses collaborate with physicians and other medical professionals on patient care, treatments, and examinations, and they administer medications.

RNs work closely with physicians to care for patients. It is their job to implement the doctor's orders regarding the treatment of a patient. In addition to interacting with patients, RNs also have a lot of contact with patients' families, so they must have good "bedside manner" and put people at ease.

Specific work responsibilities vary from one RN to the next. An RN's duties and title are often determined by his or her work setting, such as *emergency room nurses,* who work in hospital emergency rooms, or *radiology nurses,* who administer x-rays and other body scans to patients or care for those undergoing radiation treatments for cancer. These nurses generally work in hospitals, clinics, or outpatient care facilities. RNs can also work outside of health care facilities, in settings such as schools, workplaces, and summer camps.

Other nurses are defined by the types of patients served. *Hematology nurses,* for example, help patients with blood disorders. *Oncology nurses* specialize in treating patients with cancer. These nurses are employed virtually anywhere, including physicians' offices, outpatient treatment facilities, home health care agencies, and hospitals. Those that specialize in a disease or condition may also specialize in the age of the patients served. Some examples include *neonatal nurses* (newborns), *pediatric nurses* (children and adolescents), and *geriatric nurses* (the elderly).

Finally, other RNs specialize in working with one or more organs or systems, such as *respiratory nurses,* who care for those with respiratory illnesses such as cystic fibrosis or asthma. RNs specializing in treatment of a particular organ or body system usually are employed in hospital specialty or critical care units, specialty clinics, and outpatient care facilities.

RNs can be one or a combination of these nursing types, such as a *geriatric dialysis nurse,* who specializes in care for elderly patients with kidney failure.

Registered nurses who pursue advanced degrees and certification are called *advanced practice nurses (APNs).* There are four advanced practice nursing specialties: *clinical nurse specialists, nurse anesthetists, nurse-midwives,* and *nurse practitioners.* For detailed information on these specialties, see the article, Advanced Practice Nurses, in this book.

Instead of working in teams under the direction of a physician, APNs work relatively independently. Clinical nurse specialists provide specialized expertise in a specific area of nursing, such as rehabilitation, mental health, or geriatrics. Nurse anesthetists administer anesthesia and provide pain management services before and after surgical, therapeutic, diagnostic, and obstetric procedures. Nurse-midwives provide primary care to women, including gynecological exams, prenatal and neonatal care, and direct assistance in labor and delivery. Finally, nurse practitioners serve as primary and specialty care providers, providing a blend of nursing and health care services to patients and families. Specialties include pediatrics, family practice, and women's health, among others.

In addition to caring for patients with existing conditions and illnesses, nurses also perform a valuable service by providing education and preventive care to healthy populations. A good example of this type of nurse includes an *occupational health nurse,* who seeks to prevent job-related injuries and illnesses and supports employers in implementing health and safety standards.

Books to Read

Ackley, Betty J., Gail B. Ladwig, et al. *Nursing Diagnosis Handbook: An Evidence-Based Guide to Planning Care.* 11th ed. Philadelphia: Mosby, 2016.

Catalano, Joseph T. *Nursing Now: Today's Issues, Tomorrow's Trends.* 7th ed. Philadelphia: F. A. Davis Company, 2015.

Dewit, Susan C. *Saunders Student Nurse Planner: A Guide to Success in Nursing School.* 12th ed. Philadelphia: W. B. Saunders Co., 2016.

Evangelist, Thomas, et al. *McGraw-Hill's Nursing School Entrance Exams.* 2nd ed. New York: McGraw-Hill, 2013.

Lewis, Sharon L., and Linda Bucher. *Medical-Surgical Nursing: Assessment and Management of Clinical Problems.* 10th ed. Philadelphia: Mosby, 2016.

Skidmore-Roth, Linda. *Mosby's 2017 Nursing Drug Reference.* 30th ed. Philadelphia: Mosby, 2016.

Taylor, Carol, Pamela Lynn, and Carol Lillis. *Fundamentals of Nursing.* 8th ed. Philadelphia: Lippincott Williams & Wilkins, 2014.

Some RNs work in applied nursing jobs, or positions that require the medical knowledge of a nurse without the traditional hands-on work with patients. The following paragraphs detail some popular applied nursing specialties:

Nurse educators evaluate existing or create new professional development plans for student nurses and RNs. They teach a variety of nursing classes to students.

Forensic nurses provide legal testimony in investigations of accidents or crimes.

Legal nurse consultants are registered nurses with considerable nursing experience and knowledge of the legal system. They use these skills to assist lawyers in health-care-related cases. According to the American Association of Legal Nurse Consultants (www.aalnc.org), legal nurse consultants offer support to the law profession in the following practice areas: personal injury, product liability, medical malpractice, workers' compensation, toxic torts, risk management, medical licensure investigation, criminal law, elder law, and fraud and abuse compliance.

Nursing informatics specialists organize a database of patients' medical information in an accessible format. They may customize and test the database according to the needs of different medical departments or specialties. Nursing informatics specialists also train nurses on computer charting, which consists of adding information to or retrieving it from the database. They may also write and install new programs or software applications to help nursing staffs work more efficiently.

As the types of nursing varieties are numerous, so are the settings in which nurses work. In addition to hospitals, doctor's offices, and medical clinics, nurses work in patients' homes, schools, large corporations, community centers, and other locations. Hospitals or other 24-hour facilities must be staffed around the clock, so some nurses work holidays, weekends, and overnight shifts.

Nurses follow strict guidelines in handling hazardous medical waste or dangerous instruments such as needles. They are also exposed to patients with contagious diseases, so they must wear protective gear such as masks and gloves. Hand washing is constant and methodical in nursing to prevent the transmission of communicable diseases.

While their jobs may be stressful, most nurses find caring for others enjoyable and rewarding.

Useful Website: DiscoverNursing.com

This Web site, created by Johnson & Johnson, is a comprehensive tool for aspiring nurses. It provides information on more than 100 nursing specialties (and the academic steps you'll need to take to prepare for these jobs); offers an overview of entry- and graduate-level educational requirements for nursing students; and provides a database of nearly 400 nursing scholarships (searchable by state, GPA, gender, ethnicity, and academic level). The site also features video profiles of nurses in a variety of practice areas and information for men who are interested in entering the field of nursing.

REQUIREMENTS

HIGH SCHOOL

Take health, mathematics, biology, anatomy and physiology, chemistry, physics, English, speech, and computer science classes in high school to prepare for a career in nursing.

POSTSECONDARY TRAINING

Prospective RNs have the option of pursuing one of three training paths: associate's degree, diploma, and bachelor's degree. Associate's degree programs in nursing last two years and are offered by community colleges. Diploma programs in nursing typically last three years and are offered by hospitals and independent schools. Bachelor of science in nursing programs are offered by colleges and universities. They typically take four— and sometimes five—years to complete. Graduates of all three paths are known as graduate nurses and must take a licensing exam in their state to obtain the RN designation. Visit www.discovernursing.com for a database of nurse training programs.

Other Nursing Careers

- ✔ Camp Nurses
- ✔ Community Health Nurses
- ✔ Correctional Facility Nurses
- ✔ Critical Care Nurses
- ✔ Gastroenterology Nurses
- ✔ Health Policy Experts
- ✔ Hospice Nurses
- ✔ Labor and Delivery Nurses
- ✔ Nephrology Nurses
- ✔ Nurse Attorneys
- ✔ Nurse Entrepreneurs
- ✔ Nurse Researchers
- ✔ Nursing Historians

- ✔ Nursing Writers
- ✔ Ophthlamic Nurses
- ✔ Orthopaedic Nurses
- ✔ Plastic Surgery Nurses
- ✔ Poison Information Specialists
- ✔ Psychiatric Nurses
- ✔ Rehabilitation Nurses
- ✔ Reproductive Nurses
- ✔ Rheumatology Nurses
- ✔ School Nurses
- ✔ Substance Abuse Nurses
- ✔ Transcultural Nurses
- ✔ Wound and Ostomy Nurses

Students who are interested in becoming nurse managers should earn at least a bachelor's degree. Those interested in becoming nursing educators, advanced practice nurses, or advancing as an RN should earn at least a master's degree in nursing, plus industry certifications.

CERTIFICATION AND LICENSING

Certification or credentialing, while voluntary, is highly recommended. It is an excellent way to stand out from other job applicants and demonstrate your abilities to prospective employers. Certification is offered by the American Nursing Credentialing Center, the National League for Nursing, and many other nursing organizations.

Nurses must be licensed to practice nursing in all states and the District of Columbia. Licensure requirements vary by state but typically include graduating from an approved nursing school and passing the National Council Licensure Examination, which is administered by the National Council of State Boards of Nursing.

OTHER REQUIREMENTS

To be a successful registered nurse, you should be detail oriented, have excellent communication skills, be sympathetic and caring, be calm under pressure, have leadership skills, and be willing to continue to learn throughout your career. You will need to be emotionally strong, since you will encounter many heartbreaking cases and emergency situations. You will also need to be physically fit, since you will spend many hours on your feet and often bend and stoop, and lift patients, as needed.

EXPLORING

Read books about nursing, talk with your counselor or teacher about setting up a presentation by a nurse, take a tour of a hospital or other health care setting, or volunteer at one of these facilities. Nursing websites, including those of professional associations, can also be a good source of information. Here are two suggestions: Discover Nursing (www.discovernursing.com) and Nurse.com (www.nurse.com). You should also join Future Nurses organizations or student health clubs at your school.

EMPLOYERS

More than 2.7 million registered nurses are employed in the United States. The U.S. Department of Labor reports that 58 percent of registered nurses work at hospitals, 7 percent in offices of physicians, 6 percent in home health care services, 6 percent in nursing care facilities, and 4 percent in outpatient care centers. Other RNs are employed by colleges and universities, prisons, corporations, government agencies (such as the Veterans Health Administration and the Indian Health Service), and social assistance agencies. Some RNs with advanced education work as nursing professors.

GETTING A JOB

Many aspiring RNs learn about job openings as a result of contacts made through college internships, clinical rotations, networking events, or social media sites. Additionally, professional associations, such as the American Nurses Association, provide job listings at their websites. See For More Information for a list of organizations. Information on job opportunities at federal agencies is available at www.usajobs.gov.

ADVANCEMENT

There are many advancement opportunities for registered nurses. Those who start their careers as staff nurses can become nurse managers or head nurses. Those already in management positions can advance from assistant unit manager or head nurse to more senior-level administrative roles such as assistant director, director, vice president, or chief of nursing. Registered nurses can earn a master's degree and industry certifications and become advanced practice nurses. Some nurses become college professors. Others work in research or serve as consultants for insurance companies, pharmaceutical manufacturers, and law firms.

EARNINGS

Median annual salaries for registered nurses were $67,490 in May 2015, according to the U.S. Department of Labor (USDL). Salaries ranged from less than $46,360 to $101,630 or more. The USDL reports the following mean annual earnings for registered nurses by employer: outpatient care centers, $73,620; general medical and surgical hospitals, $72,980; home health care services, $68,510; offices of physicians, $65,350; and nursing care facilities, $63,490.

Employers offer a variety of benefits, including the following: medical, dental, and life insurance; paid holidays, vacations, and sick days; personal days; 401(k) plans; profit-sharing plans; retirement and pension plans; and educational assistance programs. Self-employed workers must provide their own benefits.

EMPLOYMENT OUTLOOK

Job opportunities for registered nurses are expected to grow by 16 percent from 2014 to 2024, according to the USDL, a rate that's much faster than the average for all careers. Approximately 439,300 new positions for registered nurses will become available from 2014 to 2024. Employment for registered nurses will be strongest in the following health care subsectors:

✔ home health care services: +60.7 percent
✔ offices of health practitioners, excluding physicians, dentists, and chiropractors: +59.0 percent
✔ offices of health practitioners: +59.0 percent
✔ outpatient care centers: +55.0 percent
✔ ambulatory health care services: +44.3 percent
✔ offices of physicians: +22.5 percent
✔ nursing and residential care facilities: +21.4 percent
✔ services for the elderly and people with disabilities: +18.7 percent
✔ social assistance services, +13.4 percent.

The career outlook for nurses is good, although an influx of new nurses in recent years has created competition for jobs in some geographic areas. The USDL predicts that more than 439,300 new and replacement nurses will be needed by 2024 to care for the growing—and aging—U.S. population. Registered nurses with a bachelor of science degree in nursing and certification will have the best job prospects.

Many nursing specialties are experiencing strong growth. One of the fastest-growing areas is the care of geriatric populations. As baby boomers continue to reach their mid-60s and beyond, there will be increasing demand for nurses with specialized training in geriatric care. According to *Who Will Care for Each of Us?: America's Coming Health Care Crisis,* the ratio of potential caregivers to those who need care (including the growing elderly population) will decrease by 40 percent between 2010 and 2030, creating a strong need for health care professionals, including nurses. In addition, the USDL reports that clinical nurse specialists, nurse practitioners, nurse-midwives, and nurse anesthetists will be in strong demand. Opportunities should also be good for nurses who "provide specialized long-term rehabilitation for stroke and head injury patients."

Many students are interested in studying nursing, but they are finding it hard to land a coveted spot in nursing school. The AACN notes that "U.S. nursing schools turned away 68,938 qualified applicants from baccalaureate and graduate

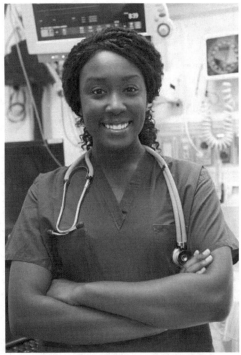

Employment for RNs at hospitals is expected to increase by 9 percent during the next decade, according to the U.S. Department of Labor. (Photos.com)

nursing programs in 2014 due to an insufficient number of faculty, clinical sites, classroom space, clinical preceptors, and budget constraints."

What is causing the faculty shortages? Earnings and age are two of the most significant factors. According to the *New York Times*, nursing educators earn 40 to 50 percent less than nurses employed in clinical settings, which keeps qualified nurses who might be interested in pursuing a career in academe on the sidelines due to financial considerations. Additionally, many nurses are becoming educators late in their careers— the average ages of doctorally-prepared nurse faculty holding the ranks of professor, associate professor, and assistant professor were 61.6, 57.6, and 51.4 years, respectively, in 2013-14 (the most recent years for which data is available)—and many educators are retiring without being replaced.

To address these shortages, professional nursing organizations are working to secure federal funding for faculty development programs, creating scholarship programs for doctoral education (the typical educational requirement for top positions in nursing education), and attempting to develop a more direct route to the Ph.D. to encourage students to pursue nursing education at a younger age.

FOR MORE INFORMATION

The following organizations provide a wealth of resources and information related to registered nursing. For a list of advanced practice nursing associations, see the For More Information section of the Advanced Practice Nurses article in this book.

For information on opportunities for men in nursing, contact
American Assembly for Men in Nursing
859-977-7453
info@aamn.org
www.aamn.org

For information on careers in assisted living facilities, contact
American Assisted Living Nurses Association
707-622-5628
www.alnursing.org

To learn more about accredited nursing programs, contact
American Association of Colleges of Nursing
202-463-6930
www.aacn.nche.edu

The ANA is the largest nursing organization in the United States. Visit its website for information about education, careers, and credentialing.
American Nurses Association (ANA)
800-274-4262
www.nursingworld.org

For certification information, contact
American Nurses Credentialing Center
c/o American Nurses Association
800-284-2378
www.nursecredentialing.org

For industry news, visit the society's website.
American Society of Registered Nurses
415-331-2700
gro.nrsa@nrsa
www.asrn.org

For information on licensing, contact
National Council of State Boards of Nursing
312-525-3600
info@ncsbn.org
www.ncsbn.org

To learn more about careers in nursing, contact
National League for Nursing
www.nln.org

The OADN serves as an advocate for registered nurses who have earned an associate degree. Visit its website for more information.
Organization for Associate Degree Nursing (OADN)
877-966-6236
oadn@oadn.org
www.oadn.org

For information on membership, contact
National Student Nurses' Association
718-210-0705
www.nsna.org

For resources for aspiring and current nurses with disabilities, visit
ExceptionalNurse.com
www.exceptionalnurse.com

For information on careers in Canada, contact
Canadian Nurses Association
613-237-2133
www.cna-aiic.ca

Interview: Mary Rita Hurley

Mary Rita Hurley is a gerontological nurse and the Past-President of the National Gerontological Nursing Association.

Q.   What made you want to become a gerontological nurse?

A.   I have always had a passion for the care of older adults. I grew up in a very large Italian matriarchal family. I developed a respect and great appreciation for what our elders bring to our lives. I personally saw how one can live not only long, but can live well. It inspired me.

Q.   What are some of the pros and cons of your job?

A.   Most everything is a "pro." I have had the honor and privilege of meeting and caring for the most amazing people across the country for more than 35 years. If there was a "con" it would be the myth in the nursing community that caring for older adults is not rewarding and almost a "default" career. In reality, geriatric nursing is one of the most challenging specialties because older adults are very complex mentally and psychosocially.

> "Geriatric nursing is one of the most challenging specialties because older adults are very complex mentally and psychosocially. "

Q.   What are the most important personal and professional qualities for gerontological nurses (GNs)?

A.   A passion for the care of older adults; an understanding that it is a specialty; and a respect for the continued contributions of people as they age.

Q.   What is the future employment outlook for GNs?

A.   Fantastic! There are more than 10,000 Baby Boomers turning 65 every day. There are not enough gerontological nurses to handle these explosive numbers. Also, the fastest-growing segment of our population is 85+. And, this demographic is typically the frailest and requires very skilled nursing care.

Q.   Can you tell us about the the National Gerontological Nursing Association (NGNA)?

A.   The National Gerontological Nursing Association works to improve the nursing care given to older adults and believes in the contribution of every nursing team member in every setting relating to the care of older adults. NGNA provides its members with numerous continuing education opportunities, access to resources, networking opportunities, and policy and legislative updates. It is made up of a growing, dynamic, and dedicated group of nursing professionals who share ideas and information to improve nursing care for older adults. NGNA is recognized as a leader in gerontology and actively collaborates with other organizations to ensure the best outcomes for our patients; and is the place where compassion meets purpose—especially if your passion involves caring for older adults.

Interesting Career: Horticultural Therapist

If you take a walk in a local park or a forest preserve, you'll probably feel an immediate calming effect as you're overwhelmed by the sights, smells, and sounds of nature—the green wash of the grass and plants, the towering leafy trees, the beautiful fragrant flowers, and the sounds of the wind and songbirds. For thousands of years, people have sought out nature to calm their nerves and heal themselves after serious life challenges. This practice is ancient, but it was not until the early 19th century that Dr. Benjamin Rush, a signer of the Declaration of Independence, observed and documented the benefits to his patients when they were exposed to nature. *Horticultural therapists* are specially trained therapists who use nature to help people cope with physical, mental, and social disabilities. As a horticultural therapist, you might work with individuals with developmental disabilities; senior citizens who face cognitive or physical decline or who are recovering from stroke, cancer, surgery, or other conditions; at-risk children; substance abusers; and people who have been physically, mentally, and/or sexually abused. Contact the American Horticultural Therapy Association (888-294-8527, info@ahta.org, www.ahta.org) for more information.

Only a few horticultural therapy programs in the United States are accredited by the American Horticultural Therapy Association (www.ahta.org/%20education/education-programs).

Typical courses in a horticultural therapy program include: Intro to Horticultural Science; Horticulture for Special Populations; Case Management; Field Techniques; Human Issues in Horticultural Therapy; Horticultural Therapy Techniques and Practices; Horticultural Therapy Management; Herbaceous Plant Materials; Introductory Floral Design; and Floriculture Techniques.

Major employers of horticultural therapists include:
- ✔ Hospitals
- ✔ Rehabilitation centers
- ✔ Government social service agencies
- ✔ Correctional facilities
- ✔ Schools
- ✔ Botanical centers
- ✔ Nursing homes
- ✔ Mental health settings
- ✔ Special education programs
- ✔ Youth and community services organizations.

Interview: Susan E. Lowey

Susan E. Lowey, Ph.D., RN, CHPN is an Assistant Professor and Advisement Coordinator at The College at Brockport in Brockport, New York. She is also the author of *Nursing Beyond the Bedside: 60 Non-Hospital Careers in Nursing.*

Q.   What made you want to enter this career, and what do you like best about working in nursing?

A.   I have wanted to be a nurse since I was six years old. I cannot think of any other career I would rather do. When I was very young, I remember visiting my grandmother in the intensive care unit of the hospital. The hospital was a very scary place, and I did not like it. There was a nurse who, at that time in the 1970s, was dressed in all white and wore a nursing cap. She came over and gave me a paper nurse's cap with a Red Cross symbol on it. Her kindness made me feel better, plus I got a nice paper cap to play with. Ever since then, I wanted to be nurse.

Although it may sound cliché, the best thing I like about working in nursing is helping to make patients feel better. By feel better I mean helping to answer their questions and helping them understand how to manage and cope with their illness, providing them support and encouragement, and providing an ear to listen to their concerns. In home health nursing, which is the care setting I am most familiar with, I really enjoy being able to go to a patient's home on a weekend or afterhours and help them. They usually have a medical condition or symptom that needs to be addressed then and there, and it is a great feeling to be able to really affect change and provide a positive outcome in regards to their concern or need.

Q.   What is one thing young people may not know about a career in nursing?

A.   My response to this question is the reason I decided to write my book, *Nursing Beyond the Bedside: 60 Non-Hospital Careers in Nursing.* Most young people, and the public, have an impression that nurses mainly work in the hospital and that is not the case at all. There are so many career options for nurses outside of the hospital setting that young people are not aware of. The overall goal of nursing care is to restore health and promote optimal healing and functioning of patients. The hospital is not the only care setting that this can be accomplished. Nurses work in schools, clinics, shelters, rehabilitation centers, home health, public health, occupational health, military bases, cruise ships, etc. People who are not hospitalized still have health-related needs that require care.

Q.   What are a few of the most-popular non-hospital careers for registered nurses?

A.   *Home health nursing* is a popular non-hospital career and growing rapidly considering the changing health care system from predominantly acute to community-based. *Telemedicine nursing* is a fairly new career choice and is also rapidly growing alongside the increased use of technology to assess patients who are in distant settings and/or used for cost reduction by utilizing technology in the patient's home for routine physical assessments. *Genetics nursing* is also a popular career choice considering recent advances in the field to improve the care of persons affected by genetic disorders. *Pediatric palliative care nursing* might not be a career for everyone, but it is also a rapidly developing field that is a combination of pediatric and palliative/hospice nursing. Registered nurses who work in most of these popular non-hospital careers can obtain certification in these specialty areas, which can be beneficial in advancing their careers.

"The nursing profession loses many qualified individuals who do not understand that hospital nursing is not their only option."

Q. Can you tell us about your book, *Nursing Beyond the Bedside: 60 Non-Hospital Careers in Nursing?*

A. *Nursing Beyond the Bedside* was specifically written for anyone interested in pursuing a nursing career and/or is already in nursing but researching career options. The nursing profession loses many qualified individuals who do not understand that hospital nursing is not their only option. The book focuses on describing 60 different non-hospital career options in nursing and is organized by population (infants and children, adults, older adults, etc.) instead of by a disease or a particular setting. A basic job description, work hours/setting, education/skills required, specialty certification, and online resources are provided for each of the 60 careers. I wanted to have a current resource available for nursing students and practicing nurses and for those who are advising young people about the profession, such as guidance counselors or college career counselors. What makes this book unique is that a registered nurse (RN) license is the basic educational requirement for most of the careers described in the book. Other books of this nature focus on careers that require advanced educational preparation (such as a master's degree), and I wanted to gear this book specifically for RNs (who are at the associate's or bachelor's educational levels).

REHABILITATION COUNSELORS

OVERVIEW

Rehabilitation counselors help people with disabilities deal with any associated personal, social, or employment effects. They work with people with both physical and emotional disabilities resulting from birth defects, illness, accidents, or other causes. Rehabilitation counselors collaborate with the individual's families or loved ones, physicians, psychologists, employers, and physical therapists to determine the client's strengths and weaknesses and develop a rehabilitation plan for their client. They arrange training to help clients develop job or life skills or even help them find a job. Their main goal is to help their clients live happy and independent lives. You will need a master's degree in rehabilitation counseling or a related field to become a rehabilitation counselor. Approximately 101,630 rehabilitation counselors are employed in the United States. Employment in the field is expected to be good during the next decade.

FAST FACTS

High School Subjects
Psychology
Sociology

Personal Skills
Communication
Helping
Technical

Minimum Education Level
Master's degree

Salary Range
$20,000 to $34,000 to
$60,000+

Employment Outlook
Faster than the average

O*NET-SOC
21-1015.00

NOC
4153

THE JOB

Rehabilitation counselors help people with many different kinds of disabilities, including cognitive or learning limitations, psychological conflicts, and physical or functional disabilities. Many times these disabilities are caused by injuries, accidents, birth defects, stress, trauma caused by crime or war, or the process of aging. Rehabilitation counselors work with clients on a one-on-one basis or as part of group counseling. They teach patients how to cope with the challenges of everyday life, find and succeed in a job, or bridge gaps with family and friends, with the ultimate goal of having clients live independent and meaningful lives.

Fast-Growing Health Care Careers

The U.S. Department of Labor reports that the following careers will enjoy strong employment growth from 2014 to 2024:

✔ Occupational Therapist Assistants and Aides: +40 percent
✔ Genetic Counselors: +29 percent
✔ Optometrists: +27 percent
✔ Phlebotomists: +25 percent
✔ Dispensing Opticians: +24 percent
✔ Massage Therapists: +22 percent
✔ Health Specialties Professors: +19 percent
✔ Chiropractors: +17 percent
✔ Dietitians and Nutritionists: +16 percent
✔ Clinical Laboratory Technologists and Technicians: +16 percent
✔ Podiatrists: +14 percent
✔ Recreational Therapists: +12 percent
✔ Respiratory Therapists: +12 percent
✔ Exercise Physiologists: +11 percent
✔ Pharmacy Technicians: +9 percent

When working with a new client, rehabilitation counselors begin by conducting a complete assessment of the individual. They evaluate the patient's strengths and identify any weaknesses or limitations. For example, if working with a client who has Down syndrome, rehabilitation counselors will take into account any cognitive or learning disabilities, as well as any physical limitations, which could hamper employment opportunities. They may suggest personal and vocational counseling such as physical therapy programs or training to help their client master certain job skills. Rehabilitation counselors provide constant support in all areas and often schedule reviews to keep up with clients' therapy or training progress. Rehabilitation counselors are on call to provide intervention in crisis situations.

If working with a client who has recently suffered an injury or become disabled, rehabilitation counselors may arrange for medical care or treatment. They often take into account their client's financial situation and can arrange for financial assistance if the client qualifies.

Rehabilitation counselors help clients master basic daily living skills and tasks such as cleaning, self-care and grooming, preparing meals, making a household budget, and shopping. They can also help clients develop skills needed to interact with others in the outside world.

While the client is undergoing counseling or training, rehabilitation counselors can search for possible employment opportunities. Certain organizations, such as Goodwill, offer training and placement opportunities for people with disabilities. The rehabilitation counselor often works with a list of such organizations and can suggest placement.

Rehabilitation counselors also tackle any social or environmental barriers that prohibit people with disabilities from living full lives. These barriers can include prejudice, stereotypes, inaccessible information, inaccessible buildings or transportation, as well as companies with inflexible practices. If not already covered by federal law, rehabilitation counselors fight for accessible walkways and stairs, wider entrance ways or hallways, or even accessible forms of public transportation—practically anything that would help disabled people improve their mobility. If counseling someone with impaired vision, rehabilitation counselors might lobby a company to provide signs in Braille or ask a school to purchase audio versions of textbooks or other materials.

Rehabilitation counselors may also interview the client's family, friends, coworkers, and employer to identify any problems or issues regarding his or her disability. They provide education to help others better understand their client's disability. Oftentimes, rehabilitation counselors can act as a bridge between the client and society.

Rehabilitation counselors spend a great deal of time conferring with the client's family, physician, social workers, and other health care professionals. They often participate in team meetings to discuss the client's progress and make provisions for extra services or training, if needed.

Full-time rehabilitation counselors work 40 hours a week, with some time scheduled in the evenings and on weekends. They work indoors in comfortable, well-lit offices, as well as in the field visiting patients and viewing their work or school environment. A reliable vehicle is usually necessary for travel to and from field sites.

REQUIREMENTS

HIGH SCHOOL

In high school, take courses in psychology, health, computer science, English, and speech.

POSTSECONDARY TRAINING

Some organizations hire rehabilitation counselors with only a bachelor's degree in rehabilitation services, counseling, psychology, sociology, or a human services-related field, but these hires typically work as rehabilitation aides, not as counselors. Most rehabilitation counselors need a master's degree in rehabilitation counseling, general counseling, or counseling psychology to enter the field. Both the Council on Rehabilitation Education and the Council for Accreditation of Counseling and Related Educational Programs accredit counseling educational programs. (See For More Information for contact information for these organizations.) According to the American Medical Association, rehabilitation counselor education programs "typically provide between 18 to 24 months of academic and field-based clinical training. Clinical training consists of a practicum and a minimum of 600 hours of supervised internship experience." Students receive training in counseling theory, skills, and techniques; individual and group counseling; principles of psychiatric rehabilitation; vocational evaluation and work adjustment; career counseling; job development and placement; and other topics.

CERTIFICATION AND LICENSING

Certification and licensing requirements vary greatly based on whether the counselor works for a private or public employer and by state law (although most states have laws requiring counselors to have some form of licensure).

Some counselors choose to become certified by the National Board for Certified Counselors (NBCC). This organization awards a general practice credential of national certified counselor. The NBCC also offers specialty certifications in clinical mental health, addiction, and school counseling.

Voluntary national certification for rehabilitation counselors is available from the Commission on Rehabilitation Counselor Certification. This certification is required by many local and state governments. Contact the Commission for information on certification requirements.

OTHER REQUIREMENTS

Rehabilitation counselors need excellent communication skills, since they spend a great deal of time speaking with patients and their families, lobbying employers, and writing reports. Rehabilitation counselors also confer with physicians, social workers, and therapists regarding the condition and goals of the patient. Successful counselors should be able to work well under pressure, since they may have to deal with the needs of multiple clients at one time. They should also be patient and have a pleasant personality in order to deal with clients who can sometimes be irritable, angry, or depressed. Other important traits for rehabilitation counselors include empathy, a strong desire to help others, good listening skills, strong ethics, and the ability to work independently or as part of a team.

EXPLORING

There are many ways to learn more about a career as a rehabilitation counselor. You can visit the websites of college rehabilitation counseling programs to learn about typical classes and possible career paths, read books and journals about the field, and ask your teacher or school counselor to arrange an information interview with a rehabilitation counselor. Professional associations can also provide information about the field. Contact the associations listed at the end of this article for more information on education and careers.

EMPLOYERS

Approximately 101,630 rehabilitation counselors are employed in the United States. State and federal rehabilitation agencies, as well as commu-

A Closer Look: Herbalism

As the public's interest in the use of various types of alternative and complementary medicine has increased, so have students' interests in academic programs that incorporate such subject matter. Practitioners of herbal medicine use herbs to improve health and treat illness. The oldest type of medicine known to humans, herbal medicine is still used in some form by the majority of people in the world. Although an herbal medicine program will focus primarily on developing students' knowledge of herbs and how they are used to promote health and well-being, modern science is also emphasized. Knowledge of human anatomy and physiology, plant biology, nutrition, and medical terminology all come into play. Students with an interest in holistic health—especially the study of herbs and their medicinal properties—should investigate herbal medicine programs. For more info:

✔ **Academy of Integrative Health & Medicine:** www.aihm.org

✔ **American Association of Integrative Medicine:**
www.aaimedicine.com

✔ **American Botanical Council:** www.abc.herbalgram.org

✔ **American Herbal Products Association:** www.ahpa.org

✔ **American Herbalists Guild:** www.americanherbalistsguild.com

✔ **American Holistic Health Association:** http://ahha.org

✔ **Herb Research Foundation:** www.herbs.org

✔ **Herb Society of America:** www.herbsociety.org

nity rehabilitation agencies, are major employers of counselors. Other employers include universities and other academic settings, substance abuse rehabilitation centers, correctional facilities, halfway houses, insurance companies, and independent-living centers.

There are many opportunities for rehabilitation counselors in related careers such as job placement specialist, general counselor, rehabilitation consultant, independent living specialist, and case manager.

GETTING A JOB

Many rehabilitation counselors obtain their first jobs as a result of contacts made through networking events, college internships, and career fairs. Others seek assistance in obtaining job leads from college career services offices, employment websites, and newspaper want ads. Additionally, the National Clearinghouse of Rehabilitation Training Materials provides job-search resources at its website, RehabJobs.org.

ADVANCEMENT

Rehabilitation counselors advance by receiving salary increases and taking on managerial duties. Some counselors choose to work for their state's department of human services or work as supervisors or administrators. Others go into private practice or become college professors.

EARNINGS

Salaries for rehabilitation counselors vary by type of employer, geographic region, and the worker's experience, education, and skill level. Median annual salaries for rehabilitation counselors were $34,390 in May 2015, according to the U.S. Department of Labor (USDL). Salaries ranged from less than $20,950 to $60,750 or more. The USDL reports the following mean annual earnings for rehabilitation counselors by employer:

✔ general medical and surgical hospitals, $50,470;

✔ state government agencies, $48,570;

✔ local government agencies, $43,780;

✔ individual and family services, $34,930;

✔ vocational rehabilitation services, $34,900; and

✔ residential intellectual and developmental disability, mental health, and substance abuse facilities, $32,170.

Rehabilitation counselors usually receive benefits such as health and life insurance, vacation days, sick leave, and a savings and pension plan. Self-employed workers must provide their own benefits.

FOR MORE INFORMATION

For information on certification and the job search, contact
American Counseling Association
www.counseling.org

For information about rehabilitation counseling, contact
American Rehabilitation Counseling Association
www.arcaweb.org

To learn more about accredited programs, contact
Council for Accreditation of Counseling and Related Educational Programs
American Counseling Association
www.cacrep.org

For information on approved programs, contact
Council on Rehabilitation Education
www.core-rehab.org

For information on rehabilitation counseling, contact the following organizations
National Clearinghouse of Rehabilitation Training Materials
https://ncrtm.ed.gov

National Rehabilitation Association
www.nationalrehab.org

National Rehabilitation Counseling Association
http://nrca-net.org

EMPLOYMENT OUTLOOK

Employment for rehabilitation counselors is expected to grow faster than the average for all careers during the next decade, according to the U.S. Department of Labor. The increasing number of elderly people (who typically become disabled or injured at a higher average rate than people in other demographic groups) will create good employment prospects for rehabilitation counselors. Growth will also occur as more elderly people are treated for mental health-related disabilities.

In addition to opportunities in geriatric care, rehabilitation counselors will be needed to work with disabled veterans and people who have learning disabilities, autism spectrum disorders, or substance abuse problems.

Interview: Tarea Stout

Tarea Stout is a rehabilitation counselor and the Past-President of the National Rehabilitation Association. She has worked in the rehabilitation field for 25 years.

Q. What made you want to enter this career?

A. I became a counselor because I knew I wanted to help people in some way; counseling was a natural fit for my personality and goals. Another influencing factor in my career choice was the servant-hearted philosophy toward people that my parents lived. After completing my undergraduate degree in psychology, I worked as a residential counselor for a year. It was then I confirmed that I wanted to work in the field, so I pursued my master's in counselor education. After completing my master's, I began working for Vocational Rehabilitation and loved the work. I have worked in mental health, vocational rehabilitation, and most recently as transition coordinator for Madison County Schools.

Q. What are some of the pros and cons of your job?

A.   Pros:
- ✔ The ability to have a long-lasting impact on people's lives for the better is what keeps you coming back.
- ✔ People in this profession are great, and you make lifelong friends.
- ✔ It can be a lot of fun! I really enjoy working with clients in their life pursuits. Because of this it really isn't like work, it's like a calling.

Cons:
- ✔ Funding is always needed. There are more needs of people than there are funds to help them.
- ✔ It is easy to get absorbed in the work, due to the nature of helping others. Maintaining a work/life balance is a skill to learn early in your career.

Q. What are the most important personal and professional qualities for rehabilitation counseling professionals?

A. Integrity, critical thinking skills, and creativity are qualities that I believe are essential to the success of the counselor. While these may seem basic to any job, helping people overcome and deal with barriers and challenges takes a level of critical thinking and creativity that you typically don't think about when discussing the counseling profession. In the field of rehabilitation counseling, when you add disability issues along with independent living and vocational issues you have to find solutions beyond the traditional answers. This is where critical thinking and creativity collide for the good. Integrity is essential. Without a high level of integrity a person should not work with people as a rehabilitation counselor.

Q. What is the employment outlook for rehabilitation counselors? What are some popular career paths?

A. The employment outlook is good. There are more jobs for qualified rehabilitation counselors than there are rehabilitation counselors. Almost every public vocational rehabilitation agency has counselor vacancies. Private rehabilitation has career options including worker's compensation, insurance, and Social Security vocational expert to name a few.

> "It's rewarding any time a client is successful in attaining his or her goals. That is what keeps you coming back to work every day."

Q. What has been one (or more) of the most rewarding experiences in your career, and why?

A. It's rewarding any time a client is successful in attaining his or her goals. That is what keeps you coming back to work every day. There are many rewarding experiences with clients through my years. One client early in my career as a rehabilitation counselor, has a special place for me. He was 28 years old, had little family support, and was totally deaf with no language skills. He had grown up in an era when you "hid" your kids with disabilities at home. The family had not learned sign language or ever really tried to communicate with him. We worked as a team to help develop language and vocational skills with AbilityWorks, a local community rehabilitation center. We also utilized the EH Gentry Center in Alabama for a couple of month to assist with language development. With the provision of the services, his attitude, and a great employer, he was able to go work in a great job and live on his own. While it took several years to get that point, we helped to change his life for the better.

Q. Can you tell us about the National Rehabilitation Association? What are the benefits of membership?

A. The National Rehabilitation Association (NRA) is the oldest professional member organization in the United States, protecting civil rights of persons with disabilities while also promoting high-quality, ethical, and collaborative practice across the rehabilitation profession. The NRA, comprised of counselors, educators, researchers, and diverse agents of community integration, is committed to continuously impacting and improving upon the multifaceted conditions across our society necessary to enhance quality of life of persons with disabilities, their families, and our communities. Imperative to our mission is providing leadership toward legislative and social advocacy, improving cultural and community awareness, advancements through research and practice, and promotion of careers for professionals throughout the field of rehabilitation.

SPEECH-LANGUAGE PATHOLOGISTS AND AUDIOLOGISTS

OVERVIEW

Speech-language pathologists, also known as *speech therapists,* assess, diagnose, and treat people with voice disorders including speech, language, cognitive-communication, and fluency irregularities. *Audiologists* work with people who have hearing, balance, and other related ear problems. Speech-language pathologists need a master's degree in speech-language pathology to work in the field. Audiologists must have a doctorate in audiology to become certified. More than 131,400 speech-language pathologists and 12,000 audiologists are employed in the United States. Job opportunities for speech therapists and audiologists are expected to be excellent during the next decade.

THE JOB

People who suffer from illnesses and injuries involving hearing loss, and those with speech rhythm and fluency problems, developmental delays, or phys-

FAST FACTS

High School Subjects
Biology
Health
Speech
Personal Skills
Communication
Complex problem solving
Helping
Technical
Minimum Education Level
Master's degree
(speech-language pathologists)
Doctorate (audiologists)
Salary Range
$46,000 to $73,000 to
$114,000+ (speech-language
pathologists)
$49,000 to $74,000 to
$111,000+ (audiologists)
Employment Outlook
Much faster than the average
O*NET-SOC
29-1127.00 (speech-language
pathologists)
29-1181.00 (audiologists)
NOC
3141

ical delays or disorders, often seek out the services of speech-language pathologists. These include patients with brain injury or deterioration, developmental delays or disorders, stroke, learning disabilities, cleft palate, voice pathology, cerebral palsy, mental retardation, and emotional problems. These problems can be acquired, developmental, or congenital.

Interesting Career: Speech-Language Pathology Assistant

Speech-language pathology assistants work under the supervision of a certified speech-language pathologist to perform speech-language screenings and to carry out tasks related to a patient's speech and language development. The assistant does not diagnose patients, but follows the supervising pathologist's orders to administer therapies. These professionals have the opportunity to work in school settings with children or in health care settings with individuals of all ages, with an emphasis on the aging population. The speech-language pathologist assistant also documents each patient's progress, submits reports to the speech language pathologist, and performs a variety of administrative tasks.

Speech-language pathologists assess, diagnose, treat, and in some cases, prevent further damage or delays.

When working with a new patient, speech-language pathologists use written and oral tests to assess the nature and extent of the impairment. They also use special technology such as electronic speech fluency rating instruments for patients with fluency irregularities such as stammering or stuttering.

After diagnosis, speech-language pathologists create an individualized plan of care. They start patients on a regular therapy treatment schedule, the length and scope depending on the patient and his or her condition. Some treatments include breathing exercises or oral motor exercises to strengthen muscles that are used in swallowing and speaking. Speech therapists also teach patients how to form their mouth and tongue, by demonstration, in order to achieve different sounds. Patients with hearing loss or cochlear implants can be trained to use special audio devices for the telephone. Others may be taught to use sign language or other alternative communication methods. Treatments are also tailored to the patient's age. For example, when working with young children with cognitive communication disorders or speech delays, speech-language pathologists may incorporate games with repetitive exercises specially designed to hold a child's interest and attention span.

Many speech-language pathologists also work with patients who want to correct their speech rhythm and fluency problems. Some patients who depend on their voices for a living may seek help to erase an accent or reduce harshness in their voices. Others, such as transgender patients, often use speech therapy to change the pitch of their voices. Some speech-language pathologists are employed by businesses to help employees improve communication with their customers.

Speech-language pathologists in medical settings often consult with doctors, nurses, psychologists, and other therapists and health care workers when evaluating a new patient. In schools, they work closely with teachers, social workers, interpreters, and other professionals. Speech therapists stay in close contact with them throughout the course of therapy, as well as with patients and their families. Speech-language pathologists keep detailed records of patients' diagnosis, treatments and therapies, and continuing progress.

Audiologists work with people who have hearing loss, balance problems, or other issues concerning the ear. These conditions can be the result of injury, illness, infections, birth defects, exposure to loud noises, or simply advanced age. They use audiometers, computers, and other devices to test the hearing and balance of patients.

When working with a new patient, audiologists use a battery of hearing tests to determine the level of impairment. They often consult with doctors, nurses, teachers, and family members to get a clearer picture of the patient's situation. Treatments include a thorough cleaning of the ear canal, as sometime excess wax may hinder hearing. Audiologists may suggest hearing devices or cochlear implants to improve a patient's hearing level. Audiologists also help patients adjust for hearing impairment by training them in the use of various hearing instruments or providing them with strategies to improve their listening skills. Some patients may be trained in lip reading. Audiologists may also encourage patients to use large area amplification devices or alerting devices in their homes.

Some people suffer from hearing loss due to their work environment. Patients include musicians and factory workers with work-related hearing problems. Audiologists try to prevent such injuries by measuring noise levels at the workplace. With extreme situations, they may suggest that clients wear protective ear devices to reduce excessive noise.

Speech-language pathologists and audiologists also are responsible for completing paperwork, billing, and supervising assistants and other staff. In addition to their clinical work, some speech-language pathologists and audiologists teach at the university level or conduct research in a particular specialty.

Full-time speech-language pathologists and audiologists work 40 hours a week, though most work longer hours in order to accommodate high patient loads. Some evening and weekend hours should be expected. Speech-language pathologists and audiologists who work part-time at several facilities need a reliable vehicle in order to travel from site to site.

Speech-language pathologists and audiologists who work in private practice have the added expense of overhead costs, including office space, furniture and equipment, and staff salary and benefits.

Speech-language pathologists and audiologists work in a wide range of settings, including schools, hospital rooms, rehabilitation centers, clinics, doctor's offices, and private practice (in office settings and in a patient's home). Their offices are located indoors and are clean and comfortable. A quiet atmosphere is often needed when working with patients. Speech-language pathologists and audiologists must relate to patients and their families, often explaining complicated medical terminology or treatments, or updating them on the patient's development and progress. They also consult with other health care professionals regarding patients.

REQUIREMENTS

High School

In high school, take courses in biology, anatomy and physiology, physics, mathematics, the social sciences, speech, English, languages, and psychology.

Postsecondary Training

The minimum educational requirement to work as a speech therapist is a master's degree in speech-language pathology. The Council on Academic Accreditation (CAA) Audiology and Speech-Language Pathology has accredited approximately 270 graduate-level academic programs in speech-language pathology.

Audiologists need a doctorate in audiology (known as the Au.D.) to become certified. The CAA accredits approximately 75 doctoral programs in audiology. Typical classes for audiology students include Acquisition and Development of Speech and Language, Electrophysiology, Audiological Assessment and Diagnosis, Acoustic Phonetics, Auditory Disorders, Application of Hearing Aids to Auditory Disorders, Sign Language, and Ethical Issues in Audiology.

Both speech therapists and audiologists participate in clinical rotations during their college study, which become progressively more challenging and involve less direct supervision as the student proceeds in the program.

The American Speech-Language-Hearing Association offers a list of schools that award degrees in speech pathology and audiology at its website, www.asha.org/edfind.

Certification and Licensing

Certification for speech-language pathologists and audiologists is available from the American Speech-Language-Hearing Association. Applicants must meet educational requirements, complete a supervised clinical practicum, and pass an examination, among other requirements. Speech therapists who complete these requirements are awarded the certificate of clinical competence in speech-language pathology, while audiologists receive the certificate of clinical competence in audiology. In addition, board certification in audiology is offered by the American Board of Audiology (www.boardofaudiology.org). The Board also offers specialty certification in cochlear implants and pediatric audiology. Those who obtain professional credentialing may satisfy some or all state licensing requirements. Speech-language pathologists with advanced training can become board certified in child language and language disorders, fluency and fluency disorders, intraoperative monitoring, and swallowing and swallowing disorders. Visit www.asha.org/certification/specialty for more information.

Nearly all states require speech-language pathologists to be licensed. To become licensed, applicants must have at least a master's degree and supervised clinical experience. Contact your state's regulatory board for information on regulation and eligibility requirements. Speech-language pathologists who work in public schools may need to meet additional licensing requirements. Check with your state's department of education for more information.

All states require audiologists to be licensed. Approximately 20 states require applicants to have a doctoral degree in audiology as a condition of licensure. Some states may also require audiologists to acquire a separate hearing-aid dispenser license. Contact your state's medical or health board for information on licensing requirements.

Did You Know?

In the United States, hearing loss affects:

- ✔ 1 out of every 25 children
- ✔ 1 out of every 14 adults aged 18 to 44
- ✔ 1 out of every 7 adults aged 45 to 65
- ✔ 1 out of every 3 adults over age 65

Ninety-five percent of people with hearing loss can be helped with hearing aids.

Some of the risk factors for hearing loss include childhood infectious diseases (such as measles and mumps), recurrent ear infections, exposure to extremely loud noises, use of certain medications, and concussion and skull fracture.

Source: Audiology Foundation of America

OTHER REQUIREMENTS

Since they work with patients of all ages, speech-language pathologists and audiologists must be able to work with people who have a variety of personalities and attention spans. Successful professionals are able to stay patient and focused, with great attention to detail. They need excellent communication skills in order to write reports, interact with coworkers, and discuss test results and treatment plans with patients and their families. Other important traits include strong organizational skills, scientific aptitude, an empathetic personality, good listening skills, and a willingness to continue to learn about new diagnostic and treatment technologies throughout one's career.

EXPLORING

There are many ways to learn more about a career as a speech therapist or audiologist. You can read books and journals about the field, ask your teacher or school counselor to arrange an information interview with a speech therapist or audiologist, and visit the websites of college speech-language pathology or audiology programs to learn about typical classes and possible career paths. Professional associations can also provide information about the field. The American Speech-Language-Hearing Association provides a wealth of information on education and careers, as well as profiles of workers, at its website, www.asha.org/students. You should also try to land a part-time job in a setting that employs speech-language pathologists or audiologists.

Emerging Health Care Tech Sectors

Consumer Health Technology

This sector creates apps, wearable devices, and handheld devices (such as glucose monitors) that help people take control of their health and reduce costs. *Inc.* says those seeking to enter this industry should have experience as Big Data engineers, physicians, medical researchers, or designers and must know how to create products that "bring sleek, user-friendly design to even the most intimidating and opaque areas of health care, such as cancer screening." Industry growth may slow as a result of government regulations regarding consumer privacy and health claims, and certain apps may require approval by the Food & Drug Administration. Major companies in this sector include Aetna and Jawbone.

Mobile Health

Mobile devices and software (sometimes known as mHealth products) provide medical information, help monitor patient health, and perform other tasks. The market for mHealth products and services is expected to enjoy strong growth because of an aging population, rising health costs, increasing consumer demand, and regulatory reforms. One promising niche: remote patient monitoring apps that monitor patients at home and reduce doctor visits. Major companies include HealthTap, Patient Conversation Media, and Informatics Group.

EMPLOYERS

More than 131,000 speech-language pathologists are employed in the United States. Forty-four percent work for elementary and secondary schools. Others work for health maintenance organizations; hospitals; public health departments; research agencies; nursing care facilities; home health care services; individual and family services; outpatient care centers; child day care centers; long-term care facilities; rehabilitation centers; and corporate speech-language pathology programs. Some work for government agencies such as the U.S. Public Health Service, U.S. Department of Veterans Affairs Administration for Children and Families, U.S. Department of Education, U.S. Department of Health and Human Services National

Institute of Neurological Disorders and Stroke, National Institutes of Health, and National Institute for Deafness and Other Communication Disorders. About 6 percent of speech therapists are self-employed.

About 12,000 audiologists are employed in the United States. Approximately 72 percent work in health care facilities. These include offices of physicians or other health practitioners, outpatient care centers, and hospitals. About 9 percent work in educational services. Other employment settings include health and personal care stores and government agencies. Some audiologists work as audiology professors, as designers of hearing instruments and testing equipment, and in industrial settings (such as factories) creating hearing protection/conservation programs for workers.

GETTING A JOB

Many speech-language pathologists and audiologists obtain their first jobs as a result of contacts made through college internships, career fairs (which are offered by the American Speech-Language-Hearing Association, ASHA, and other organizations), or networking events. Others seek assistance in obtaining job leads from college career services offices, newspaper want ads, and employment websites. Additionally, the ASHA provides job listings and career advice (such as preparing a résumé, acing a job interview, and negotiating a salary) at its website, www.asha.org/careers. Those interested in positions with the federal government should visit the U.S. Office of Personnel Management's website, www.usajobs.gov.

ADVANCEMENT

Speech-language pathologists and audiologists advance by receiving pay raises, by taking on managerial or administrative duties, by becoming college professors, and by becoming experts in certain populations (such as youth or the elderly) or disorders (such as learning disabilities). Others open their own practices.

EARNINGS

Salaries for speech-language pathologists and audiologists vary by type of employer, geographic region, and the worker's experience, education, and skill level. Median annual salaries for speech-language pathologists were $73,410 in May 2015, according to the U.S. Department of Labor (USDL). Salaries ranged from less than $46,000 to $114,840 or more. The USDL reports the following mean annual earnings for speech-language pathologists by employer: home health care services, $97,410; nursing care facilities, $91,560; continuing care retirement communities and assisted living facilities for the elderly, $90,030; offices of other health practitioners, $82,770; general medical and surgical hospitals, $80,810; and elementary and secondary schools, $68,150.

Speech-language pathologists who worked in health care earned average salaries of $70,000 in 2015, according to the American Speech-Language-Hearing Association. Those employed in administration earned $93,534.

Salaries for audiologists ranged from less than $49,760 to $111,450 in May 2015, according to the USDL. They earned a median annual salary of $74,890.

Employers offer a variety of benefits, including the following: medical, dental, and life insurance; paid holidays, vacations, and sick and personal days; 401(k) plans; profit-sharing plans; retirement and pension plans; and educational-assistance programs. Self-employed and part-time workers must provide their own benefits. Approximately 20 percent of speech-language pathologists work part-time.

EMPLOYMENT OUTLOOK

Employment for speech-language pathologists is expected to grow by 21 percent from 2014 to 2024, according to the U.S. Department of Labor (USDL)—or much faster than the average for all careers. Increases in elementary- and secondary-school enrollments, the aging of the large Baby Boomer generation (which will have a growing number of neurological disorders and associated language, speech, and swallowing impairments), and medical advances that are increasing survival rates for trauma and stroke victims and premature infants (who may require speech therapy) are all increasing demand for speech-language pathologists. Demand will be best for speech-language pathologists who speak a second language, such as Spanish, and who are willing to relocate to areas of the United States where demand is higher for speech therapists.

FOR MORE INFORMATION

For information on hearing and balance disorders, contact
American Auditory Society
877-746-8315
amaudsoc@comcast.net
www.amauditorysoc.org

For a wealth of information on education and careers in speech-language pathology and audiology, visit
American Speech-Language-Hearing Association
800-638-8255
www.asha.org

To learn more about the Au.D. degree, contact
Audiology Foundation of America
480-219-6000
www.audfound.org

For information on audiologists who work in education and other settings, contact
Educational Audiology Association
800-460-7322
admin@edaud.org
www.edaud.org

This association is for undergraduate and graduate students studying normal and disordered human communication. Visit its website for more information.
National Student Speech Language Hearing Association
www.nsslha.org

To learn more about career opportunities in Canada, contact
Speech-Language and Audiology Canada
www.sac-oac.ca

Job opportunities for audiologists are expected to grow much faster than the average for all occupations during the next decade, according to the USDL. But since only a small number of people are employed in the field, it will be difficult to land a job. Those who have the Au.D. degree will have the best job prospects. As school enrollments continue to grow, there will be good job prospects for audiologists who work at elementary and secondary schools. Areas that have a large number of retirees (who typically have more hearing problems than other demographic groups) will also offer strong prospects for audiologists.

Interview: Diane Paul

Dr. Diane Paul, the Director of Clinical Issues in Speech-Language Pathology at the American Speech-Language-Hearing Association

Q. What made you want to enter this career?

A. I heard a camp counselor talking about the field of speech-language pathology. When I needed to select a major, I was going through the course catalogue and came across some speech-language pathology courses. Although my entry into the field may have been based more on a need to find a major rather than a life calling, my interest and desire to stay in the field has been sustained because of my passion for the varied, interesting, and rewarding work.

Q. What is one thing that young people may not know about a career as a speech-language pathologist?

A. The settings (school, hospital, university, private-practice clinic), clients (children and adults across the life span), types of communication disorders (speech-articulation, voice, fluency; language-understanding and expression in the areas of vocabulary, grammar, use of words in social situations, reading, and writing; and swallowing disorders), and nature of work (clinic, research, teaching, administration) are so varied, that the work can easily maintain a person's interest for a lifetime.

Q. What are the most important personal and professional qualities for people in your career?

A. Energy, enthusiasm, skills in spoken and written communication, enjoyment interacting with different people, sensitivity to the needs of persons with communication disorders, and organization

Q. What do you like most and least about your job?

A. Most: Each day is different and I have the opportunity to do creative, intellectually stimulating, meaningful work that makes a difference. Least: Not enough time in the day to accomplish all that I'd like to do.

Q. What advice would you give to young people who are interested in the field?

A. The population in our country is increasingly diverse. Knowing at least one other language besides English would be helpful to serve a broader population. Developing cultural competence is necessary to serve a broad population as well.

Q. **What is the employment outlook for your field? How will the field change in the future?**

A. We are serving individuals across the age span with more severe medical needs. For example, more infants are surviving with lower birth weights and resulting complications, including language and learning problems. People are living longer and may have communication needs resulting from strokes, injuries, or other health conditions.

We also are serving individuals without communication disorders who want to improve the effectiveness of their communication in the workplace or other settings.

Technological advances are changing the way we provide services: there are opportunities for telepractice; individuals with more severe disabilities are benefiting from the new computers and other speech-generating devices as an augmentative or alternative form of communication.

Services are becoming more collaborative: speech-language pathologists work on teams with parents, teachers, and other professionals. They collaborate on the development and implementation of the individualized education program.

Our scope of practice has expanded over the years and likely will continue to change. We've moved from a field focused primarily on speech correction to one with a much greater focus on language, communication, swallowing, literacy, social interactions, learning and learning disabilities, severe disabilities, and other specialized areas.

Currently, we are experiencing shortages of speech-language pathologists in the United States. The Bureau of Labor Statistics indicates that speech-language pathology is one of the best professions for seeking a job.

Interview: Pamela Mason

Pamela Mason, M.Ed., CCC-A, the Director of Audiology Professional Practices at the American Speech-Language-Hearing Association

Q. **What made you want to enter this career?**

A. I learned about the profession of audiology when I enrolled in an undergraduate program in speech-language pathology. It was then that I realized that I might have what it takes to become a good audiologist. I have always enjoyed music and was never afraid of audio technology; back then I felt confident setting up a stereo and understood (somehow through my music interest) how to set the frequency equalizer and volume for best fidelity.

I also have good communication skills and love to teach. Both of these qualities are necessary to become a good audiologist and to enjoy the profession. Audiologists must be able to communicate with and teach individuals (patients and clients) with hearing or balance issues. It takes empathy as well. An audiologist understands the impact of hearing loss on the quality of life. The audiologist must have good listening skills, which are part of counseling. If you are working with infants and young children, and hearing loss has been identified at birth during universal newborn hearing screening programs in hospitals, these skills are paramount because it can be difficult news to accept when your baby is only one day old. Young families need support and information. Audiologists also need to be objective in interpreting test results and in their support of patients/clients. Decisions are never based just upon the audiologist's thoughts; options are discussed, and the families with knowledge makes the decision.

Q. **What is the one thing that young people may not know about a career in audiology?**

A. Wow! What a question! Our services are necessary across a lifetime. More than 95 percent of infants born in the United States receive a hearing screening before they are discharged from the hospital. Infants identified [with hearing loss] through the screening are followed through a process called Early Hearing Detection and Intervention (EHDI). Pediatric audiologists work with families, infants, pediatricians, and other health professionals in the EHDI programs in each state. On the other end of the age continuum, the baby boomers are approaching retirement, and hearing loss in the older population is greater than in younger individuals. And over the past decade or so, the scope of practice has grown and will continue to grow. Audiologists are also expert in understanding the balance system, which is situated in the inner ear next to the cochlea, the end organ for hearing. Audiologists help people with balance concerns. Through a battery of tests, audiologists can assist in the medical diagnosis of the cause of balance disorders.

Employment opportunities are expected to grow. A four-year post-baccalaureate degree is required. Detailed career information is available at www.asha.org; look in the Careers tab.

Q. **What are the most important personal and professional qualities for people in your career?**

A.   ✔ Work with people of all ages
   ✔ Enjoy technology
   ✔ Work in a variety of settings
   ✔ Assess, diagnosis, and treat individuals with non-medical hearing and balance problems
   ✔ Good communication skills
   ✔ Good listening skills
   ✔ Objective when faced with difficult situations

Q. **What do you like most about your job?**

A. Every day is different! Each patient brings a new set of unique characteristics—both as an individual and as an individual with a hearing or balance concern. I like helping people. Audiology is not a life-saving profession, but it is a life-changing profession.

Q. **What advice would you give to young people who are interested in the field?**

A. In a word: Google. And begin your Internet search at www.asha.org. Through our website, you can locate an audiologist nearby your home at www.asha.org/profind. Contact that person, and learn firsthand about the field.

Q. **How will the field change in the future?**

A. Audiology is a dynamic field with new technological advances occurring frequently. The following areas may be considered new areas of clinical practice based on a review of data sources: new treatment protocols for tinnitus treatment; caloric stimulation for balance treatment; genetic screening for hearing loss; hybrid cochlear implants; preservation of hearing using otoprotective agents.

SURGICAL TECHNOLOGISTS

OVERVIEW

Surgical technologists help surgeons, nurses, and other members of the surgical team before, during, and after surgical procedures. They are sometimes referred to as *surgical technicians* or *operating room technicians*. Training programs for surgical technologists last nine to 24 months and lead to a certificate, diploma, or associate's degree. Approximately 100,270 surgical technologists are employed in the United States. Strong employment opportunities are expected in the next decade.

THE JOB

You've probably seen enough operating-room scenes on television and in the movies to know that there are many health care professionals present during a surgery—far more than just surgeons and nurses. Surgical technologists are part of this group. Preparing the operating room, creating and maintaining the sterile field, and gathering and organizing necessary equipment and supplies are just some of the vital pre-operative responsibilities of this professional. During surgery, the surgical technologist passes instruments to the surgeon and must be skilled enough to anticipate the needs of the surgeon. He or she also handles and prepares medications and specimens. When the surgery has concluded, the surgical technologist is responsible for maintaining the sterile field until the patient is transported and for removing any instruments or equipment. The operating room can be a stressful environment, and the surgical technologist must be able to work well under pressure. The surgical technologist's role is indeed vital to a successful surgery—he or she plays a role in saving lives. The following paragraphs provide an overview of the most popular surgical technology specialties.

FAST FACTS

High School Subjects
Biology
Health

Personal Skills
Communication
Coordination
Critical thinking
Operation monitoring

Minimum Education Level
Some postsecondary training

Salary Range
$31,000 to $44,000 to $63,000+

Employment Outlook
Much faster than the average

O*NET-SOC
29-2055.00

NOC
3414

Emerging Career: Radiosurgeon

What do they do?: Radiosurgeons are radiation oncologists who use robotic high-energy radiation beams to treat cancerous tumors. This technology has been used for years to treat brain cancer, but now it is being used to attack spinal tumors, early-stage lung cancer, and other tumors.

Earnings: $200,000 to $800,000

Educational Requirements: Medical degree, board certification recommended; three-week training course in radiosurgery

Top employers: Large hospitals and research universities, as well as entrepreneurial options

Scrub surgical technologists assist the surgical team during procedures. They have a good understanding of the type and scope of the procedure being done and can anticipate the needs of the medical team. For preoperative case management, their duties include preparing the operating room. This entails making sure all supplies are readily available and equipment is functioning properly. Scrub surgical technologists wear operating gowns and gloves only after they have scrubbed—washing thoroughly with antiseptic soap. They set up the sterile table and make sure supplies, instruments, medications, and solutions are in place. They keep an accurate count of all pieces of equipment and supplies, such as forceps, sponges, or rolls of gauze. The pre-operative count must match at the end of the procedure, ensuring no foreign objects are mistakenly left in the patient's body during surgery. This count is done with another member of the surgical team.

Scrub surgical technologists help doctors and nurses into their sterile gowns and gloves. They are also responsible for exposing the sterile area by draping the patient with cloth.

During the surgical procedure, scrub surgical technologists pass instruments to the surgeon. When the surgeon asks for a particular instrument, the technologist must be able to locate and give the instrument quickly, many times anticipating the needs of the surgeon. Technologists may also prepare sterile dressing in preparation for closing the surgical site. At this time, the post-operative count of instruments and dressings is made.

After the surgical procedure, scrub surgical technologists are responsible for terminal sterilization of all instruments and equipment used. This is important to ensure the instruments and equipments are free from all traces of bacteria. The technologist also cleans the operating room and prepares it for the next procedure.

Circulating surgical technologists have many of the same pre-operative and post-operative duties as scrub surgical technologists. They obtain necessary instruments, supplies, and equipment, and they help sterilize the operating room after each procedure. However, circulating surgical tech-

Educational Requirements for Health Care Workers on the Rise

The health care industry traditionally has offered good job prospects for workers with only a high school diploma or an associate's degree. But this is changing as technology and an emphasis on cutting costs and improving patient outcomes reduces opportunities for certain mid-level health care workers. The *Wall Street Journal* reports that "positions such as licensed practical nurses and medical-records clerks are being eliminated or pushed out of hospitals into lower-paying corners of the field such as nursing homes." Additionally, there is a trend toward increasing the educational requirements for particular positions. For example, the Institute of Medicine recommends increasing the proportion of registered nurses (RNs) who hold at least a bachelor's degree to 80 percent by 2020 (today, only 50 percent of RNs have bachelor's degrees). According to the Apollo Research Institute, "employers find greater value in nurses and health care support workers who pursue bachelor's and advanced degrees because they bring to the job improved skills, including enhanced patient care, teamwork, critical-thinking and problem-solving capacities, and stronger science and mathematics knowledge." Look for this trend to continue as employers—especially hospitals—seek better-educated employees that can help them improve their bottom lines.

nologists have more patient responsibility. Before each procedure, they check the patient's chart and consent forms to match the proper patient with the surgical procedure that is scheduled. They then transport the patient to the operating room and transfer him or her to the operating table. Circulating surgical technologists often converse with the patient, and if he or she is anxious or fearful, they may provide words of reassurance and comfort.

Circulating surgical technologists set up electrosurgical grounding pads, monitors, or other equipment before the procedure begins. They also prepare the patient's skin with an antiseptic solution to ensure that bacteria does not enter the patient's body through the incision. When surgeons remove a piece of tissue for further pathology, circulating surgical technologists place the specimen in the proper solution and container. They also secure the patient's dressings while the surgeon closes the incision. Afterwards, circulating surgical technologists transfer the patient to the operating recovery room.

With advanced training and certification, surgical technologists can advance to the rank of *first assistant surgical technologist*. First assistant technologists help surgeons during procedures by carrying out many of the technical tasks. They hold instruments such as retractors or forceps, as instructed by the surgeon. They may also help in hemostasis—the process of stopping a bleed—by applying electrocautery or clamps. Some first assistant technologists may be directed by surgeons to cut suture material or apply dressings to a closed wound.

Second assistant surgical technologists handle technical tasks that do not involve cutting, clamping, and suturing tissue. They may hold retractors or instruments, use suction or sponges on the operative site, connect drains to suction apparatus, apply dressings to closed wounds, and perform other duties.

Full-time surgical technologists work 40 hours a week, with some shifts scheduled on weekends and holidays. Some surgical technologists have assigned emergency call shifts.

At times the work environment can be quite stressful, especially when assigned surgical procedures back-to-back. It is important for surgical technologists to stay alert and focused, paying special attention to key details. Surgical technologists are also exposed to many situations that may be unpleasant or uncomfortable, such as blood or open wounds. Exposure to communicable diseases is also possible.

REQUIREMENTS

HIGH SCHOOL

In high school, take courses in health, anatomy and physiology, biology, chemistry, and mathematics to prepare for the field. Speech classes will help you to develop your communication skills, which you will need when interacting with coworkers and patients.

POSTSECONDARY TRAINING

Training programs for surgical technologists last nine to 24 months and lead to a certificate, diploma, or associate's degree. Typical classes include Surgical Instrumentation, Equipment and Supplies, Principles of Asepsis and Sterile Technique, Surgical Procedures, Medical Terminology, Anatomy and Physiology, Microbiology, Surgical Pharmacology and Anesthesia Techniques, Safety Standards in the Operating Room, General Patient Care and Safety, Preoperative and Postoperative Considerations, and Legal, Moral, and Ethical Issues. Students also participate in clinical experiences under the supervision of trained surgical technologists. The Commission on Accreditation of Allied Health Education Programs (CAA-HEP) has accredited approximately 435 surgical technology programs. Visit its website, www.caahep.org, for a list of programs.

CERTIFICATION AND LICENSING

Certification is available from the National Board of Surgical Technology and Surgical Assisting (www.nbstsa.org). Those who graduate from a CAAHEP-accredited program and pass a national certification examination can use the designation, certified surgical technologist. The certified surgical first assistant designation is also available. Surgical technologists can also become certified by the National Center for Competency Testing (www.ncctinc.com). Applicants

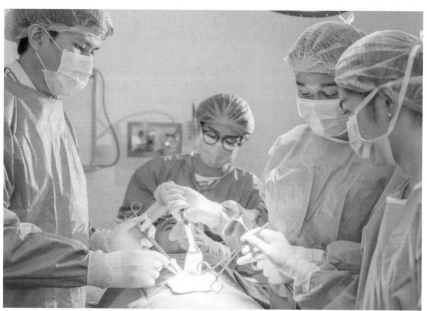

To be successful, surgical technologists must have excellent teamwork and communication skills. (Adobe Stock)

who meet education and experience requirements and pass an examination may use the designation, tech in surgery-certified. Certification, while voluntary, is highly recommended. It is an excellent way to stand out from other job applicants and demonstrate your abilities to prospective employers. The National Commission for the Certification of Surgical Assistants and the American Board of Surgical Assistants also provide certification.

OTHER REQUIREMENTS

To be a successful surgical technologist, you should be very organized and attentive to detail. You will need excellent manual dexterity, and you should be in good physical shape, since you'll be on your feet for long periods of time and be required (in the case of circulating technologists) to move quickly back and forth between operating rooms and supply areas during surgeries. You must be able to respond quickly to requests for instruments; many experienced technologists are able to anticipate the instruments needed by a surgeon before they are even requested. Finally, you should be willing to continue to learn throughout your career via seminars, educational conferences, and other methods of continuing education.

EXPLORING

Does the career of surgical technologist sound interesting to you? If so, there are many ways to learn more about a career as a surgical technologist. You can read books and journals (such as *The Surgical Technologist*, www.ast.org/Publications/The_Surgical_Technologist) about the field, visit the websites of college surgical technology programs to learn about typical classes and possible career paths, and ask your teacher or school counselor to arrange an information interview with a surgical technologist. Here are some sample questions to ask:

✔ What do you like best and least about your job?

✔ What's the work environment like at your employer?

✔ What are the most important personal and professional qualities for people in your career?

✔ What's the best way to network in the health care industry?

✔ What's the best way today for people to land jobs in the industry?

✔ What advice would you give to job seekers in terms of applying to and interviewing for jobs?

Finally, the Association of Surgical Technologists provides a wealth of information on education and careers at its website, www.ast.org.

EMPLOYERS

Approximately 100,270 surgical technologists are employed in the United States—with 70 percent employed by hospitals, mainly in delivery and operating rooms. Other employers include outpatient care centers, offices of physicians and other medical professionals, and the U.S. military. Some surgical technologists work as college educators; others pursue careers in medical equipment sales.

GETTING A JOB

Many surgical technologists obtain their first jobs as a result of contacts made through college internships, career fairs, or networking events. Others seek assistance in obtaining job leads from college career services offices, newspaper want ads, and employment websites. Additionally, the Association of Surgical Technologists provides job listings at its website, http://careercenter.ast.org/jobseekers. Information on job opportunities at federal agencies is available at www.usajobs.gov.

ADVANCEMENT

Surgical technologists advance by receiving salary increases and by specializing in a particular area of surgery, such as neurosurgery. Others become managers of surgical technologists or supervise central supply departments in hospitals. Surgical technologists who earn graduate degrees can become college professors. Many technologists complete additional education to become physician assistants.

EARNINGS

Salaries for surgical technologists vary by type of employer, geographic region, and the worker's experience, education, and skill level. Median annual salaries for surgical technologists were $44,330 in May 2015, according to the U.S. Department of Labor (USDL). Salaries ranged from less than $31,410

FOR MORE INFORMATION

For education and career information, contact

Association of Surgical Technologists
800-637-7433
www.ast.org

---

to $63,410 or more. The USDL reports the following mean annual earnings for surgical technologists by employer: offices of physicians, $46,720; outpatient care centers, $46,700; general medical/surgical hospitals, $45,590.

Surgical technologists usually receive benefits such as health and life insurance, vacation days, sick leave, and a savings and pension plan. Some employers offer tuition reimbursement and child care benefits. Part-time workers must provide their own benefits.

EMPLOYMENT OUTLOOK

According to the U.S. Department of Labor, the demand for surgical technologists is expected to increase much faster than the average for all occupations during the next decade. An aging population along with advances in medical technology (such as fiber optics and laser technology) are creating demand for skilled surgical technologists. Hospitals, the largest employers of surgical technologists, will continue to offer a large number of job openings, but employment will grow fastest at offices of physicians and in outpatient care centers, including ambulatory surgical centers. Employment prospects will be best for surgical technologists who are certified and who are willing to relocate to areas of the country where there is a shortage of workers.

Interview: Sharon Rehn

Sharon Rehn, MA, BS, RN, CST, the Chair of the Surgical Technology Program at Southeast Community College in Lincoln, Nebraska

Q. Can you tell us about the career of surgical technologist?

A. Surgical technologists are important members of the surgical team. They are highly trained individuals who focus their attention on the surgical procedure with the emphasis placed on the required instrumentation needed for each procedural step. The surgical technologist is called on to deliver instruments and supplies to the surgeon and his or her assistants with precision and speed. When the surgical technologist is not in the handing role, they take on the role of assisting the surgeon with any tasks that do not require a medical license such as retracting tissues, sponging and suctioning blood, and cutting suture.

Q. What is one thing that young people may not know about the field?

A. What most people are unaware of is that the surgical technologist is the only professional on the team who has specific education in sterile technique, which is vital for maintaining an infection-free surgical experience for all their patients.

Q.   What high school classes should students focus on to be successful in this career?

A.   For the high school student who is planning on a career in surgical technology, the following courses are highly recommended to help with a successful outcome within an associate degree surgical technology program. The science courses of biology, anatomy, and physiology are essential to lay the groundwork. English, social science, and math are some of the general education courses that are highly recommended, with the understanding that a student will find better success in college math if they continue to take math courses throughout their high school years. The longer it has been since a student has taken a math course the more difficult it may be to succeed in a college math course. If your high school offers a medical terminology course, that would be an excellent addition to your course work.

Q.   What are the most important personal and professional skills for surgical technologists?

A.   When looking at the best things a student can offer when coming into a surgical technology program, I feel that a highly motivated, self-driven, responsible, and mature individual will find success within such an important profession.

After graduation, a surgical technologist will be called upon to have great manual dexterity to handle instruments quickly, and this will require excellent hand-to-eye coordination. A successful surgical technologist will need to be emotionally stable to be able to handle the stressful conditions that come with surgery. Surgical technologists must have good critical-thinking skills that will help them to concentrate and respond to the needs of the surgeon.

All surgical team members must have good interpersonal relations skills, physical strength, and stamina but most of all they must possess a surgical conscience that requires them to protect their patients at all times.

Q.   What is the employment outlook for surgical technologists?

A.   When looking at the employment outlook for the area that I teach in, the Midwest cannot fill all the surgical technologist positions that are needed for all surgical departments to practice safely with well-trained surgical technologists. The rural areas tend to suffer the most at getting educated surgical technologists to stay within their areas. Surgical technologists who have experience and choose to work for contracting companies are still filling the gaps at a much higher cost to the hospitals for the time being.

Q.   Can you please tell us about your program?

A.   Southeast Community College is where my program graduates surgical technologists with an associate's degree in applied science. My program requires nine pre-requisites to be completed with a GPA of 2.5 prior to getting accepted into the program. The Surgical Technology Program courses take 15 months to complete. The first six months of the program are spent within the classroom and LAB with a few visits to the hospital for observation. The final nine months of the program includes classroom coursework and 700 hours of time in the surgical department spent at the surgical field learning to hand instruments proficiently to the surgeon. My students sit for their board exam on their last day of the program with the intent on continuing our record of 100 percent pass rate of our graduates.

HEALTH CARE SCHOLARSHIPS

The following professional associations, government agencies, nonprofit organizations, and companies provide scholarships to high school and college students who are studying health care-related majors at colleges and universities. In addition to these resources, don't forget to check out financial aid that is provided by state and local health care associations, nonprofits, and hospitals (which sometimes provide scholarships for aspiring nurses or allied health professionals).

AMERICAN ACADEMY OF ORTHOTISTS & PROSTHETISTS (AAOP)

202-380-3663, ext. 212

scholarship@oandp.org

www.oandp.org/education/professional_development/scholarships.asp

Scholarship Name: The AAOP offers several named scholarships for orthotic and prosthetic students. **Academic Area:** Orthotics and prosthetics. **Who May Apply?:** College students. **Eligibility:** Applicants must demonstrate financial need, display leadership qualities (for certain scholarships), and contribute to their own education financially. **Application Process:** Students must submit a completed application (available at the AAOP website), a letter of recommendation from someone currently working within the orthotic and/or prosthetic profession, and a 200-word essay on why they want to work in the orthotic and/or prosthetic professions. **Amount:** $500 to $1,000. **Deadline:** Varies by scholarship.

AMERICAN ART THERAPY ASSOCIATION (AART)

www.arttherapy.org

Scholarship Name: The AART offers more than five named scholarships for art therapy students. **Academic Area:** Art therapy. **Who May Apply?:** College students. **Eligibility:** Applicants must be members of the AART, demonstrate financial need, be a strong academic performer, and be attending or accepted to an AART-approved graduate art therapy program. **Application Process:** Applicants must submit a completed application form (available at the AART website), academic transcript, two academic or work-related signed letters of recommendation, financial information, and a brief biography and a statement of how they view their role in the future as an art therapist. **Amount:** $500 to $900. **Deadline:** Typically in April.

AMERICAN ASSOCIATION FOR MEN IN NURSING (AAMN) FOUNDATION

859-977-7453

www.aamn.org/about-us/scholarships

Scholarship Name: The AAMN Foundation sponsors more than five named scholarships for men who are pursuing nursing degrees. **Academic Area:** Nursing. **Who May Apply?:** College students. **Eligibility:** Applicants must be current AAMN members, male students who are currently enrolled in an accredited nursing program; and meet other requirements. **Application Process:** Visit the AAMN's website to learn about each scholarship and to download applications. **Amount:** $1,000 to $5,000. **Deadline:** Varies by scholarship.

AMERICAN ASSOCIATION OF COLLEGES OF NURSING (AACN)

202-463-6930

sbradfield@aacn.nche.edu (address questions to Sonja Bradfield)

www.aacn.nche.edu/students/scholarships

Scholarship Name: The Geraldine "Polly" Bednash Scholarship is provided by the AACN and its partner, Castle Branch. **Academic Area:** Nursing. **Who May Apply?:** High school seniors, college students. **Eligibility:** Applicants must maintain at least a 3.20 GPA in their current program or at last school attended, be admitted or enrolled in a baccalaureate or higher degree nursing program at an AACN-member institution affiliated with CastleBranch (see www.aacn.nche.edu/students/scholarships/CBSchools.pdf), OR have submitted their application to a nursing school through NursingCAS (see https://portal.nursingcas.org). **Application Process:** Visit www.aacn.nche.edu/students/scholarships for links to the various scholarship applications. **Amount:** Two $5,000 scholarships. **Deadlines:** January 31, April 30, July 31, and October 31.

AMERICAN ASSOCIATION OF COLLEGES OF NURSING (AACN)

202-463-6930

www.aacn.nche.edu/students/scholarships

Scholarship Name: Students pursuing a baccalaureate, master's, or doctoral degree in nursing are eligible for four scholarships provided by the AACN and its partners. **Academic Area:** Nursing. **Who May Apply?:** College students. **Eligibility:** Varies by scholarship. **Application Process:** Visit the website above for links to the various scholarship applications. **Amount:** $2,500 to $5,000. **Deadline:** Varies by scholarship.

AMERICAN DENTAL ASSISTANTS ASSOCIATION (ADAA)

www.adaausa.org/Membership/Awards-and-Scholarship-Information/JASInfo

Scholarship Name: Juliette A. Southard Scholarship Program. **Academic Area:** Nursing. **Who May Apply?:** College students. **Eligibility:** "Candidates must be high school graduates; or hold a GED; or be 18 years of age to be eligible for consideration. Applicant must be a student member of ADAA." **Application Process:** Applicants must submit a completed application, academic transcripts, two letters of reference, and a statement of intent. **Amount:** Varies. **Deadline:** Typically in mid-March.

AMERICAN DENTAL ASSOCIATION FOUNDATION

adaf@ada.org

www.adafoundation.org/en/what-we-do/dental-student-resources

Scholarship Name: The foundation offers a variety of scholarships for dental, dental hygiene, dental assisting, and dental laboratory technology students (including ones specifically for minorities). **Academic Area:** Dentistry. **Who May Apply?:** College students. **Eligibility:** Applicants must be enrolled full-time in a dental program, be U.S. citizens, and demonstrate financial need. **Application Process:** Varies by scholarship. **Amount:** Varies by scholarship. **Deadline:** Varies by scholarship.

AMERICAN DENTAL HYGIENISTS' ASSOCIATION (ADHA) INSTITUTE FOR ORAL HEALTH

institute@adha.net

www.adha.org/ioh-scholarships-main

Scholarship Name: Students interested in pursuing full-time study in dental hygiene are eligible for several scholarships. **Academic Area:** Dental hygiene. **Who May Apply?:** College students. **Eligibility:** Applicants must be enrolled in an accredited dental hygiene program in the United States, have completed—or about to complete—a minimum of one year in a dental hygiene curriculum, have a minimum GPA (varies by scholarship), and be a professional member or student member of the ADHA. **Application Process:** Apply at the website above. **Amount:** Varies by scholarship. **Deadline:** Typically in early February.

AMERICAN HEALTH INFORMATION MANAGEMENT ASSOCIATION (AHIMA) FOUNDATION OF RESEARCH AND EDUCATION

info@ahimafoundation.org

www.ahimafoundation.org/education/MeritScholarships.aspx

Scholarship Name: Merit Scholarships. (Note: A Veterans Scholarship is also available). **Academic Area:** Health information management (HIM) or health informatics. **Who May Apply?:** College students. **Eligibility:** Applicants must be currently attending an approved associate or baccalaureate program of study or a graduate program in a field related to HIM or health informatics. They also must have a GPA of at least 3.5 and be members of AHIMA. Scholarships are awarded based on the applicant's academic achievement, volunteer and work or leadership experience, commitment to the profession, and quality of references. **Application Process:** Applicants must submit a completed application (available for download at the Foundation's website), two letters of reference, and academic transcripts. **Amount:** $1,000 to $2,500. **Deadline:** Typically late September.

AMERICAN INDIAN SCIENCE AND ENGINEERING SOCIETY (AISES)

www.aises.org/scholarships/bnsf

Scholarship Name: Burlington North Santa Fe (BNSF) Foundation Scholarship. **Academic Area:** Medicine, health administration, engineering, education, business, mathematics, natural/physical sciences, technology. **Who May Apply?:** High school seniors. **Eligibility:** Applicants must be American Indian high school seniors who reside in one of the 13 states serviced by the Burlington Northern and Santa Fe Pacific Corporation and its affiliated companies: Arizona, California, Colorado, Kansas, Minnesota, Montana, New Mexico, North Dakota, Oklahoma, Oregon, South Dakota, Texas, and Washington. Scholarship recipients must maintain a 2.5 GPA during their freshman and sophomore years and a 3.0 GPA during their junior and senior years. Applicants must be members of the AISES. **Application Process:** Applicants should submit a completed application, official transcripts, a resume, three essays, and proof of tribal enrollment. Visit the association's website for membership information and to download an application. **Amount:** $2,500 per academic year for up to four years. **Deadline:** Typically in early May.

The AISES also provides health- and STEM-related educational scholarships for undergraduates and graduate students. Visit its website for more information.

AMERICAN MEDICAL TECHNOLOGISTS (AMT)

847-823-5169

www.americanmedtech.org

Scholarship Name: Student Scholarship. **Academic Area:** Medical technology/laboratory science/assisting. **Who May Apply?:** High school seniors, college students. **Eligibility:** Students who plan to or who are currently pursuing college education that will result in a career as a medical assistant, medical laboratory assistant, medical administrative specialist, medical technologist, medical laboratory technician, phlebotomist, allied health educator, clinical lab consultant, or dental assistant may apply. **Application Process:** Applicants must submit official academic transcripts, two letters of personal reference, a typed statement that explains why they are interested in the career, and a completed application. Visit the AMT website to download an application. **Amount:** Five $500 scholarships. **Deadline:** Typically in early April.

Tips on Reducing the Cost of College, Part I

✔ **File the FAFSA.** Be sure to complete and submit the Free Application for Federal Student Aid (which is available on October 1) to ensure your eligibility for as much federal financial aid as possible.

✔ **Attend a public college in your state to save money.** Tuition at these schools will traditionally be lower than tuition at out-of-state colleges and universities.

✔ **Consider attending a community college for the first two years of postsecondary education.** Tuition is significantly less expensive at community colleges than at four-year institutions. The College Board reports that students who attend a community college for the first two years of their education—instead of enrolling in a typical private college—will save nearly $70,000. If you plan to go on to pursue a bachelor's degree at a four-year institution, make sure that your academic credits transfer to that school.

AMERICAN MUSIC THERAPY ASSOCIATION (AMTA)

www.musictherapy.org/careers/scholars

Scholarship Name: The AMTA offers several named scholarships. **Academic Area:** Music therapy. **Who May Apply?:** College students. **Eligibility:** Applicants must be members of the AMTA and enrolled in a college or university program in music therapy approved by the AMTA. **Application Process:** Visit the AMTA's website to download an application. **Amount:** $500 to $1,000. **Deadline:** Varies by scholarship.

AMERICAN OCCUPATIONAL THERAPY FOUNDATION (AOTF)

240-292-1034

scholarships@aotf.org

www.aotf.org/scholarshipsgrants

Scholarship Name: The Foundation offers more than 50 annual scholarships to students enrolled in occupational therapy programs at all educational levels. **Academic Area:** Occupational therapy. **Who May Apply?:** College students. **Eligibility:** Applicants must be currently enrolled full-time in an occupational therapy educational program, have completed at least one year of occupational therapy-specific coursework, and be a member of the American Occupational Therapy Association. **Application Process:** Applicants complete one application at the AOTF website, which is used toward all applicable scholarships. **Amount:** $150 to $5,000. **Deadline:** Typically in late October.

AMERICAN SOCIETY FOR CLINICAL LABORATORY SCIENCE (ASCLS)

www.ascls.org/alpha-mu-tau-scholarships

Scholarship Name: Alpha Mu Tau is a national fraternity that promotes clinical laboratory science careers. It offers more than 10 scholarships. **Academic Area:** Clinical laboratory sciences. **Who May Apply?:** College students. **Eligibility:** Applicants must be U.S. citizens; be accepted into an accredited program in clinical laboratory science, to include clinical laboratory science/medical technology, clinical laboratory technician/medical laboratory technician); and be entering their last year of undergraduate study. Applicants for graduate-level scholarships must be ASCLS members. **Application Process:** Download an application at the ASCLS's website. **Amount:** $2,000 to $3,000. **Deadline:** Typically in mid-March.

AMERICAN SOCIETY OF HUMAN GENETICS

dnaday@ashg.org

www.ashg.org/education/dnaday.shtml

Contest Name: DNA Day Essay Contest "aims to challenge students to examine, question, and reflect on the important concepts of genetics." **Academic Area:** Science. **Who May Apply?:** High school students. **Eligibility:** High school students from the United States and other countries may enters. **Application Process:** Essays are "expected to contain substantive, well-reasoned arguments indicative of a depth of understanding of the concepts related to the essay question," which is available at the society's website. The essay must be no longer than 750 words. Essays must be submitted electronically through the submission site of the society. Only classroom teachers or primary instructors of homeschooled children may submit student essays. **Amount:** First place, $1,000; second place, $600; third place, $400; honorable mention, 10 prizes of $100. **Deadline:** Typically in mid-March.

ASE FOUNDATION

American Society of Echocardiography (ASE)

www.asefoundation.org/why-donate/sonographer-and-career-development-grants

Scholarship Name: Alan D. Waggoner Student Scholarship Award. **Academic Area:** Sonography. **Who May Apply?:** High school seniors, college students. **Eligibility:** Sonographer students enrolled in a Commission on Accreditation of Allied Health Education Programs (CAAHEP)-accredited cardiac or echocardiography ultrasound educational programs "who exhibit a passion for the discipline of echocardiography and demonstrate leadership abilities" may apply. Applicants also must be members of the ASE. **Application Process:** Students must be nominated by their sonography program director. Visit the Foundation's website for details about the application process. **Amount:** $1,000. **Deadline:** Typically in late-September.

ASSOCIATION OF PERIOPERATIVE REGISTERED NURSES FOUNDATION

303-368-6278

foundation@aorn.org

www.aorn.org/foundation

Scholarship Name: The AORN Foundation provides scholarships to students who are pursuing a career in perioperative nursing and to registered nurses who are continuing their education in perioperative nursing by pursuing a bachelor's, master's, or doctoral degree. **Academic Area:** Perioperative nursing. **Who May Apply?:** College students, nursing professionals. **Eligibility:** Nursing students (applicants must be in an accredited program leading to initial licensure as an R.N.), baccalaureate, master, and doctoral candidates with a cumulative G.P.A. of 3.0 or higher. **Application Process:** Scholarships are awarded based on the quality of academics/transcripts, essay, financial need, and accurate completion of the scholarship application. Visit the Foundation's Web site for further details and to download an application. **Amount:** Varies. **Deadline:** Typically mid-June.

BIOCOMMUNICATIONS ASSOCIATION

office@bca.org

www.bca.org/resources/grants/effe_scholarships.html

Scholarship Name: Endowment Fund for Education Scholarship. **Academic Area:** Scientific/biomedical visual communications. **Who May Apply?:** College students. **Eligibility:** Full-time undergraduate or graduate students pursuing a career in scientific/biomedical visual communications may apply. **Application Process:** Applicants must submit a completed application (which is available at the Association's website), academic transcript, portfolio, and an essay that explains what inspired them to pursue a course of study in scientific/biomedical visual communications. **Amount:** Two $500 scholarships. **Deadline:** Typically in early-February.

DAUGHTERS OF THE AMERICAN REVOLUTION (DAR)

www.dar.org/national-society/scholarships

Scholarship Name: DAR is a volunteer women's service organization that promotes patriotism and the preservation of American history. It offers a variety of scholarships to aspiring nurses, doctors, and occupational, physical, art, and music therapists. **Academic Area:** Health care. **Who May Apply?:** High school seniors, college students. **Eligibility:** Eligibility requirements vary by scholarship, but all require applicants to be accepted by a postsecondary training program, be citizens of the United States, and demonstrate strong academic performance. **Application Process:** Visit the DAR website to download an application. **Amount:** $2,000 to $5,000. **Deadline:** Typically in mid-February.

Tips on Reducing the Cost of College, Part II

✔ **Don't be pessimistic about your chances of landing financial aid.** Many students think their parents earn too much money to be eligible for financial aid. This is untrue in many instances. In fact, a survey by The College Board found that about 75 percent of families earning more than $100,000 a year applied for financial aid for the current academic year.

✔ **Be sure to apply for private scholarships.** Foundations and corporations award approximately $11 billion in private scholarships each year, according to The College Board, although only about 8 percent of students receive these awards (which average about $3,400, but can range up to the full cost of tuition).

✔ **Get a job.** Working during school will help you to offset the cost of college tuition. But be careful: don't work so much that your studies suffer. A study led by Gary Pike of Indiana University Purdue University Indianapolis found that college students who worked more than 20 hours a week had lower grades than students who did not do so.

✔ **Graduate on time.** Only about 60 percent of college students earn a bachelor's degree in four years—those extra years add up to a lot of extra tuition, room and board, and other costs.

FOUNDATION OF THE NATIONAL STUDENT NURSES' ASSOCIATION

nsna@nsna.org

www.forevernursing.org

Scholarship Name: Students currently enrolled and matriculated in a state-approved nursing program leading to an associate degree, baccalaureate, diploma, generic pre-licensure doctorate, or generic pre-licensure master's degree; or enrolled in an RN to BSN completion, RN to MSN completion, or LPN/LVN to RN program are eligible for general scholarships. **Academic Area:** Nursing. **Who May Apply?:** College students. **Eligibility:** Scholarships are awarded based on academic achievement, financial need, and involvement in student nursing associations and community health activities. **Application Process:** Visit the Foundation's Web site to download an application. **Amount:** $1,000 to $7,500. **Deadline:** Typically in January.

HEALTH RESOURCES AND SERVICES ADMINISTRATION (HRSA)

U.S. Department of Health and Human Services

800-221-9393

https://nhsc.hrsa.gov

Scholarship Name: National Health Service Corps (NHSC) Scholarship Program. **Academic Area:** Health care. **Who May Apply?:** College students. **Eligibility:** Applicants must be committed to primary care and accepted to or enrolled in an accredited U.S. school in one of the following primary care disciplines: physicians (M.D. or D.O.), dentists, nurse practitioners (post-graduate degree with clinical practice focus), certified nurse-midwives, and physician assistants. They also must be U.S. citizens or U.S. nationals and attend school full time. Those who receive scholarships must commit to work at least two years at an NHSC-approved site in a medically underserved community. **Application Process:** Visit the HRSA website to complete an application. **Amount:** Tuition, fees, and other educational costs, plus a living stipend. **Deadline:** Typically in the spring.

HEALTH RESOURCES AND SERVICES ADMINISTRATION (HRSA)

U.S. Department of Health and Human Services
800-221-9393
https://bhw.hrsa.gov/loansscholarships/nursecorps/scholarship

Scholarship Name: NURSE Corps Scholarship Program. **Academic Area:** Nursing. **Who May Apply?:** High school students, college students. **Eligibility:** Students accepted to or enrolled in a diploma, associate's, baccalaureate, or graduate nursing program can apply for funding for tuition, fees, and other educational costs in exchange for working at an eligible critical shortage facility for at least two years after they graduate. Scholarship recipients also receive a monthly stipend. Applicants must be U.S. citizens (born or naturalized), nationals, or lawful permanent residents; be enrolled or accepted at an accredited school of nursing in the U.S.; and begin classes no later than September 30 of the year in which they apply. Applicants with the greatest financial need will be given preference. **Application Process:** Apply at the HRSA's website. **Amount:** Full tuition, required fees, monthly stipend, and other reasonable costs. **Deadline:** Typically early May.

HISPANIC DENTAL ASSOCIATION FOUNDATION

512-904-0252
support@HDAssoc.org
http://hdassoc.org/hda-foundation/scholarship-program

Scholarship Name: The Foundation—in cooperation with Colgate-Palmolive, Proctor & Gamble, and other companies and individuals—offers scholarships to Hispanic high school and college students. **Academic Area:** Dental sciences. **Who May Apply?:** High school seniors, college students. **Eligibility:** Applicants must have been accepted into or currently attending an accredited dental hygiene, dental assisting, dental technician, or dental program; be current student members of the Hispanic Dental Association; have a GPA of at least 3.0 (for high school students); and meet other requirements. Scholarships will be awarded based on the applicant's "commitment and dedication to improving the oral health of the Hispanic community, community service (i.e., volunteer efforts in school, medical facilities, church, etc.), leadership skills, and scholastic achievement." **Application Process:** Visit the Foundation's website for an application. **Amount:** $500 to $4,000. **Deadline:** Typically in mid-September.

HISPANIC SCHOLARSHIP FUND (HSF)

www.hsf.net/scholarships

Scholarship Name: The Fund offers dozens of scholarships (including the HSF General College Scholarship) to help students pay for their college education. **Academic Area:** Varies by scholarship. **Who May Apply?:** High school seniors, college students. **Eligibility:** Applicants must be Hispanic/Latino U.S. citizens or eligible non-citizens and have a GPA of at least 3.0 on a 4.0 scale; other requirements vary by scholarship. **Application Process:** Applicants can apply online at the Fund's website. **Amount:** $500 to $5,000. **Deadline:** Typically in late March.

IMAGINE AMERICA FOUNDATION

http://imagine-america.org/scholarships-education

Scholarship Name: The Imagine America Foundation is a nonprofit organization that provides scholarships to students who plan to attend a career college. These scholarships can be used at more than 1,000 career colleges in the United States. **Academic Area:** Many majors (including those that prepare students for careers in health care); visit the IAF website for a listing of the academic majors that are typically offered by career colleges. **Who May Apply?:** High school students. **Eligibility:** Applicants must demonstrate financial need, have a GPA of at least 2.5 on a 4.0 scale, and have participated in voluntary community service during their senior year. **Application Process:** High schools must be enrolled in Imagine America before scholarship applications can be submitted; there is no fee for enrollment. Counselors can enroll their schools by calling 571-267-3015 or sending an email to studentservices@imagine-america.org with the following information: high school name, address, and phone number; full name of guidance counselor or contact; and guidance counselor/contact email address. Visit Imagine America's Web site for complete details. **Amount:** $1,000. **Deadline:** Typically in late December.

The Foundation also offers $1,000 Adult Skills Education Awards for students 19 and over pursuing career education.

INDIAN HEALTH SERVICE (IHS)

www.ihs.gov/scholarship/scholarships

Scholarship Name: The IHS offers three scholarships for American Indian and Alaska Native students in order to educate health professionals to staff Indian health programs. **Academic Area:** Medicine. **Who May**

Apply?: High school seniors, undergraduate students. **Eligibility:** Applicants must be Native American, be U.S. citizens, have a GPA of at least 2.0, and plan to serve Native American people at the completion of their training. **Application Process:** Visit the IHS website for an application. **Amount:** Full tuition and related fees, plus a stipend for daily living needs. **Deadline:** Typically in late March.

MEDICAL LIBRARY ASSOCIATION (MLA)

www.mlanet.org

Scholarship Name: MLA Scholarship for Minority Students. **Academic Area:** Medical librarianship. **Who May Apply?:** College students. **Eligibility:** Applicants must have a strong interest in health sciences librarianship; be a member of a minority group, defined as Black or African-American, Hispanic or Latino, Asian, Aboriginal, North American Indian or Alaskan Native, or Native Hawaiian or other Pacific Islander; must be entering a master's program at an American Library Association-accredited graduate library school or, at the time of the granting of the scholarship (February), have completed no more than one-half of the academic requirements of the graduate program; and be U.S. or Canadian citizens or have permanent residence. **Application Process:** Applicants must submit a completed application, academic transcripts, and two letters of reference. **Amount:** Up to $5,000. **Deadline:** Typically in early December.

NATIONAL ASSOCIATION OF HEALTH SERVICES EXECUTIVES (NAHSE)

NAHSEawards@gmail.com

www.nahse.org/student-scholarships.html

Scholarship Name: The NAHSE offers scholarships to minority students pursuing careers in health care management or a related field. **Academic Area:** Health care management. **Who May Apply?:** High school seniors, college students. **Eligibility:** Applicants must be accepted or enrolled in an accredited college or university program, pursuing a bachelor of science, master of science, or doctorate degree, majoring in health care administration or a related field. They also must have a minimum GPA of 2.5 (for undergraduates) and 3.0 (for graduate students) and be NAHSE members. **Application Process:** Applicants should submit a completed application (available at the Association's website), academic transcripts, and other application materials. **Amount:** $2,500. **Deadline:** Typically in early May.

NATIONAL ASSOCIATION OF HISPANIC NURSES

919-573-5443

info@thehispanicnurses.org

www.nahnnet.org/NAHNScholarships.html

Scholarship Name: Hispanic nursing students are eligible for a variety of academic scholarships. **Academic Area:** Nursing. **Who May Apply?:** College students. **Eligibility:** Applicants must be currently enrolled in an accredited LVN/LPN, associate, diploma, baccalaureate, or graduate nursing program. The Association says that "selection of recipients is based on need, current academic standing, whether they are a U.S. citizen or legal resident of the United States, and other criteria." **Application Process:** Visit the Association's website for details. **Amount:** Varies. **Deadline:** Contact the Association for the latest deadline.

NATIONAL DENTAL ASSOCIATION FOUNDATION (NDAF)

www.ndafoundation.org/dental-scholarships.html

Scholarship Name: African American and other underrepresented minority students who are interested in careers in dentistry, dental hygiene, and dental assisting are eligible for two merit-based (academic performance/community service) scholarships from the NDAF. **Academic Area:** Dentistry, dental hygiene, and dental assisting. **Who May Apply?:** College students. **Eligibility:** Applicants must be U.S. citizens or have permanent resident status, be enrolled in a postsecondary program (or, in the case of dental students, be accepted to dental school), be in good academic standing, demonstrate evidence of community service, and demonstrate financial need (for some scholarships). **Application Process:** Applicants must submit a letter of request for consideration, a financial aid report, and two letters of recommendation. **Amount:** $500 to $10,000. **Deadline:** Typically in mid-May.

NATIONAL INSTITUTES OF HEALTH (NIH)

www.training.nih.gov/programs/ugsp

Scholarship Name: Undergraduate Scholarship Program. **Academic Area:** Behavioral science, biomedical science, social science health. **Who May Apply?:** High school seniors, undergraduate students. **Eligibility:** Low-income or disadvantaged students interested in studying behavioral, biomedical, or health science may apply. Applicants must be enrolled or accepted as full-time students and have a GPA of 3.3 (on a 4.0 scale) or be in the top 5 percent of their classes. They also must be U.S. citizens or nationals or qualified noncitizens. Scholarship recipients must participate in a 10-week Summer Laboratory Experience and work one year full-time for each year of scholarship. **Application Process:** Visit the NIH's website to download an application. **Amount:** Up to $20,000 a year to cover tuition, educational expenses, and reasonable living expenses (scholarships can be renewed for up to four years). **Deadline:** Typically mid-March.

PA FOUNDATION

571-319-4510

https://pa-foundation.org/scholarships-fellowships/pa-student-schol-arships

Scholarship Name: The PA Foundation, the philanthropic arm of the American Academy of Physician Assistants (AAPA), offers five named scholarships. **Academic Area:** Physician assisting (PA). **Who May Apply?:** College students. **Eligibility:** Applicants must be student members of the AAPA, attend an ARC-PA-accredited PA program, have successfully completed at least one term of PA studies and be in good academic standing, and be enrolled in PA school at the time the application period closes. **Application Process:** Contact the foundation for details. **Amount:** $1,000 to $2,000. **Deadline:** Typically in spring.

SNMMI

703-708-9000

www.snm.org

Scholarship Name: Paul Cole Scholarship. **Academic Area:** Nuclear medicine technology. **Who May Apply?:** High school seniors, undergraduate students. **Eligibility:** Applicants must be active members of the SNMMI and enrolled in or accepted for enrollment in associate, baccalaureate, or certificate programs in nuclear medicine technology. Applicants will be judged based on their financial need, statement of goals, academic performance, and program director recommendations. They must also have a GPA of at least 2.5 (on a 4.0 scale) or a B average in a nuclear medicine technology core curriculum. **Application Process:** Applicants must submit a completed application (available at SNMMI's website), an applicant statement, academic transcripts, and a letter of recommendation from the nuclear medicine technology program director verifying acceptance to or enrollment in the program. **Amount:** A limited number of $1,000 scholarships are awarded. **Deadline:** Typically in March.

SOCIETY FOR VASCULAR ULTRASOUND (SVU)

jwedge@svunet.org

www.svunet.org/membershipmain/students/annejonesscholarship

Scholarship Name: Anne Jones Scholarship. **Academic Area:** Ultrasound. **Who May Apply?:** College students. **Eligibility:** Applicants must attend a CAAHEP-accredited program, with a concentration in vascular or non-invasive vascular study; have a cumulative grade point average of at least 3.5; be either a U.S. citizen or a permanent resident of the United States; and be a student member of the SVU. **Application Process:** Applicants must submit a completed application (available at the SVU website), two letters of professional recommendation, and an essay that details their career objectives, why they chose to study vascular ultrasound, where they see themselves in five years, and why you they deserving of this scholarship. **Amount:** Up to $2,500; runner-ups receive $1,000. **Deadline:** Typically in February.

SOCIETY OF DIAGNOSTIC MEDICAL SONOGRAPHY (SDMS)

foundation@sdms.org

www.sdms.org/foundation/programs/scholarships

Scholarship Name: Sonography Student Scholarship Program. **Academic Area:** Sonography, cardiovascular technology. **Who May Apply?:** High school seniors, college students. **Eligibility:** Applicants must be accepted to or currently enrolled in an educational program in diagnostic medical sonography or cardiovascular technology that is accredited by the Commission on Accreditation of Allied Health Educational Programs and be a member of the SDMS. **Application Process:** Applicants must submit a completed application (available at the Society's website), answers to three essay questions (available at the SDMS website), official transcripts, and a Federal Student Aid Report. **Amount:** Two awards of $2,500. **Deadline:** Applications are accepted throughout the year.

TOGETHER WE CARE NURSE
PRACTITIONER SCHOLARSHIP PROGRAM

www.cvs.com/minuteclinic/resources/jj-together-we-care

Scholarship Name: Together We Care Nurse Practitioner Scholarship Program. **Academic Area:** Nurse practitioner. **Who May Apply?:** College students. **Eligibility:** Applicants must be legal U.S. residents enrolled in a nationally accredited, master's of science in nursing (MSN) or doctor of nursing practice (DNP)-level preparation nurse practitioner program. They also must demonstrate strong involvement in community and leadership activities and achieve high academic performance, with a GPA of 3.2 or higher. **Application Process:** Apply online at the website listed above. **Amount:** 20 MSN scholarships at $2,500 each, and 20 DNP scholarships at $2,500 each. **Deadline:** Typically in March.

TYLENOL FUTURE CARE SCHOLARSHIP

866-851-4275

Tylenol@applyists.com

www.tylenol.com/news/scholarship

Scholarship Name: Tylenol Future Care Scholarship. **Academic Area:** Various health care areas such as public health/health education, medical school, nursing, and pharmacy. **Who May Apply?:** College students. **Eligibility:** Applicants must demonstrate academic excellence, exemplary leadership and community involvement, and be dedicated to a career of caring for others. They also must be residents of the United States. **Application Process:** Visit the Tylenol website for more information. **Amount:** $500 to $10,000. **Deadline:** Typically in June.

COLLEGE SUMMER EXPLORATION PROGRAMS

Colleges and universities offer a variety of experiential programs for high school students who want to do more on their summer vacations than just hang out with friends, play video games, update their Facebook status, and head to the beach. These programs offer excellent opportunities for students to learn about college majors and careers, meet people with similar interests, interact with college professors, visit college campuses, and get a feel for college life. Residential and commuter programs are available.

Programs, which last anywhere from a few days to two months, are available in many health care fields—from nursing and medicine, to sonography and dentistry, to psychology and biomedical engineering. Some colleges offer these programs for college or high school credit, while others are available only for self-enrichment. And some of these programs are offered year-round.

The colleges and universities listed on the following pages offer great summer and year-round programs for those interested in learning more about health care fields. Many of these schools attract students from all over the United States—and even the world. If you don't find your local colleges on the list, contact schools in your area. Even if they don't currently offer health care-related programs, your interest may prompt them to create such a program.

Here are a few things to keep in mind as you review the listings:

✔ Eligibility requirements vary by program. For example, some are selective and require applicants to have a high GPA, while others are open to students regardless of their academic achievement.

✔ Programs often fill up fast, so it's important to register as soon as possible.

✔ Program costs range from free, to a small fee, to very expensive. If your family's finances are tight, it's a good idea to start your search early to find a free or affordable program before classes or programs fill up.

✔ A term we often use in relation to grade level is "rising," as in "rising senior"—someone who will be a senior when the next school year begins.

✔ Program information (available classes, costs, session dates, etc.) changes often. The information provided on the subsequent pages is the most recent available from the program websites at the time of publication. Be sure to visit the websites of these programs for the latest information.

ARIZONA STATE UNIVERSITY (PHOENIX, AZ)

Summer Health Institute @ ASU
https://chs.asu.edu/prehealth/summer-health-institute-asu
What: Week-long residential program that allows students to explore careers in health care
Eligibility: Students who have completed their junior year of high school

ARIZONA STATE UNIVERSITY (PHOENIX, AZ)

Collegiate Scholars Academy
480-965-6060
collegiatescholars@asu.edu
https://eoss.asu.edu/collegiate-academy
What: The Collegiate Scholars Academy "offers high-achieving current high school students the opportunity to fast-track their college experience by enrolling in ASU courses and earning college credit. Courses are available in a variety of topics and are offered during the fall, spring, and summer."
Eligibility: High school students
What's Available: Introduction to Health and Wellness; General Biology Lecture & Lab; General Chemistry Lecture & Lab; Culture and Health

BOSTON UNIVERSITY (BOSTON, MA)

High School Honors Program
summerhs@bu.edu
www.bu.edu/summer/high-school-programs/honors
What/Eligibility: The High School Honors program "offers academically motivated rising juniors and seniors the opportunity to earn college credit while they get a taste of undergraduate life." Commuter or residential options are available.
What's Available: More than 80 undergraduate courses, including Biology; Human Infectious Diseases: AIDS to Tuberculosis; General Chemistry; Foreign Languages; Photography; Psychology

BOSTON UNIVERSITY (BOSTON, MA)

Summer Challenge Program
summerhs@bu.edu
www.bu.edu/summer/high-school-programs/summer-challenge
What/Eligibility: 12-day residential summer programs for rising high school sophomores, juniors, and seniors
What's Available: Anatomy and Physiology; Business: From the Ground Up; Chemistry of Medicine; Infectious Diseases; Nutrition; Photography; Visual Arts

BRIAR CLIFF UNIVERSITY (SIOUX CITY, IA)

Summer Nursing Camp
712-279-1662
www.briarcliff.edu/academics/departments/nursing/nursing-camp

What: Three-day residential camp that explores the field of nursing
Eligibility: Open to high school sophomores, juniors, and seniors

BROWN UNIVERSITY (PROVIDENCE, RI)

Summer@Brown
www.brown.edu/academics/pre-college/pre-college-courses.php

What: Noncredit courses in the liberal arts and sciences that allow high schools students to take courses in health care-related subjects and other fields. One- to four-week sessions. Residential program.
Eligibility: Students in grades 9 through 12
Available Classes: More than 200 courses are available, including Hands-On Medicine: A Week in the Life of a Medical Student; Introduction to Medicine: Do You Want to Be a Doctor?; Techniques in DNA-Based Biotechnology; and The Body: An Introduction to Human Anatomy and Physiology

CORNELL UNIVERSITY (ITHACA, NY)

Summer College for High School Students
summer_college@cornell.edu
www.sce.cornell.edu/sc/programs

What: Summer College "offers academically motivated high school students an unparalleled opportunity to take courses at a great Ivy League university while earning college credit."
Eligibility: Must be current high school sophomore, juniors, or seniors at the time of application.
What's Available: Cornell Engineering Experience; Fabricating the Future: Robotics and Artificial Intelligence; Biological Research and the Health Professions; and Research Apprenticeship in Biological Sciences

DARTMOUTH UNIVERSITY (HANOVER, NH)

Health Careers Institute at Dartmouth
603-646-1225
www.tdi.dartmouth.edu/hcid#&panel1-3

What: Week-long, residential, summer program for students interested in learning more about health care careers; classroom and field work opportunities are provided
Eligibility: Incoming 10th, 11th, and 12th grade students

HARVARD UNIVERSITY (CAMBRIDGE, MA)

Pre-College Program

summer@dcemail.harvard.edu
www.summer.harvard.edu/high-school-programs

What: A two-week residential experience featuring more than 100 non-credit courses

Eligibility: High school students ages 15 to 18

Available Courses: Psychopharmacology: Drug Action in the Brain; Fundamentals of Epidemiology; Genome Editing; The Promises of Regenerative Medicine

HARVARD UNIVERSITY (CAMBRIDGE, MA)

Secondary School Program
summer@dcemail.harvard.edu
www.summer.harvard.edu/high-school-programs

What: Provides the opportunity to take college courses (there are more than 200 courses in 60+ subjects to choose from) for credit in a seven-week session; participants can live on campus, commute, or study online

Available Classes: Introduction to Molecular and Cellular Biology; Introduction to Biochemistry; Principles of Genetics; Stem Cell and Regenerative Biology; Introduction to Biomedical Ethics

JOHNS HOPKINS UNIVERSITY (BALTIMORE, MD)

Discover Hopkins
http://pages.jh.edu/summer/experiencehopkins

What: 10- to 12-day summer sessions in which students register for one course per session, and may enroll in up to three sessions. Open to both residential and commuter students.

Eligibility: Applicants must have completed their sophomore, junior, or senior year of high school

What's Available: Introduction to Lab Research; The Hospital; Medical School Intensive; Physiology & Disease: Brain, Muscle, and Cardiopulmonary; Introduction to Biology & Medicine; Physiology & Disease: Renal, Digestive, Immune, Endocrinology, and Reproduction

JOHNS HOPKINS UNIVERSITY (BALTIMORE, MD)

Summer University
http://pages.jh.edu/summer/precollege/summer

What: A five-week program that "offers qualified high school students the opportunity to take freshman- and sophomore-level credit classes in arts and sciences and engineering." Open to both residential and commuter students.

Eligibility: Applicants must have completed their sophomore, junior, or senior year of high school

What's Available: Classes in Biology; Chemistry; Computer Science; Neuroscience; Psychological and Brain Sciences; Public Health Studies

LOYOLA UNIVERSITY CHICAGO (CHICAGO, IL)

Pre-College Summer Scholars Program
773-508-7381
summerscholars@luc.edu
www.luc.edu/summerscholars

What: A one-week seminar and six-week academy that allow high school students the opportunity to explore different fields of study and career opportunities through seminars that involve hands-on activities and field trips.
Eligibility: Current high school freshmen, sophomores, and juniors
What's Available:

✔ One-Week Seminar: From Brain to Behavior: An Introduction to the Inner Workings of the Human Brain; Psych 101: An Introduction to the Field of Psychology; Exercise & Nutrition 101; Nursing...Yesterday, Today, and Your Tomorrow

✔ Six-Week Academy: College Algebra; Precalculus; General Psychology; Spanish; French

MIAMI UNIVERSITY (OXFORD, OH)

Junior Scholars Program
summerscholars@MiamiOH.edu
http://miamioh.edu/admission/high-school/summer-scholars

What/Eligibility: Two-week, summer, residential program that "provides a rich, early college experience for academically-talented rising high school juniors and seniors from across the globe."
What's Available: Understanding the Human Brain; The Dynamics of Nutrition and Dietetics; Health and How to Change the World; The Discovery of Novel Antibiotics; Basics of Business; Genetic Engineering in Society

MICHIGAN TECHNOLOGICAL UNIVERSITY (HOUGHTON, MI)

Pre-College Explorations
906-487-2219
www.syp.mtu.edu

What: Week-long, summer programs that allow high school students to explore various career areas. Residential and commuter options are available.
Eligibility: Applicants must have completed 9th, 10th, or 11th grade as of June of the summer they plan to participate in the program.
Available Programs: Mechanical Engineering: Engineering the Human Body; Genetic Modification and Biotechnology; Medical Physiology; Psychology in the Real World; Digital Photography; Computer Graphics and Design; Wild World of Chemistry

MULTIPLE COLLEGES

EXPLO Focus

www.explo.org/explo-focus

What: Two-week, summer program at Yale University (New Haven, CT), Wellesley College (Wellesley, MA), and Wheaton College (Norton, MA).
Eligibility: Students ages nine to 17
What's Available: ExploOrtho and ExplorE.R.

NEW YORK UNIVERSITY (NEW YORK, NY)

Pre-College Program
university.programs@nyu.edu
212-998-2292
www.nyu.edu/admissions/high-school-programs/precollege.html

What: Six-week program in which high school students take college-level courses with current college students to obtain academic credit toward a future degree. (Note: Other programs for high school students are available; see www.nyu.edu/admissions/high-school-programs.html.)
Eligibility: Rising high school juniors and seniors
Available Classes: Intro to Psychology; Introduction to Cell and Molecular Biology; Introduction to Engineering and Design

NORTH CAROLINA STATE UNIVERSITY (RALEIGH, NC)

Pre-College Programs
https://emas.ncsu.edu/precollege

What: Pre-College Programs "give students the opportunity to develop academic skills, conduct research, investigate careers, build a portfolio, experience college life, and prepare for college enrollment. Disciplines include cultural education, design, engineering, leadership, math, science, technology, writing, and more."
Eligibility: Elementary through high school students
What's Available: More than a dozen programs, including NC-MSEN Summer Scholars Program; Science and Technology Enriching Lifelong Leadership In Tomorrow's Endeavors; Summer College in Biotechnology and Life Sciences

NORTHWEST ASSOCIATION FOR BIOMEDICAL RESEARCH (SEATTLE, WA)

Camp BIOmed
info@nwabr.org
www.nwabr.org/events-programs/student-events/camp-biomed-0

What: A five-week, commuter science camp held at Seattle Pacific University and Bellevue College
Eligibility: Students in grades 9 to 12
What's Available: Cancer Laboratory and Basics of Biology; Molecular Biology of Cancer; Next Gen Science: Origami of Life & Bioinformatics; Genetic Engineering: Recombinant DNA Technology; Crime Scene Investigation

PENNSYLVANIA STATE UNIVERSITY (UNIVERSITY PARK, PA)

Science Camps
www.sciencecamps.psu.edu

What: Five-day to week-long camps that allow participants to explore a variety of scientific areas
Eligibility: Opportunities are available for students in grades 5-12
Available Camps: Kinesiology: The Limitations of Human Performance; Pre-Med Experience; Infection!

ROCHESTER INSTITUTE OF TECHNOLOGY (ROCHESTER, NY)

College & Careers Program
www.rit.edu/emcs/admissions/careers

What: Two-day, summer career workshops
Eligibility: Rising high school seniors
Available Workshops: Medical Illustration; Biomedical Engineering: Engineering Solutions for the Human System; Biomedical Photographic Communications: The Magnified Image; Exercise Science and Nutrition: How Fit are You?; Hands-On Biotechnology; Imaging Science: See What Your Eyes Can't; Medical Science: Medical Detective-You Make the Call!, Medical Ultrasound; Premedical Studies and Biomedical Sciences: What's Up Doc?

SMITH COLLEGE (NORTHAMPTON, MA)

Summer Science and Engineering Program
www.smith.edu/summer/programs_ssep.php

What: A four-week residential program for young women with strong interests in science, engineering, and medicine. Since its inception, nearly 1,800 high school students have participated, representing 46 states, the District of Columbia, Puerto Rico, and 53 countries. Participants choose two two-week research courses.
Eligibility: Female high school students
Available Courses: The Chemistry of Herbal Medicine: A Complex Molecular Story; Your Genes, Your Chromosomes: A Laboratory in Human Genetics; Biomedical Ethics; Anatomy in Motion: An Inquiry Into Exercise Science; Science & Nature Writing

SOUTHWEST LOUISIANA AREA HEALTH EDUCATION CENTER

Future Docs
800-435-2432
www.swlahec.com/programs/health-careers/career-a-professional-education/future-docs

What: Future Docs is a one- to two-week "intense and immersive program that offers high school students who are seriously considering becoming a doctor, an opportunity to experience hands-on activities taught by doctors and other health personnel, along with tours, field trips, speaking with doctors, and much more." A commuter program.

Eligibility: Students who will be entering 11th or 12th grade or entering college in the fall

SYRACUSE UNIVERSITY (SYRACUSE, NY)

Summer College for High School Students
sumcoll@syr.edu
http://summercollege.syr.edu

What: 2-, 3-, 4- and 6-week programs exploration programs; residential and commuter options are available

Available Programs: More than 35 programs, including those in Photography and Spanish Immersion

UNIVERSITY OF CALIFORNIA AT DAVIS

COSMOS
cosmos@ucdavis.edu
http://cosmos.ucdavis.edu

What/Eligibility: Monthlong, residential program for students in grades 8-12 "who are interested in exploring science, technology, engineering, and mathematics fields. Students work side-by-side with university researchers and faculty in labs, focusing on current research at the University of California."

Available Clusters: Introduction to Engineering Mechanics; Computers in Biophysics & Robotics; Mathematics; Biomedical Sciences; The Chemistry of Life; Mathematical Modeling of Biological Systems

UNIVERSITY OF CALIFORNIA AT LOS ANGELES

Summer Discovery
info@summerdiscovery.com
www.summerdiscovery.com/u-texas-austin

What: The Summer Discovery Program "combines academics, athletics, and activities to give high school students a taste of college life." Residential and commuter options are available. Program lengths: 2, 3, 5, and 6 weeks.

Eligibility: Open to students completing grades 9, 10, 11, and 12.

What's Available: Students can choose from more than 100 classes, including Chemistry/Chemical Structure; Precalculus; Introduction to Psychology

UNIVERSITY OF COLORADO AT BOULDER

Summer Discovery
info@summerdiscovery.com
www.summerdiscovery.com/u-texas-austin

What: Students in the three- or four-week Summer Discovery Program "choose between STEM Research and one of 10 STEM Academies that focus on topics in science, technology, engineering, and mathematics—or choose one of five CU Scholars Credit Academies." Residential and commuter options are available.

Eligibility: Open to students completing grades 9, 10, 11, and 12

What's Available: Frontiers in Biotechnology; Neuroscience: Inside the Brain; Exploring Engineering

UNIVERSITY OF DENVER (DENVER, CO)

Early Experience Program
www.du.edu/apply/admission/apply/earlyexperience.html

What: Courses for college credit taken throughout the year
Eligibility: High school juniors and seniors
Available Classes: A variety of science and health care-related classes

UNIVERSITY OF FLORIDA (GAINESVILLE, FL)

Explorations in Biomedical Research
352-392-2310
ebr@cpet.ufl.edu
www.cpet.ufl.edu/students/explorebiomed/Explorations in Biomedical Research

What/Eligibility: A two-week summer program for high school students entering 11th and 12th grade. The program "focuses on translational research, from discovery-based research to clinical therapeutics. During the program, students engage in an experimental sequence in basic science. Visits to research and clinical lab spaces help to illustrate scientific content, research methods, career options, and interrelationships within translational research."

UNIVERSITY OF KENTUCKY (LEXINGTON, KY)

Health Reserchers Youth Academy Camp
859-323-8018
https://ahec.med.uky.edu/summer-health-career-camps

What: A 2.5-week residential program for students interested in health care careers, either in clinical practice or in the area of health care research.
Eligibility: Open to rising high school seniors

UNIVERSITY OF KENTUCKY (LEXINGTON, KY)

Summer Enrichment Program Camp
859-323-8018
https://ahec.med.uky.edu/summer-health-career-camps

What: A 2.5-week residential program for students interested in health care careers, either in clinical practice or in the area of health care research.
Eligibility: Open to rising high school juniors

UNIVERSITY OF IOWA

Secondary Student Training Program
800-336-6463
www2.education.uiowa.edu/belinblank/students/summer/Classes.asp
x?P=SSTP

What: Five-and-a-half-week residential summer research program. In this program, "students conduct scientific research under the guidance of a faculty mentor." The University of Iowa Colleges of Engineering, Liberal Arts and Sciences, Dentistry, Medicine, Nursing, Pharmacy, Public Health, and the Graduate College participate in the program.
Eligibility: Students entering grades 11 and 12 in the fall

UNIVERSITY OF MARYLAND (COLLEGE PARK, MD)

Terp Young Scholars
https://oes.umd.edu/young-scholars

What: Two-and-a-half-week summer program for high school students who are interested in "pursuing academic interests, discovering career opportunities, earning three university credits, and exploring university life." Residential or commuter options are available. (Note: Terp Discovery is a similar program for middle-school students.)
Eligibility: Rising high school freshmen, sophomores, juniors, or seniors
Available Courses: Kinesiology (Movement & The Human Body); Biopharmaceutical Production; Engineering Design

UNIVERSITY OF MINNESOTA (MINNEAPOLIS, MN)

Girls Solve It! With Mathematical Biology
csek12@umn.edu
https://cse.umn.edu/r/summer-camps

What: A week-long day camp that "introduces the role of mathematical modeling in the study of biology and the treatment of disease. Topics may include designing radiation schedules in cancer treatment using mathematical models, analyzing flu epidemic data from the Centers for Disease Control and optimal designing vaccination policies, predicting the spread of infectious diseases through a network of relationships, and predicting the dynamics of predator-prey populations in a national park." Other programs available from the university include Discover STEM; IMA-MathCEP Math Modeling Camp; Eureka! (STEM); and Kids' University.
Eligibility: Girls entering grades 11 and 12

UNIVERSITY OF MISSOURI (COLUMBIA, MO)

Pre-College Opportunities
https://musis1.missouri.edu/precollege/summer_program.cfm

What: The University of Missouri offers a variety of summer career exploration programs.

Eligibility: High school students
Available Programs: Pharmacy Camp; High School Mini Medical School; MU Health Professions Summit; Scrub-in to a Health Career; Engineering High School Summer Camp; Life Sciences Quest

UNIVERSITY OF SOUTH CAROLINA (COLUMBIA, MO)

Carolina Master Scholars Adventure Series
pups@mailbox.sc.edu
https://sc.edu/about/offices_and_divisions/continuing_education/yout
h_and_teen_preuniversity_programs/carolina_master_scholars_adve
nture_series

What: Five-day, summer career exploration programs with residential and commuter options.
Eligibility: Open to rising 6th-12th grade students
Available Camps: Adventures in Medicine-Ultrasound; Adventures in Engineering; Adventures in Pharmacy; Adventures in Speech Pathology; Adventures in Women in Engineering

UNIVERSITY OF TEXAS AT AUSTIN

Summer Discovery
info@summerdiscovery.com
www.summerdiscovery.com/u-texas-austin

What: The three-week Summer Discovery Program "combines academics, athletics, and activities to give high school students a taste of college life." Residential and commuter options are available.
Eligibility: Open to students completing grades 9, 10, 11, and 12
What's Available: Students can choose from more than 20 classes, including Introduction to Medicine; Anatomy and Pathology; Foundations of Psychology

UNIVERSITY OF WISCONSIN

Wisconsin Precollege Programs
www.precollege.wlearn.com

What: This is a database of pre-college programs at Wisconsin's public colleges-for example, the Discovery Summer Science Camp at the University of Wisconsin (UW) at Madison and the Life's A Lab Camp at UW at Green Bay. Opportunities are available in Health Sciences, Engineering, Business, Languages, and other areas.
Eligibility: Grades 1-12, plus adults

VANDERBILT UNIVERSITY (NASHVILLE, TN)

Vanderbilt Summer Academy
https://pty.vanderbilt.edu/students/vsa

What: The Vanderbilt Summer Academy (VSA) is a residential academic

experience that introduces young people to college life. VSA students "live on campus and take accelerated courses with Vanderbilt professors, lecturers, and graduate students." Programs last anywhere from six to 20 days.
Eligibility: Students entering grades 8 through 12

WORCESTER POLYTECHNIC INSTITUTE (WORCESTER, MA)

Frontiers
www.wpi.edu/academics/pre-collegiate/summer/stem-residential/frontiers

What: 12-day, on-campus, summer residential program "that challenges participants to explore the outer limits of their knowledge in science, technology, engineering, and math with current laboratory techniques and exploring unsolved problems across a wide spectrum of disciplines."
Eligibility: Students entering grades 11 and 12
Available Workshops: Biomedical Engineering; Biology, Biotechnology, and Bioinformatics; Chemistry and Biochemistry; Pre-Health; Psychology
Available Classes: Diabetes Research and Treatment; Med School 101; Addiction in the Modern Age; Alzheimer's Treatment and Research

YALE UNIVERSITY (NEW HAVEN, CT)

EXPLO 360 Summer
781-762-7400
www.explo.org/explo-360/yale/academics

What: Three-week summer courses and workshops
Eligibility: Entering grades 10 through 12
What's Available:

✔ Courses: Anatomy+Physiology; First Aid Training+Certification; Genetic Engineering; Infectious Disease+Immunology

✔ Workshops: Team Building+Leadership Skills; Chemistry Lab; CPR/AED Certification; Heart Science

INDEX